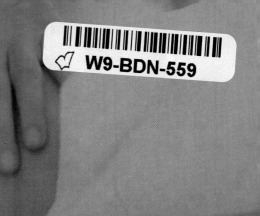

Professional Foundations
for Massage Therapists

PATRICIA J. BENJAMIN, PH.D., NCTMB

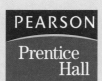

PEARSON

Prentice
Hall

Upper Saddle River, New Jersey 07458

Library of Congress Cataloging-in-Publication Data

Benjamin, Patricia J.
  Professional foundations for massage therapists / Patricia Benjamin.
    p. ; cm.
Includes bibliographical references and index.
ISBN-13: 978-0-13-171736-7
ISBN-10: 0-13-171736-7
1. Massage therapy. 2. Massage therapy—Vocational guidance.
  [DNLM: 1. Massage. 2. Ethics, Professional. 3. Professional Practice. WB 537 B468p
2009] I. Title.
  RM722.B48 2009
  615.8'22023—dc22

                                                            2007041297

Publisher: Julie Levin Alexander
Publisher's Assistant: Regina Bruno
Executive Editor: Mark Cohen
Associate Editor: Melissa Kerian
Editorial Assistant: Nicole Ragonese
Media Editor: John J. Jordan
Development Editor: Lynda Hatch
Managing Production Editor: Patrick Walsh
Production Liaison: Christina Zingone
Production Editor: Jessica Balch, Pine Tree Composition, Inc.
Manufacturing Manager: Ilene Sanford
Manufacturing Buyer: Pat Brown
Design Director: Maria Guglielmo
Design Coordinator: Christopher Weigand
Interior/Cover Designer: Karen Quigley
Director of Marketing: Karen Allman
Marketing Manager: Harper Coles
Marketing Specialist: Michael Sirinides
Media Project Manager: Stephen Hartner
Director, Image Resource Center: Melinda Patelli
Manager, Rights and Permissions: Zina Arabia
Manager, Visual Research: Beth Brenzel
Manager, Cover Visual Research & Permissions: Karen Sanatar
Image Permission Coordinator: Ang'john Ferreri
Composition: Pine Tree Composition, Inc.
Printer/Binder: Quebecor World Dubuque
Cover Printer: Phoenix Color Corp.
Cover Photos: PhotoDisc/Getty Images, Inc.
Interior Photos: Chapter opener/Practical Application: Media Images/Getty Images, Inc;
Case for Study: Eye Wire Collection/PhotoDisc/Getty Images, Inc.; Critical Thinking: Digital Vision/Getty Images, Inc.

Credits and acknowledgments borrowed from other sources and reproduced, with permission, in this textbook appear on the appropriate pages within text.

Pearson Education, LTD.
Pearson Education Singapore, Pte. Ltd.
Pearson Education, Canada, Ltd.
Pearson Education–Japan
Pearson Education Australia PTY, Limited

Pearson Education North Asia Ltd.
Pearson Educación de Mexico, S.A. de C.V.
Pearson Education Malaysia, Pte. Ltd.
Pearson Education, Upper Saddle River, New Jersey

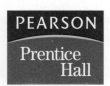

10 9 8 7 6 5 4 3 2 1
ISBN-13: 978-0-13-171736-7
ISBN-10:   0-13-171736-7

Brief Contents

Appendices

Contents

PART I   MASSAGE THERAPY OVERVIEW

1   A Career in Massage Therapy   3

2   The Massage Therapy Profession   19

3   A History of Massage as a Vocation   39

PART II PERSONAL AND COMMUNICATION SKILLS

4 Personal Development and Professionalism 69

5 Social and Communication Skills 107

PART III PLANNING AND DOCUMENTATION

6 Goal-Oriented Planning 135

7 Documentation and SOAP Notes   159

PART IV PROFESSIONAL ETHICS

8 Foundations of Ethics   183

9 Therapeutic Relationship and Ethics   199

Appendices

Preface

Massage therapists today are expected to be caring and competent professionals. This means more than skill in performing manual techniques. It involves having a deeper understanding of the field as a whole, and acting ethically at all times. It includes communicating well with clients, and meeting their goals. It means interacting with other health professionals, and keeping updated on new information and the latest trends.

Building a thriving massage therapy practice takes some basic business knowledge, and good communication and social skills. Getting a job as a massage therapist depends on developing a professional image and interviewing well. Personal characteristics like a strong work ethic, the ability to concentrate, and emotional intelligence support career success.

Professional Foundations for Massage Therapists covers aspects of the field not usually found in massage technique textbooks. It complements technical books by painting a broad picture of the massage therapy profession. It delves into the softer skills needed by massage therapists such as intuition, critical thinking, and behaving ethically. This book covers the many varied aspects of being a competent massage therapist and the competencies needed by massage therapists starting on their careers.

In *Professional Foundations for Massage Therapists*, massage therapy is approached as a wellness profession. Wellness encompasses everything from relaxation, to health promotion, to work with special populations, to treatment for medical conditions, to all of the many other reasons clients come for massage. The background knowledge and skills presented here are needed by professional massage therapists in all settings.

Professional Foundations for Massage Therapists presents massage therapy education as a holistic process. It recognizes that students grow in many ways while becoming massage therapists. They use their minds, hands, and hearts in acquiring the foundation skills needed to start their new careers. Professional knowledge and skills cannot be downloaded into a student like a computer software program. It takes effort by students to transform themselves from the inside out. This book is intended to be a guide to that transformation.

The topics presented here are sometimes found in introductory classes, or, alternately, scattered throughout the curriculum in different courses. Wherever they are covered, these topics lay the foundation for a bright future as a massage therapist.

ORGANIZATION OF THE BOOK

Professional Foundations for Massage Therapists is divided into five parts that reflect broad areas of foundation knowledge for massage therapists. Each part has two or more chapters that focus on a particular topic within that area.

PART I: MASSAGE THERAPY OVERVIEW offers a survey of massage therapy as a career—today and yesterday. It lays the groundwork for understanding massage therapy as a wellness profession, and celebrates the diversity of the field. It shows how massage therapy has evolved over the years to the emerging profession that it is today.

> *Chapter 1: A Career in Massage Therapy* focuses on current work settings for massage therapists in personal care, sports and fitness, health care, and private practice.
>
> *Chapter 2: The Massage Therapy Profession* looks at educational standards, credentials, licensing, associations, the body of knowledge and research, and growing acceptance of massage therapy by the general public and other health professionals.
>
> *Chapter 3: A History of Massage as a Vocation* describes the work of massage therapists in different time periods in such diverse places as public baths, salons and spas, sports clubs, and in Western medicine and natural healing settings.

PART II: PERSONAL AND COMMUNICATION SKILLS explores the softer skills of successful massage therapists—those personal characteristics that underpin the more technical skills. It guides students through development of professionalism. It lays out personal and interpersonal skills necessary for doing the work of massage therapy and building good relationships.

> *Chapter 4: Personal Development and Professionalism* outlines the essentials of looking and acting like a health professional, as well as the importance of abilities such as concentration and intuition. Personal competencies like emotional intelligence, physical condition, and ethical behavior in school are discussed.
>
> *Chapter 5: Social and Communication Skills* reviews basic social behaviors for maintaining good relationships and projecting professionalism, as well as skills for interpersonal communications inherent in developing a massage therapy practice.

PART III: PLANNING AND DOCUMENTATION gives instructions for the important processes of planning and then writing notes about massage therapy sessions. It comes from the belief that no matter where massage therapists work, they owe it to their clients to tailor sessions to meet client expectations. Writing notes is practical in all settings and essential in more clinically oriented practices.

> *Chapter 6: Goal-Oriented Planning* leads students through a step-by-step approach to organizing massage sessions to meet client goals. Detailed instructions are given for gathering useful information used in determining what to do and evaluating results of sessions.
>
> *Chapter 7: Documentation and SOAP Notes* covers the content of the SOAP note format for recording massage sessions in writing and offers tips for developing a practical and readable writing style.

PART IV: PROFESSIONAL ETHICS lays the groundwork for understanding ethical behavior, and delves into specific issues of ethics in relationships with clients and in business practices. It presents ethics as perhaps the most basic of foundations in a helping profession based on person-to-person interaction with touch as the major mode of contact. It explores common pitfalls and ways of avoiding unethical behavior.

> *Chapter 8: Foundations of Ethics* explores the nature of professional ethics and the process of making ethical decisions based on knowledge and good judgment.
>
> *Chapter 9: Therapeutic Relationship and Ethics* looks closely at specific ethical issues involving relationships with clients and presents models for dealing with common ethical situations.

Chapter 10: Business Ethics focuses on the commercial aspects of massage therapy, especially issues related to money, the buying and selling of health services, and advertising. It considers ethical issues from the point of view of clients as customers.

Part V: CAREER DEVELOPMENT describes what it takes to get started in a successful massage therapy career—from envisioning a future practice to making that dream come true. It identifies the nuts and bolts of putting a practice plan into action. It covers the many possibilities for massage therapy practices from employment to building a private practice.

Chapter 11: Career Plans and Employment leads students to imagine their dream massage therapy practices for the first year after graduation and to develop their identities as massage therapists. Strategies for getting employment are discussed.

Chapter 12: Private Practice and Finances outlines in detail the development of a business plan for a private massage therapy practice and provides information on financial matters from budgeting to bookkeeping to paying taxes.

The APPENDICES contain reference information too extensive to include in the chapters.

Appendix A: **25 Forms of Therapeutic Massage and Bodywork**
Appendix B: **Personal Care and Health Professionals**
Appendix C: **Summary of Competencies for Massage Therapists**
Appendix D: **Massage Licensing Laws in North America**
Appendix E: **Goal-Oriented Planning**
Appendix F: **Intake and Health History Forms**
Appendix G: **Code of Ethics and Standards of Practice for Massage Therapists**
Appendix H: **List of Figures and Tables**
Appendix I: **References and Additional Resources**

The **INTERACTIVE GLOSSARY** provides definitions for terms used in the textbook and suggests relationships between terms.

The **INDEX** gives page numbers for important terms, concepts, people, and places appearing in the textbook.

CHAPTER FORMAT

Chapters follow a consistent organization to help students locate information easily. Each chapter has the following:

Learning Outcomes describe the chapter focus and what students will have information to do once they have studied the chapter contents.
Key Terms identify important words and ideas that students can study for better understanding major points of information in the chapter.
Headings and Subheadings organize the text logically and assist in locating information easily.
Exam Review presents several different strategies for learning the chapter content and preparing for exams. *Learning Outcomes* point to major areas of study and intended goals, while *Key Terms* provide a focus for learning definitions. *Memory Workout* enhances recall through fill-in-the-blanks sentences, and *Test Prep* presents

multiple-choice questions in a format used often in standardized tests. *Video Challenge* directs students to find major concepts illustrated in the video CD-ROM accompanying the text. *Comprehension Exercises* provide the opportunity for verbal or written expression of important ideas. *For Greater Understanding* exercises lead the student to real world applications of chapter ideas.

SPECIAL FEATURES

Special features present exercises that students can do to deepen their understanding of material presented in the text and to develop the competencies required for a successful career in massage therapy.

Case for Study exercises use fictitious stories to bring the theoretical material in the text to life. They give the massage therapists a name, and describe situations commonly encountered in massage therapy practices. They ask students to apply the concepts and guidelines explained in the chapter to analyze the case and to solve the problems presented.

Practical Application exercises provide opportunities for students to relate chapter material to their own development as massage therapists. They involve observation, role play, creativity, and planning. They ask students to apply lessons learned in school to their own transformation into massage therapy professionals and to their future massage therapy practices.

Critical Thinking exercises pose questions for students to consider thoughtfully and situations to analyze and evaluate. They lead students to ask intelligent questions, discover the truth, and make informed decisions.

VIDEO CD-ROM

The video CD-ROM included with *Professional Foundations for Massage Therapists* is divided into segments according to chapters in the book. This video CD-ROM can be viewed in class as an introduction to a chapter and for discussion by the class as a whole. It can also be viewed at home by students as a study tool and review of chapter material.

STUDY TIPS FOR STUDENTS

Knowing your own learning style is a key to success in school. Are you primarily a visual, auditory, or kinesthetic learner? Do you learn best alone or in a study group? Do you study better in the morning or at night? Do you have a learning disability, and if so, have you gotten help to learn compensation techniques? Develop a learning strategy that works best for you, and take responsibility for using it in school and beyond.

Big Picture versus Details

Research indicates that learners fall into two camps: (1) "right-brain" learners who process information by focusing on the big picture and relationships between ideas and (2) "left-brain" learners who process information in a sequential step-by-step fashion focusing on details. Each style of learning has strengths and drawbacks. For example, right-brain learners can miss important details, while left-brain learners may get so bogged down in details that they miss the big picture. Be aware of your natural style, but incorporate methods that help you get both the big picture as well as the details.

Better Study Habits

Here are some simple things you can do to improve your study habits:

▶ Understand the learning outcomes for a class, and keep your attention on material that helps you achieve them. Be selective and focused.

▶ Read assigned material before a lecture so that you are not hearing about the subject for the first time in class. The lecture will sink in more deeply if you are already somewhat familiar with the terminology and concepts presented. You will be less likely to get lost in class.

▶ Underline, highlight, and write in the margins of reading material to identify important terms and concepts. Be selective in finding the most important ideas. Mark passages directly related to topics from classes. Don't highlight too much.

▶ Pick out key terms and write out their definitions. Identify related concepts and subtopics.

▶ Become familiar with the features in your textbooks. The table of contents, figures, tables, appendices, glossary, and index provide valuable information, and help you find what you are looking for more quickly.

▶ Within 24 hours after a class, review and rewrite your class notes. Write summaries of major topics in your own words, noting where ideas covered in class are found in your textbooks.

▶ If you learn best by hearing (auditory learner), ask permission to tape lectures so that you are not distracted from what the teacher is saying by taking notes. Replay the tapes after class, and then make notes of the most important ideas.

▶ If you learn best by doing (kinesthetic learner), write out concepts and definitions, draw pictures and diagrams, and outline chapters in your textbooks. Do things like handle bones of the skeleton when learning anatomy, palpate muscles as you memorize their locations and attachments, and combine doing massage techniques with memorizing their effects.

▶ In study groups, explain basic concepts to each other, ask each other questions, and discuss important topics. Listen to what others have to say, and also practice saying your ideas out loud to others. This helps you clarify your thoughts.

▶ Use study guides and supplemental materials that come with your textbooks.

Take Time

Set aside enough time to read, discuss, think about, and test yourself on material you are learning. The more you review the material and interact with it in different ways, the better your grasp of it will be. A general rule is to study 3 hours for every hour you are in class. Finally, tell the instructor or a counselor if you are getting lost or behind in class. Be open to suggestions and to trying new learning methods.

Remember the old adage, "you can lead a horse to water, but you can't force him to drink." The school and teachers are responsible for setting up a good learning environment, but you must do your part for learning to take place.

TAKING TESTS

Written examinations are a fact of life in school and in attaining certification and licensing. Some people find exams a positive experience. They enjoy testing their knowledge, and approach them like game shows on TV. Others find exams anxiety provoking and decidedly unpleasant. Following some simple guidelines can maximize the chances that your test results will truly reflect what you have learned.

Get Focused

First, arrive early and get organized and settled into your seat. Get out your pencil and other items you will need for the test. Put your other things away and out of sight so that you have a clear space to work and think. Do whatever works for you to calm down, focus, and concentrate; for example, quiet sitting or deep breathing.

If you get distracted easily, find a quiet place in the room away from doors and windows. Sit in the front row near a wall if possible. Ask the monitor if you can wear earplugs or a headset that drowns out sound.

Understand the Test

Read and understand the test directions before you start. Ask the monitor for an explanation of directions you do not understand. Quickly look over the entire test to see how long it is and what types of questions are on it, so that you can plan your time.

Read each question carefully before answering. Reading too quickly can cause you to miss important words. Be sure you fully understand what the question is asking.

Don't panic if you have a momentary lapse of memory. If you draw a blank on a question, skip over it and go back to it later. Don't be disturbed if others finish before you do. Focus on what you are doing and take the time allowed to finish. If you have extra time, check over your answers to catch careless mistakes, or reread and improve essay answers.

Answer Questions Thoughtfully

Essay Questions. First determine what level of knowledge the question is asking for. Action words like *list*, *define*, *compare*, *analyze*, and *explain* tell you how to approach your answer. Outline your answer on a scratch sheet to organize your thoughts and identify important points.

Do not write everything you remember about the topic. Be sure that your answer addresses the specific question asked. Be concise and direct in your answer. Don't ramble. Write legibly, and in complete sentences. Use good grammar and correct spelling. Come back to your answer later if you have time to recheck for accuracy, completeness, clarity, and to correct grammatical and spelling errors.

If you run out of time, quickly outline an answer. Providing some information is better than leaving the question blank.

Objective Test Questions. The most common objective test questions are multiple choice, true/false, and matching. Answer the questions in order, marking the ones you are not sure of in the margin. Do not spend too much time on any one question. Give it your best guess and move on. You can go back to it later if you have time.

Watch out for negative wording such as *not* or *least*, "double negatives," and qualifying words like *always*, *seldom*, *never*, *most*, *best*, *largest*. Read each question thoroughly for full understanding of what it says.

Multiple-choice questions are designed so that only one choice is correct. A good strategy is to find the correct answer by the process of elimination of the incorrect ones. Grammatical inconsistencies may tip you off to the right answer or to a wrong one. Read the question and your choice together to make sure it makes grammatical sense.

True/false questions need to be read very carefully. One incorrect detail makes the whole statement false. If a sentence has two parts (compound sentence), both parts need to be true for the whole question to be true.

For matching questions, use one column as your reference. For each item in that column, go through all items in the second column until you find a match. Match all the ones you are sure of first, and then go back to match the others with your best guess.

Do not change your answers without good reason. First "guesses" tend to be better than "second guessing." If you are not guessing, but have a good reason to change your mind, go ahead and change an answer.

YOUR RESOURCE FOR LEARNING

Professional Foundations for Massage Therapists is intended to be a useful resource for learning. Every feature is designed to lead you to success in laying the foundations for your career in massage therapy. By keeping your career goals in sight, you can find motivation to do what it takes to get the most out of your time in school. I sincerely hope that this textbook can provide guidance and inspiration to make your massage therapy education an exciting and transformational period of growth for you personally and professionally.

Patricia J. Benjamin

Acknowledgments

Professional Foundations for Massage Therapists is a testament to the many teachers, colleagues, mentors, and role models who over the years have helped me understand what it means to be a professional and to strive for excellence in all endeavors, and especially in our chosen work.

I am humbled when I watch my colleagues and see the knowledge and skill evident in their practices. I learn from them as I listen to their stories of being massage therapists, and I appreciate the comfort they bring to the world and the challenges they face to be good people and to make a living doing the work that they love. My clients have provided experiences that bring theory to life and underscore the reason we do this work at all.

I would like to acknowledge a former business partner, Patricia Portman, who took a risk to open a massage therapy practice with me in a conservative suburb of Chicago in the mid 1980s. I learned a little about politics and a lot about the business of being in practice from our modest massage center.

I was fortunate to be involved as a volunteer at the national level at the American Massage Therapy Association during a time of tremendous growth in the late 1980s and early 1990s, and I am active at the chapter level today. I owe a debt of gratitude to everyone I have worked with on boards, committees, and projects, hammering out programs that lead massage therapy forward to a new level of professionalism. The way is not always easy, but it is educational and has sharpened my thinking and social skills in so many ways.

I would like to thank Frances Tappan, who had faith in me to carry on her work in *Tappan's Handbook of Healing Massage Techniques*. I was blessed to get to know her before she passed away and to hear stories of her history with massage. I hope that she approves of how things have turned out.

To everyone who writes for professional magazines and journals, and to fellow book authors—thank you for your part in the great conversation within the profession of massage therapy. I know we learn from each other and push each other to greater excellence.

To the schools in which I have worked as an administrator and teacher, I am grateful for the experiences and insights provided. There is not a more exciting place to be than at the center of learning. And as every teacher knows, I learned more from my students than they can ever imagine. They taught me to be organized, to be clear, to be kind, and challenged me on every front. They truly are great teachers in their own way.

Thanks to reviewers who took the time and effort to comment on preliminary drafts. Your expertise is essential to making this an accurate and useful educational tool. And thanks to the massage therapists and students who appear in the video and text illustrations. Special gratitude is extended to the Fox Institute of Business, Parisi Gym, and The Center for Optimal Living, Inc. where much of the footage was shot.

I am indebted to the editorial and production team at Prentice Hall, especially Mark Cohen, Executive Editor, who is in charge of this project. They make it all happen and keep me on the path to meeting deadlines.

Finally I'd like to acknowledge the support of my family and friends, who have journeyed with me from start to finish of this project. Especially the many varied contributions of Martha Fourt who critiqued drafts, posed for photos, kept my computer running, and performed many little tasks I needed done to keep the wheels of progress turning.

So thank you everyone. I dedicate this book to you and to the students of massage therapy who want to be the best and to be successful in this honorable profession.

Patricia J. Benjamin

January 6, 2008

Reviewers

Tom Adams, AA
Medical Coordinator
Omega Institute
Pennsauken, New Jersey

Robert Allen
Falls River Community College
Narragansett, Rhode Island

Patricia A. Coe, DC
Message Therapy Clinic Supervisor
National University of Health Sciences
Lombard, Illinois

Theresa J. Ford, BS, LMT
Instructor
East West College
Portland, Oregon

Sandy Friedland, BA, LMT
Seminar Leader
Educating Hands School of Massage
Miami, Florida

Debra Fronek, CMT
Education Department Coordinator and Instructor
Lakeside School of Massage Therapy
Milwaukee, Wisconsin

Lisa Jakober
Corporate Director of Education
National Massage Therapy Institute
Philadelphia, Pennsylvania

Lorinda Krinke, CMT
Instructor/Clinical Coordinator
Blue Sky School of Massage
Poynette, Wisconsin

Janice Luzzi, LMT
Instructor
Greenfield Community College
Greenfield, Massachusetts

Lisa Mertz, PhD, LMT
Program Coordinator
Queensborough Community College
Bayside, New York

Linda L. Moore, RN, ADN, BA, LMT
Coordinator, Therapeutic Massage Program
Morton College
Cicero, Illinois

Roger Olbrot, BS
Director of Education
Myotherapy College of Utah
Salt Lake City, Utah

Debra Rilea
Co-Director
Ralston School of Massage
Reno, Nevada

Karen Schilling, MS RD LMT
Associate Director
New Hampshire Institute for Therapeutic Arts
Bridgton, Maine

Cheryl Siniakin, PhD
Director, Massage Therapy Program
CCAC–Allegheny Campus
Pittsburgh, Pennsylvania

Nancy Smeeth
Instructor
Connecticut Center for Massage Therapy
Newington, Connecticut

Elizabeth Wedge, BS, LMT
Instructor, Clinical Coordinator
Apollo College
Tucson, Arizona

Video Contributors

A special thanks to the individuals who contributed their time and expertise to assist us in the production of the video CD-ROM that accompanies this book:

Joli Behr-Cook
Massage Therapist

Dr. S.C. Benanti
The Center for Optimum Living,
    Parisi Sports Clubs USA

Cheryl Coutts
NASM Certified Personal Trainer

Christopher Coutts
Fox Institute of Business

Jennifer van Dam
Massage Therapist

Selene DelValle
Massage Therapist

Caleb Edmond
Massage Therapist

Julie Favaro
Massage Therapist

Theresa Cecylija Leszczynski
Massage Therapist

Jeff Mann
Massage Therapist
Cortiva Institute

Abby Nickerson
Massage Therapist

PART I

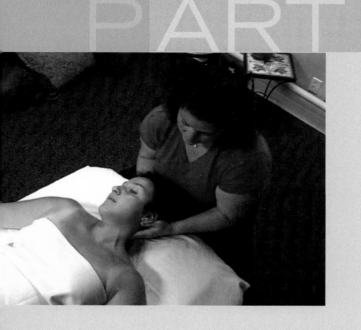

MASSAGE THERAPY OVERVIEW

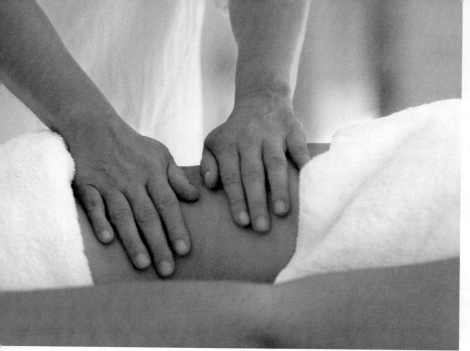

A Career in Massage Therapy

Learning Outcomes
Key Terms
The Journey
Massage Defined
Wellness Profession
Trends
Typical Work Settings
Chapter Highlights
Exam Review

→ LEARNING OUTCOMES

After studying this chapter, you will have information to:

1. Define massage therapy.
2. Use the Wellness Massage Pyramid to explain the scope of massage therapy.
3. Explain massage therapy as a wellness profession.
4. Identify trends related to massage therapy.
5. Understand the variety of career opportunities for massage therapists.
6. Describe typical work settings for massage therapists.

→ KEY TERMS

Complementary and alternative medicine (CAM)
Health care settings
Home visit practice

Integrative medicine center
Massage
Massage therapy
Personal care settings

Private practice settings
Sports, fitness, and recreation settings

Wellness Massage Pyramid (WMP)
Wellness profession

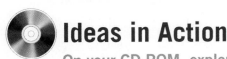

Ideas in Action

On your CD-ROM, explore:

▶ A variety of workplaces for massage therapists
▶ The Wellness Massage Pyramid
▶ Interactive video exercises

↳ THE JOURNEY

Welcome! You have begun the journey to becoming a successful massage therapist. The next several months will be a period of transformation as you learn to be a competent and caring professional. Your education will be a holistic experience as you physically master massage techniques, mentally absorb the science and theory of massage therapy, and practice the social skills needed for good relationships with clients. You will exercise your memory, develop reasoning skills, and internalize the principles of ethical behavior. You will learn how to start and maintain a massage therapy practice.

The first step in this journey is to survey the landscape of massage therapy, that is, to get the big picture of the career that you have chosen. That means understanding what massage therapy is, its broad scope as a wellness profession, trends related to its use, and where massage therapists work.

↳ MASSAGE DEFINED

Massage is the intentional and systematic manipulation of the soft tissues of the body to enhance health and healing. Massage is performed with or without lubricating substances such as oil. Joint movements and stretching are commonly performed as part of massage. Adjunct modalities within the scope of massage include the use of hot and cold packs, and hydrotherapy in the form of whirlpool bath, sauna, and steam room.

Simple hand tools are sometimes used to apply pressure during massage, as are machines that mimic massage techniques. However, massage is primarily manual therapy, that is, it is performed by hand. It is the person-to-person touch essential to massage that gives it a unique healing potential.

The most common system of massage in North America and Europe is traditional Western massage, sometimes called Swedish massage. Western massage is based on an understanding of anatomy, physiology, pathology, and other biosciences. The seven technique categories of Western massage are effleurage, petrissage, tapotement, friction, vibration, touch without movement, and joint movements. Western massage techniques are applied to improve overall functioning of the body systems, to enhance healing, and for relaxation of body and mind.

Other Western systems of soft tissue manipulation include specialized manual techniques to affect specific body systems, for example, myofascial massage, neuromuscular therapy, and lymphatic massage. Some massage therapy systems are based on unconventional theories of how the body works, for example, reflexology and polarity therapy.

Massage and bodywork traditions are found all over the globe. In addition to Western massage, major traditions include folk and native practices from different areas of the world. There are also Ayurvedic massage from India and Asian bodywork therapies based in Chinese medicine. Eclectic forms of massage combine theory and techniques from several systems.

Massage therapy is a general term used to describe all of the different systems of soft tissue manipulation. Bodywork is a term coined in the late 20th century to encompass a wide variety of manual therapies including massage, movement integration, structural integration, and energy balancing. The terms massage and bodywork are often used together to describe the occupational field of massage therapy, as in National Certification for Therapeutic Massage & Bodywork. Appendix A on page 301 is a guide to 25 different forms of massage and bodywork including their origins, techniques, theories, and websites for further information.

WELLNESS PROFESSION

Massage therapists apply massage and related modalities to help clients on their quest for high-level wellness. This includes massage therapy as a simple healthy pleasure, for stress reduction, for treatment and recovery from illness and injuries, and for a variety of other reasons. The broad scope of the field is evident in the **Wellness Massage Pyramid (WMP)** in Figure 1–1◀.

The WMP illustrates the major goals of massage therapy and its many applications. It is loosely based on Maslow's hierarchy of needs (Huitt, 2002). The goal at the top is high-level wellness, a condition of optimal physical, emotional, intellectual, spiritual, social, and vocational well-being. The concept of wellness is holistic at its core, encompassing the whole person.

The three levels at the base of the pyramid address *deficiency* needs related to illness and injury. These include applications of massage therapy for treatment of, recovery from, and prevention of illness and injury. Satisfying those needs brings one to the *neutral zone*, which is the old definition of health as the absence of disease.

Next in the WMP are the *growth* levels. These include massage therapy applications for health maintenance, personal growth, and enjoyment of life to its fullest— all aiming toward a state of high-level wellness. The upper part of the pyramid encompasses massage therapy for purposes like optimal body system functioning,

◀**Figure 1–1** Wellness Massage Pyramid.

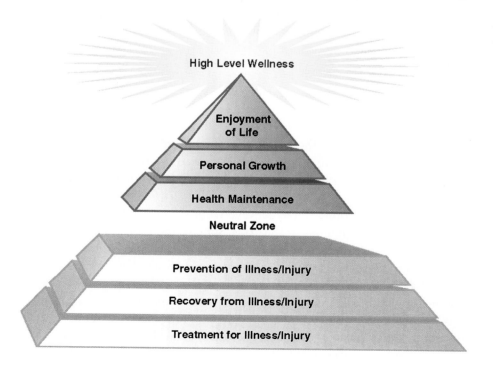

CRITICAL THINKING

Think about your current state of well-being. Note where improvements can be made and formulate some wellness goals for yourself. Now determine, using the following suggestions, how massage can help you meet these goals.

1 Analyze what percentage of a one-hour massage ideally would be spent on each level of the Wellness Massage Pyramid to help you meet your wellness goals.

2 Explain your analysis in a brief outline.

3 Compare the specific benefits you might get from massage to others in the class. Notice how unique each person's needs are.

developing greater awareness of the inner self, feeling integrated in body and mind, and enjoying the healthy pleasure of caring touch.

Massage therapy is sometimes referred to as a **complementary and alternative medicine** (**CAM**) therapy. CAM therapies are healing systems or modalities generally outside of mainstream allopathic medicine, for example, herbal remedies, acupuncture, naturopathic medicine, biofeedback, and music therapy. The White House Commission on CAM Policy (2002) cited therapeutic massage, bodywork, and somatic movement therapies as a major CAM domain. Massage therapy as a CAM domain generally refers to applications of massage at the base of the WMP.

In its fullest sense, massage therapy is best thought of as a **wellness profession**, since the work of massage therapists spans the entire wellness massage paradigm. Because of its broad scope, there are a wide variety of career opportunities for massage therapy practitioners. These include developing general practices, or more narrow specializations such as in personal care, sports and fitness, or health care. Some massage therapists focus on a particular client group like the elderly, athletes, people with cancer, children, or other special populations. Over time, massage and bodywork practitioners learn new skills, deepen their knowledge, take advanced training, and change work settings. Because it is a wellness profession, a career in massage therapy provides many opportunities for satisfying individual interests, talents, and strengths.

⟶ TRENDS

Surveys reveal trends in the popularity of massage and the reasons people seek it out. Several recent surveys indicate an increased use of massage overall, and a high percentage in the use of massage in spas and as a CAM therapy for various ailments and injuries.

The Spa Association (SPAA) surveyed more than 3,500 spas about their services and reported their findings in the 2004 State of the Industry Report. Massage was offered at 97% of the spas responding and generated the largest amount of money compared to any other spa service (American Massage Therapy Association, 2004).

A 2004 survey conducted by the Opinion Research Corporation International and commissioned by the American Massage Therapy Association questioned a sample of 1,009 adults in the continental United States about their use of massage. The survey measured the popularity of massage and looked at the factors that motivate people to receive massage. (See Figure 1–2 ◀ for survey results.) It found that 65% of those

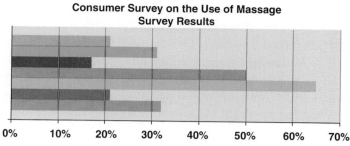

Consumer Survey on the Use of Massage Survey Results

- Therapy for an injury would motivate them to receive regular massage 65+ year olds
- Therapy for an injury would motivate them to receive regular massage 18-24 year olds
- Therapy for an injury would motivate them to receive regular massage
- Had received massage to relieve pain
- Would recommend massage
- Received massage in the last year
- Received massage in the last 5 years

◀**Figure 1–2** Data from 2004 survey conducted by the Opinion Research Corporation International and commissioned by the American Massage Therapy Association®.

polled would recommend massage to someone they know. The popularity of massage among African Americans and Hispanics was equal to or greater than the population as a whole. It also found that nearly half (49%) of those polled have had a massage at some time to relieve pain. Taking medication was the only action that ranked higher than massage for pain relief.

The National Health Interview Survey (NHIS) conducted by the National Center for Complementary and Alternative Medicine (NCCAM) and the National Center for Health Statistics gathered information in 2003 about the use of alternative and complementary therapies in the United States, including massage therapy (NCCAM *Newsletter*, 2004). CAM therapies are approaches to healing outside of conventional medicine, including acupuncture, chiropractic, naturopathy, biofeedback, energy healing, homeopathy, yoga, tai chi, qi gong, and massage therapy. Massage was cited by respondents as the ninth most used CAM therapy with 5% of the 39,000 adults surveyed reporting having received massage in the past year. (See Figure 1–3◀ for the reasons people choose massage for CAM therapy.) General findings were that women were more likely than men to use CAM, that CAM use increased with age and education level, and that those who had been hospitalized in the past year were more likely to turn to CAM.

In a survey of one particular group, military personnel, massage was cited as the most frequently used CAM therapy. Of the 291 military people and their families surveyed, 41% reported having received massage. Respondents were not sure, however, of how effective massage and other CAM therapies actually were for various medical

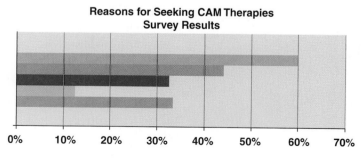

Reasons for Seeking CAM Therapies Survey Results

- Combined conventional treatment and massage
- Thought CAM would be interesting to try
- Massage was suggested by a medical professional
- Conventional treatments were too expensive
- Conventional medicine didn't help

◀**Figure 1–3** Data from the annual National Health Interview Survey (NHIS) conducted by the National Center for Complementary and Alternative Medicine (NCCAM) and the National Center for Health Statistics.

conditions. Researchers felt that the survey results indicated a desire for CAM therapies to be offered at military treatment facilities and called for further evaluation (McPherson & Schwenka, 2004).

The American Hospital Association (AHA) survey of the use of CAM therapies in U.S. hospitals sheds light on the use of massage in mainstream health care. The survey of 1,007 hospitals revealed that 82% of the hospitals reporting use of CAM therapies had incorporated massage into hospital care. Of those offering massage, 74% use it for stress management in patients, 69% for stress relief in hospital staff, 59% for cancer patients, and 55% for pregnant women. Relief of stress and pain were cited most often as the reasons for the use of massage.

The surveys discussed here point to a trend of increased desire for and use of massage therapy for a variety of reasons and in a variety of settings. The use of massage in spas for relaxation and rejuvenation and its use as a CAM therapy are particularly evident in recent surveys.

↳ TYPICAL WORK SETTINGS

Massage therapists work in a variety of settings, reflecting the broad range of the benefits of massage. Four categories of typical work settings include (1) personal care; (2) sports, fitness, and recreation; (3) health care; and (4) private practice. Table 1–1 ◀ lists examples of places where massage therapists typically work. Appendix B, on page 311 is a guide to personal care providers and health care professionals who interact with massage therapists in these work settings and are mentioned throughout this textbook.

TABLE 1-1

Typical Work Settings for Massage Therapists

Personal Care	Sports, Fitness, and Recreation	Health Care	Private Practice—Self-employed
▶ Beauty salon and barbershop	▶ Nonprofit community center	▶ Conventional health care center	▶ Massage therapy office or clinic
▶ Spa	▶ Commercial health club	Medical office or clinic	▶ Storefront business
Club spa	▶ Specialty exercise studio	Hospice service	▶ Home-based practice
Cruise ship spa	▶ Sports club or team	Hospital	▶ Home visit practice
Day spa		Nursing home	▶ On-site chair massage
Destination spa		▶ Integrative medical center	
Medical spa		Integrative medical clinic	
Mineral spring spa		Sports medicine clinic	
Resort/hotel spa		Medical spa	
		Wellness center	
		▶ Alternative health care center	
		Chiropractic office	
		Naturopathic clinic	
		Chinese medicine clinic	

Personal Care

Personal care settings focus on personal grooming, relaxation, and rejuvenation. They include beauty salons and barbershops; and day, destination, and specialty spas (see Figure 1–4◀). In these settings, massage is just one of several services offered.

Beauty salons and barbershops cater to consumers' needs related to hair, nail, and skin care. These establishments are found in storefronts, shopping malls, department stores, hotels, and other commercial spaces. Cosmetologists, beauticians, barbers, and estheticians are licensed professionals providing services in these businesses. Massage may be part of their services within their scope of practice. For example, cosmetologists are usually permitted by law to perform facials and pedicures that include some massage. In this setting, massage therapists offer full body massage for relaxation and rejuvenation.

Spas also offer a variety of personal care services. Spas are defined by the International SPA Association (ISPA) as "entities devoted to enhancing overall well-being through a variety of professional services that encourage renewal of mind, body and spirit." Seven kinds of spas recognized by ISPA include club spa, cruise ship spa, day spa, destination spa, medical spa, mineral spring spa, and resort/hotel spa. The ISPA motto summarizes the intent of the spa experience as to "relax, reflect, revitalize, and rejoice" (www.experienceispa.com).

Day spas offer many of the same services as beauty salons and barbershops, plus special services such as herbal wraps, different kinds of hydrotherapy (e.g., whirlpool, sauna, steam room), mud baths, mineral baths, exercise facilities, and therapeutic massage and bodywork. Guests come for one or more services, staying a short time or the entire day. Massage therapists are sometimes trained to perform services in addition to massage, for example, herbal wraps.

Destination spas are places with overnight accommodations that immerse guests in a healthy environment. Services include fitness activities, nutritious meals, lifestyle education, and the day spa services listed above, including massage.

Other types of spas are distinguished either by focus or location. For example, club spas are fitness facilities that also offer spa services. Medical spas integrate spa

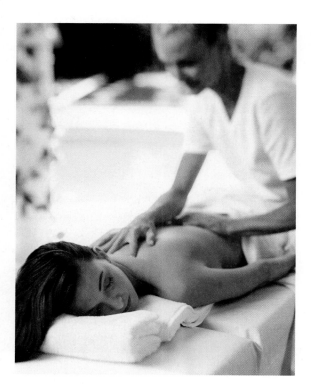

◀ **Figure 1–4** Personal care setting. (Stone/Getty Images)

services with conventional and complementary therapies for healing mind and body. Cruise ship spas are located aboard cruise ships, and mineral spring spas at mineral and hot springs. Resort and hotel spas cater to business and vacation travelers staying at their establishments. The range of services offered in different spas varies, but their common purpose is renewal and rejuvenation through personal care. Massage is an integral part of the modern spa scene.

Sports, Fitness, and Recreation

Sports, fitness, and recreation settings are facilities whose main purpose is to provide opportunities for physical exercise and sports, but that also provide support services like massage. These include nonprofit community centers like the YMCA, commercial health clubs, and specialty exercise studios such as yoga centers. Some massage therapists work with professional or amateur sports teams at their own training facilities and on the road. (See Figure 1–5◀).

Massage is offered in these settings as an adjunct to fitness and sport training regimens. Massage therapists interact with other health professionals working in these facilities, including coaches, personal trainers, exercise physiologists, and athletic trainers. The focus of massage here is to help clients achieve their fitness goals, improve athletic performance, and enhance healing from minor injuries.

Health Care

Health care settings are places where patients are treated for illnesses and injuries. They include conventional Western medical facilities such as doctors' offices and clinics, hospitals, hospice facilities, nursing homes, and rehabilitation centers. Integrative medical settings offer both conventional and complementary and alternative healing methods as options, based on the greatest potential benefit for the patient. Health care also includes alternative medicine settings such as chiropractic clinics, naturopathic offices, and Chinese medicine and acupuncture clinics.

In conventional health care settings, massage therapists work in conjunction with doctors, nurses, physical therapists, and other health care professionals within the tradition of Western medicine (Figure 1–6◀). Hospital-based massage is a specialty in which massage is integrated into regular hospital settings such as in the pediatric ward, cancer unit, or cardiac care unit. For more information visit the Hospital-Based Massage Network (www.hbmn.com).

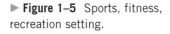

▶ **Figure 1–5** Sports, fitness, recreation setting.

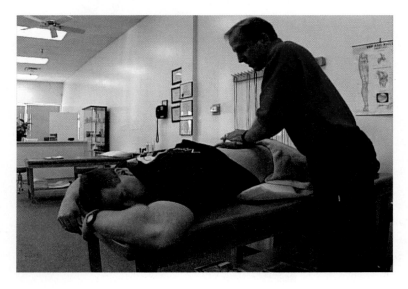

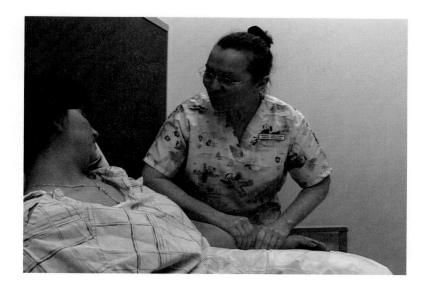

◀ **Figure 1–6** Health care setting.

Conventional health care centers may take an integrative approach by having alternative healing practitioners, including massage therapists, available to patients. An **integrative medicine center** goes one step further by offering a team approach among a variety of Western medical health care providers, traditional and indigenous healers, and CAM practitioners in a collaborative effort. Massage therapists in these settings are an integral part of a health care team.

Integrative medical settings take different forms. For example, in sports medicine centers, massage therapists team up with physical therapists and athletic trainers for rehabilitation of athletic injuries and improvement of sports performance. In medical spas, conventional and complementary therapies are available in a spa environment. Wellness centers connected to hospitals offer fitness activities, rehabilitation programs, massage therapy, and classroom instruction in preventing disease and developing a healthy lifestyle.

Chiropractors hire massage therapists to work with their patients in conjunction with regular chiropractic treatment. Massage may be given before or after a chiropractic adjustment or at a different time as part of an overall treatment plan. Chiropractors also lease space to massage therapists to whom they refer patients for ongoing massage for prevention of problems and general well-being.

Naturopathic physicians often refer patients for massage as part of a treatment strategy. They also hire massage therapists to work in their clinics, or they may lease space to massage therapists so that they are on-site at the naturopathic office.

Chinese medicine clinics hire practitioners skilled in Western massage and Asian bodywork therapy. Asian bodywork systems that complement traditional healing practices such as acupuncture and herbs include tuina, amma, shiatsu, acupressure, and Jin Shin Do®.

Private Practice

Private practice settings are the most varied. Massage therapists in private practice are self-employed and develop their businesses to suit their own interests and talents, and to respond to current consumer demands.

The most common private practice setting is the one-room massage office, or massage clinic with two or more rooms, in an office building. A storefront massage business might be on a commercial street, in a shopping mall, or in an airport. A dedicated massage room can be set aside in a residence for a home-based practice

PRACTICAL APPLICATION

Prepare an informal survey of the availability of massage in your community and the varieties of career opportunities for massage therapists there.

1 Make a list of the places in your community where massage is available.

2 Look at the types of settings, e.g., personal care, sports and fitness, health care and private practice.

3 Indicate the names and addresses of the businesses, and what types of massage they offer. Note the environ-

ment, e.g., if massage is one of many services offered like at a spa, or is unique like chair massage at a health food store, or a separate massage office.

4 Divide the list according to how close the places are to where you live. Are they within a half-mile, one mile, more than one mile?

5 Comment on the accessibility of massage in your community and the potential for career opportunities for massage therapists there.

where not prohibited by zoning laws. Clients come to the massage therapist's space for appointments in these settings, as shown in Figure 1–7 ◄).

An alternative is for the massage therapist to travel to the client's home, sometimes called a **home visit practice**. There the massage therapist creates a setting for massage in an appropriate space provided by the client. The home visit practice is convenient for busy working clients and the homebound elderly and disabled.

With the invention of the special massage chair, settings for massage have expanded to the workplace and other public places. Seated massage settings have been created in places like parks, inside grocery or department stores, and at trade shows and conferences. The traveling or on-site massage practice can be set up temporarily in a small space using portable equipment suitable for the situation.

► **Figure 1–7** Private practice setting.

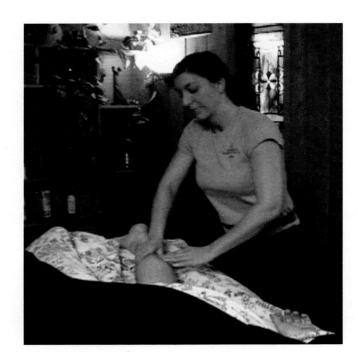

CASE FOR STUDY

Sarah and Finding the Right Massage

Sarah has read a lot about the benefits of receiving massage and has decided to try it for herself. She sees massage advertised in different places in her community and wonders where the best place to go for massage would be for her. Sarah has been feeling stressed out lately and somewhat sore from her new fitness program. She has a few health problems like mild asthma and allergies. She has a busy schedule and values convenience highly, but also wants a high quality massage experience.

Question:
How should Sarah go about finding the right place to receive massage for herself?

Things to consider:

▶ What might Sarah's initial goals be for her massage session?

▶ What might her priorities be in terms of location and setting?
▶ What types of settings might she explore for a massage that meets her current needs?

Where might Sarah go for massage in your community?
Using the information from the Practical Application exercise in this chapter, determine the two best places for Sarah to go for massage in your community. (Assume she lives near you.)

_____
_____
_____

Many massage therapists develop eclectic practices; for example, combining an office practice with making home visits or part-time employment at a spa or chiropractic office. Specialized or advanced training may be required to work in certain settings, but the examples described above portray the broad and diverse range of career opportunities for massage therapists in today's world.

Chapter Highlights

▶ The journey to becoming a successful massage therapist is a holistic experience requiring development of physical, mental, and social skills.
  ● The first step on the journey is to survey the landscape to get the big picture of massage therapy as a career choice.
▶ Simply defined, massage is the intentional and systematic manipulation of the soft tissues of the body to enhance health and healing.
  ● Massage and bodywork is a term often used to describe the occupational field of massage therapy.
▶ Massage is performed with or without oil and may include joint movements and stretches, as well as hydrotherapy.
▶ Massage is primarily a manual therapy, and the person-to-person touch essential to massage gives it a unique healing potential.
▶ The Wellness Massage Pyramid illustrates the broad scope of massage therapy. In this schematic, the goal for the client is achieving high-level wellness.

- The three base levels of the pyramid include deficiency needs related to treatment, recovery from, and prevention of illness and injury. Satisfying these needs gets one to the neutral zone.
- Above the base levels are growth levels related to health maintenance, personal growth, and enjoyment of life.
- As wellness professionals, massage therapists work within the entire wellness massage paradigm, although individuals may focus on a specific level of the WMP or with a certain client population.

▶ Recent surveys reveal a trend in increasing popularity of massage at spas and as a CAM therapy.

▶ In hospital settings, massage is used for stress reduction in patients and staff, for pregnant women, and for pain management.

▶ Typical work settings for massage therapists include:

- Personal care (e.g., beauty salons and spas)
- Sports, fitness, and recreation (e.g., health clubs, exercise centers, sports teams)
- Health care (e.g., conventional Western medical centers, integrative health care centers, chiropractic offices, naturopathic centers, and Chinese medicine clinics)
- Private practice (e.g., commercial office or storefront, home visit practice, and on-site business)

▶ Massage therapists often develop eclectic practices working in a variety of settings.

Exam Review

Learning Outcomes

Use the learning outcomes at the beginning of the chapter and shown here as a guide to the major topics covered. Perform the task given in each outcome, and share your results with a study partner. Check off the tasks as you complete them.

- ❏ Define massage therapy.
- ❏ Use the Wellness Massage Pyramid to explain the scope of massage therapy.
- ❏ Explain massage therapy as a wellness profession.
- ❏ Identify trends related to massage therapy.
- ❏ Understand the variety of career opportunities for massage therapists.
- ❏ Describe typical work settings for massage therapists.

Key Terms

To study key terms listed at the beginning of the chapter, choose one or more of the following exercises. Writing or talking about ideas helps you better remember them, and explaining them to someone else helps deepen your understanding.

1. Write a one-sentence definition of each key term. Put the term in a general category, and then distinguish it from other terms in that category. For example, "*Health-care settings* are places where patients are treated for illnesses and injuries." Or, "*Sports, fitness, and recreation settings* are facilities whose main purpose is to provide opportunities for physical exercise and sports, but which also provide support services like massage." Try to capture the essence of each term in a concise statement.

2. Make study cards by writing the key term on one side of a 3 × 5 card and a concise definition on the other side. Shuffle the cards and read one side, trying to recite either the explanation or word on the other side.

3. Pick out two or three terms and explain how they are related.

4. With a study partner, take turns explaining key terms verbally.

5. Make up sentences using one or more key terms. Variation: Read your sentences to a study partner who will ask you to explain unclear statements.

Memory Workout

The following fill-in-the-blank statements test your memory of the main concepts in this chapter.

1. Massage is the _____ and _____ manipulation of the soft tissues of the body.

2. Massage is primarily a _____ therapy, meaning it is performed by hand.

3. The seven technique categories of Western massage are _____, _____, _____, _____, _____, _____ _____ _____, and _____ _____.

4. The aim of Western massage is to improve overall functioning of the _____ _____, to enhance _____, and for _____ of body and mind.

5. The occupational field of massage therapy is often called _____ _____ and _____.

6. Because the work of massage therapists spans the entire Wellness Massage Pyramid, massage therapy is best thought of as a _____ profession.

7. Spas with overnight accommodations, and which immerse guests in a healthy environment are referred to as _____ spas.

8. The focus of massage therapy in sports and fitness settings is to help clients achieve their _____ goals, improve sports _____, and enhance healing from minor _____.

9. In _____ health care settings both conventional and CAM therapies are available.

10. Massage therapists in private practice are _____ employed, and develop their businesses to suit their own interests and _____, and to respond to current _____ demands.

Test Prep

The following multiple choice questions will help to prepare you for future school and professional exams.

1. Which of the following is not within the scope of massage therapy as practiced in the United States?
   a. Soft tissue manipulation
   b. Joint movements
   c. Chiropractic adjustments
   d. Use of hot packs

2. Which of the following would appear nearest the top of the Wellness Massage Pyramid as an aspect of seeking high-level wellness?
   a. Prevention of illness
   b. Enjoyment of life
   c. Recovery from illness
   d. Neutral zone

3. Herbal remedies, acupuncture, music therapy, and massage therapy are considered:
   a. Allopathic medicine
   b. Mainstream medicine
   c. Conventional medicine
   d. Complementary and alternative medicine

4. "Enhancing overall well-being through a variety of professional services that encourage renewal of mind, body and spirit" is the main focus of which type of setting?
   a. Health club
   b. Naturopathic physician office
   c. Spa
   d. Private practice

5. Health care settings that use a collaborative approach to healing by including a variety of Western medical health care providers, traditional and indigenous healers, and/or CAM practitioners, are referred to as:
   a. Integrative
   b. Comprehensive
   c. Conventional
   d. Alternative

6. Facilities connected to hospitals that offer fitness activities, rehabilitation programs, massage therapy, and classroom instruction in developing a healthy lifestyle are called:
   a. Sports medicine centers
   b. Medical spas
   c. Wellness centers
   d. Chiropractic offices

7. A massage practice in which seated massage is given on special massage chairs at the workplace or at events like health fairs is called:
   a. Home visit practice
   b. On-site practice
   c. Sports massage practice
   d. Integrative practice

8. Combining a massage office with some home visits and part-time employment at a spa or chiropractic office is called:
   a. Environmental practice
   b. Ecological practice
   c. Eclectic practice
   d. Eccentric practice

Video Challenge

Watch the appropriate segment of the video on your CD-ROM and then answer the following questions.

Segment 1: A Career in Massage Therapy

1. What do the massage therapists interviewed in the video say about the rewards of their careers? What settings have they worked in?

2. Give examples from the video of massage therapists working at different levels of the Wellness Massage Pyramid.

3. Can you see yourself working in any of the settings discussed in the video? Which settings appeal to you the most and why?

Comprehension Exercises

The following exercises provide questions for you to answer and tasks you can do to enhance your understanding of the material presented in this chapter.

1. Read about three different forms of massage therapy, ideally from different massage traditions. See Appendix A: 25 Forms of Therapeutic Massage and Bodywork on page 301 for ideas about different forms and where to find additional information. Think about the techniques used and the focus of the sessions; then briefly describe why they can all be called massage and bodywork.

2. Describe the variety of settings in which massage therapists work today. Discuss which settings are best suited for your interests and talents as you currently see them.

3. Starting at the base, name the six levels of the Wellness Massage Pyramid, placing the *neutral zone* in its correct place. Think about your current state of well-being, and write a list of potential benefits you could get from receiving a massage today.

For Greater Understanding

The following exercises are designed to give you a deeper understanding of the subjects covered in this chapter. Action words are underlined to emphasize the active nature of this approach to learning.

1. <u>Receive</u> at least two different forms of massage therapy, ideally from different massage traditions. <u>Compare and contrast</u> the techniques used and the overall approach of the sessions. <u>Write</u> a short report of your experiences and <u>present</u> it to the class.

2. <u>Interview</u> a successful massage therapist, and <u>describe</u> his or her practice in terms of the types of clients served and the setting in which the therapist works. <u>Write</u> a report, and <u>present</u> it to a study partner or to a class.

3. <u>Receive</u> massage in a personal care setting, a sports and fitness setting, a health care setting, and a private practice setting. <u>Compare and contrast</u> the settings, and <u>evaluate</u> which settings are best suited for your interests and talents as you see them today.

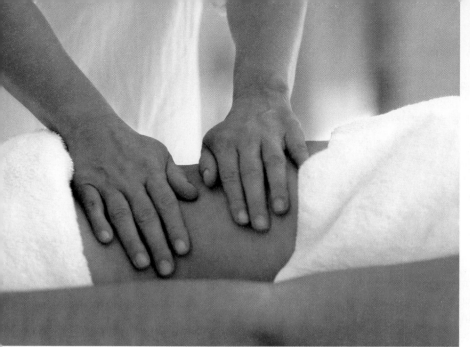

The Massage Therapy Profession

 LEARNING OUTCOMES

After studying this chapter, you will have information to:

1. Distinguish between an occupation, a job, and a profession.
2. Describe the unique knowledge base of massage therapy.
3. Discuss education standards for massage therapists.
4. Describe the types of credentials available to massage therapists.
5. Distinguish among various kinds of professional organizations.
6. Name major massage therapy organizations.
7. List major publications and other sources of information about massage therapy.
8. Describe the state of massage therapy research.
9. Evaluate the level of acceptance of massage therapists by the general public and by other professionals.

KEY TERMS

Accreditation	**Credentials**	**National certification**	**Profession**
Certification	**Ethical standards**	**Occupational licensing**	**Professional associations**
Continuing education			

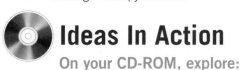

Ideas In Action

On your CD-ROM, explore:

▶ Licensing and credentials   ▶ Research
▶ Ethics   ▶ Interactive video exercises
▶ Organizations

EMERGING PROFESSION

Massage therapy is an emerging profession with a tradition as old as time. Once performed by servants, slaves, and village healers, massage therapy has evolved into a modern wellness profession and attractive career option. With an increasing level of professionalism, massage therapists contribute to the overall health and well-being of their clients and their communities.

As the benefits of massage therapy become better appreciated and the demand for massage therapy grows, there are corresponding expectations that massage therapists become increasingly professional. That means being better educated, having valid credentials, adhering to a code of ethics, and generally being held to a higher standard. Massage therapy is considered an emerging profession in that some of the hallmarks of a mature profession are still in development.

Characteristics of a Profession

An *occupation* is a type of work or livelihood, while a *job* is a specific position of employment. You can stay in one occupation for many years, while changing jobs several times. For example, you might be a massage therapist by occupation and have a job at a spa one year, and at a chiropractic office the next.

The term *profession* as commonly used can mean any highly skilled occupation or trade. In sports, someone who gets paid for playing, or who receives prize money, is considered a professional. The older, more specific definition of the term **profession** describes an occupation with a higher level of organization, standards, and ethical conduct.

This more defined concept of profession developed in Medieval Europe. The first professionals in this more specific sense were lawyers, doctors, and clergymen. Over the centuries, other occupations have been molded in the shape of these original professions, taking on certain essential characteristics.

The benchmarks of a profession in this more defined sense include having a unique body of knowledge and skills, and intensive entry-level education. It also includes valid credentials and continuing education throughout a career. The theoretical and scientific information underlying a profession develops through experience, as well as scholarship and research, and is published in professional journals. Professionals form associations that support their members, set standards, represent the profession to the public, and promote professional interests.

Ethical codes and standards of practice describe expectations of excellence and good conduct. They are the foundations of self-determination and self-regulation for a profession. The overall focus of all professions is commitment to service and the good of humanity. This latter commitment sets professions apart from other businesses and occupations. The public trust afforded to professionals is based on an expectation of honesty, integrity, and selfless service.

All of the benchmarks mentioned above set the stage for acceptance by other professionals and recognition by the general public. The professionalizing of massage therapy has occurred at a steady pace since the 1980s. Table 2–1◀ summarizes the foundation characteristics of a profession.

Since organizations have such a significant role in professions, it is important to know the major organizations in the profession you have chosen. They are typically known by their acronyms or initials, and the "alphabet soup" of organizations can be confusing. Use Table 2–2◀ as a reference for the organizations mentioned in this chapter. Some of the important aspects of professionalism in massage therapy today are explored in the following paragraphs.

TABLE 2-1
Characteristics of a Profession

- ▶ Specialized knowledge and skills
- ▶ Intensive entry-level education
  - Accreditation
- ▶ Continuing education
- ▶ Valid credentials
  - National certification
  - Specialty certification
  - Occupational licensing
- ▶ Professional associations
- ▶ Ethical codes and standards of practice
- ▶ Acceptance among other professionals
- ▶ Recognition by the general public
- ▶ Commitment to public service and the good of humanity

TABLE 2-2
Guide to Major Massage Therapy Organizations in the United States*

Acronym	Name	Type
ABMP	Associated Bodywork & Massage Professionals	Member Services Organization
AMTA	American Massage Therapy Association	Professional Association
AOBTA	American Organization for Bodywork Therapies of Asia	Specialty Association
COMTA	Commission on Massage Therapy Accreditation (USDE recognized)	School Accreditation
COS	Council of Schools (AMTA affiliate)	School Membership
IMSTAC	Integrative Massage and Somatic Therapies Accreditation Council (ABMP affiliate)	School Accreditation
MSA	Massage School Alliance (ABMP affiliate)	School Membership
MTF	Massage Therapy Foundation (formerly AMTA Foundation)	Research, Education, Outreach
NCBTMB	National Certification Board for Therapeutic Massage and Bodywork	National Certification

*Many other massage therapy organizations have been founded to serve the profession, and many others can be found in countries outside of the United States. This is a sample of the largest and most influential organizations in the United States in 2007.

↪ BODY OF KNOWLEDGE AND SKILLS

The body of knowledge and skills that define the massage therapy profession is unique in many respects, while sharing some things with other professions. The uniqueness of massage therapy lies in the primacy of touch and soft tissue manipulation in its skill base and the broad range of applications throughout the entire Wellness Massage Pyramid (see Figure 1–1 on page 5). The knowledge base for massage therapy, although occasionally borrowing from other professions, is uniquely focused on the use of soft tissue manipulation to improve the well-being of recipients. The profession is rooted in the tradition of natural healing and maintains a holistic and wellness perspective.

Examples of shared knowledge are the sciences of anatomy, physiology, and pathology that are basic to all health professions. Concepts like the therapeutic relationship and related ethical principles are common to professions with one-on-one interaction with clients and patients. The communication skills involved in health history taking and documentation are also required in other professions.

Massage skills are part of the scope of other professionals (e.g., estheticians, physical therapists, athletic trainers). However, soft tissue manipulation is only a small part of other professions, while it is the defining modality for massage therapists. Massage therapy and the professions mentioned above have overlapping histories, with separate professions branching off over time.

Massage therapists apply massage through the entire range of wellness applications as depicted in the Wellness Massage Pyramid (WMP)—from treatment, recovery, and prevention of illness and injury to health maintenance, personal growth, and enjoyment of life. Massage therapists are experts in massage applications in a variety of work settings.

This unique body of knowledge is found in the increasing number of textbooks and journals written specifically for massage therapists. It is also reflected in massage therapy program curriculum standards, core competencies, job analyses, and licensing examinations for massage therapists.

↪ EDUCATION

Entry-level education lays the foundation of knowledge and skills needed to perform massage therapy competently. The curriculum typically includes basic massage and bodywork techniques; sciences of anatomy, physiology, kinesiology, and pathology; assessment skills; client communication skills; hygiene and safety; professional standards, ethics, and law; and business practices. Basic massage techniques and their applications are learned in hands-on classes (Figure 2–1◀).

The Commission on Massage Therapy Accreditation (COMTA) has identified core competencies for massage therapists (www.comta.org). Competencies define education in terms of what a practitioner can actually do, rather than just having completed a number of hours in certain subjects. Competencies for entry-level massage therapy programs are found in Appendix C: Summary of Competencies for Massage Therapists on page 315.

Most massage therapy programs are offered in private vocational schools and community colleges. Graduates are awarded a diploma or certificate, associate degree, or in a few cases, an academic bachelor's degree. The general standard for length of entry-level programs varies from 500–1,000 clock hours. COMTA currently requires 600 clock hours of classroom instruction.

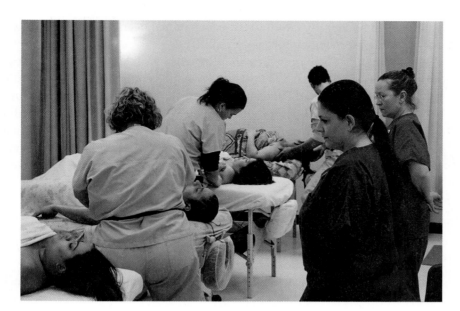

◀ **Figure 2–1** Hands-on class in a massage therapy program.

Massage programs in the United States are required to be approved by the state government agency that oversees vocational, academic, or other school programs. This ensures minimal standards of operation. In other countries, a provincial or national education agency typically approves school programs.

Massage schools, and massage programs within larger institutions like community colleges, may seek additional recognition through **accreditation**. Accreditation is awarded by a nongovernmental organization whose mission is to uphold high educational standards. Accreditation organizations develop evaluation criteria and conduct peer evaluations to confirm that their standards are met. For example, the Integrative Massage and Somatic Therapies Accreditation Council (IMSTAC), a division of Associated Bodywork and Massage Professionals (ABMP), is a body that sets standards for massage programs.

The U.S. Department of Education (USDE) publishes a list of nationally recognized nonprofit accrediting commissions determined by their criteria to be reliable. Some USDE-recognized accrediting bodies that accredit massage programs include the Accrediting Bureau of Health Education Schools (ABHES), Accrediting Commission for Career Schools and Colleges of Technology (ACCSCT), and the National Accrediting Commission of Cosmetology Arts and Sciences (NACCAS). COMTA is the only accrediting agency focused exclusively on massage therapy programs and recognized by the USDE. A complete list of USDE-recognized accrediting agencies can be found on the USDE website (www.ed.gov).

Massage schools and programs may also join member organizations that provide forums for discussion of education-related issues, publications, liability insurance, and other resources. Do not confuse membership in these organizations with accreditation. Two major school organizations in the United States are the Council of Schools, affiliated with AMTA (www.amtamassage.org) and the Massage School Alliance (www.abmp.com), affiliated with ABMP.

Continuing Education

Continuing education (CE) is education beyond entry-level training. Continuing education keeps massage therapy professionals up-to-date and offers the opportunity to gain a higher level of knowledge and skills. A certain number of hours of continuing education are generally required for occupational license and certification renewals, and by some membership organizations.

Continuing education is provided by massage schools, individual teachers, and professional associations. CE providers may be required to be approved for license or certification renewal. The National Certification Board for Therapeutic Massage and Bodywork has a list of their Approved CE Providers and the criteria for approval on their website (www.ncbtmb.org). If your state or local government licenses massage therapists, check with them for their approved providers of continuing education. See Appendix D: Massage Laws in North America on page 317 for information about state licenses.

CREDENTIALS

Credentials testify to the accomplishments of the person holding them. They are a method for the general public, other professionals, and employers to evaluate a person's background in a given field. Credentials are awarded by a school, organization, or government agency to a person meeting their criteria for the credential. Résumés and CVs (curriculum vitae) are documents that list credentials earned and provide a summary of training and experience in the profession.

Using the language of credentials properly is important as massage therapists take their place in the larger world of health professionals. Presenting credentials honestly is a basic ethical principle. Four types of credentials available to massage therapists are a school diploma or certificate, national certification, specialty certification, and occupational licensing.

School Diploma

A school diploma or certificate is a statement that a person has graduated or successfully completed a course of study. It is the piece of paper hung on the wall to show the public the education a massage therapist has had. It designates the school name, location, course of study, number of hours completed, and date of graduation, and is signed by school officials (Figure 2–2◀).

A transcript is a more detailed record of a student's performance while in school, including specific subjects studied, grades, and attendance, in addition to the information on the diploma. An original transcript carrying the school seal is usually required for official purposes such as obtaining a license to practice.

National Certification

National certification is a term usually reserved for a credential given by a nongovernmental nonprofit organization that attests to a person's competency in a given profession. It involves qualifying by virtue of education and/or experience, and passing a written examination and/or performance evaluation based on an objective analysis of job requirements. Those certified agree to abide by a specific code of ethics. National certification is renewed periodically, which usually requires a certain amount of continuing education. It is sometimes referred to as *board certification*.

How does one know if a national certification credential is based on accepted standards and will be respected by other professionals? The National Commission for Certifying Agencies (NCCA) accredits certifying programs that comply with their standards. Many certification programs in the health professions seek NCCA

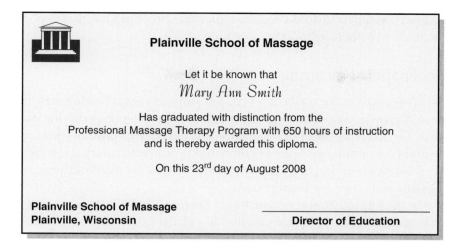

recognition. A list of NCCA-accredited programs can be found on their website
(www.noca.org/ncca/accredorg.htm). Two NCCA-accredited programs apply to
massage and bodywork practitioners.

The National Certification Board for Therapeutic Massage and Bodywork
(NCBTMB) is an organization that offers recognized credentials for massage therapists. It offers two credentials: Nationally Certified in Therapeutic Massage and Bodywork (NCTMB) and Nationally Certified in Therapeutic Massage (NCTM). Eligibility
criteria and content outlines for their exams can be found on their website
(www.ncbtmb.org). In the United States, many states use the NCBTMB examinations
as their state licensing exams.

The National Certification Commission for Acupuncture and Oriental Medicine (NCCAOM) offers a credential called Diplomate in Asian Bodywork Therapy (Dipl. A.B.T.–NCCOAM). Information about this certification and others in
oriental medicine, acupuncture, and Chinese herbology can be found on their
website (www.nccaom.org).

Specialty Certification

To be certified in a specific massage and bodywork system (e.g., polarity therapy,
reflexology, or shiatsu) involves some combination of education, skill development, internship, written and performance tests, ethical code, continuing education, and/or periodic renewal. Specialty certifications can be as rigorous as a 1,000
clock-hour program with internship and written and performance exams, or as
minimal as a weekend workshop. Therefore, determining what a specialty certification really means requires some information about who is offering it and what
is involved in getting it.

Since massage therapy is an emerging profession and retains some entrepreneurial aspects, the terms *certification* and *certified* are sometimes used with ambiguity.
For example, a course of study is sometimes called a "certification program" when
it would be more correctly referred to as a "certificate program" for which a "certificate of completion" is given. In established professions, the term *certification* is
more commonly reserved for credentials with more extensive education, examinations, continuing education, and renewal.

Some massage and bodywork systems are protected by trademark, and the
name is registered with the U.S. Patent and Trademark Office. These systems will
use the registered trademark symbol ®. Practitioners may not use a trademarked
name to describe their work unless certified by the system's organization or

properly authorized to do so. Examples are Jin Shin Do®, Rolfing®, and Bonnie Prudden Myotherapy®.

Occupational Licensing

When deemed in the public interest, governments may choose to regulate a profession. A growing number of governments are licensing or certifying massage therapists. The main purposes of occupational licensing are consumer protection and the assurance of a minimal level of competence of practitioners. However, in the case of massage, an underlying motivation may also be to weed out practitioners using massage as a cover for prostitution.

In the United States, occupational licensing is done at the state level. In some unlicensed states, jurisdictions like big cities (e.g., San Diego) may choose to license massage therapists. In Canada, occupational licenses are administered at the provincial level, and in some other countries at the federal or national level of government.

Occupational licensing is permission granted to qualified practitioners to accept compensation for massage in a specific governmental jurisdiction. Licenses are awarded by the government agency that regulates professions in the jurisdiction. It is required in order to practice, unlike the national or specialty certification described above, which is voluntary. Table 2–3◀ compares and contrasts diplomas, national certification, occupational licensing, specialty certification, and accreditation.

The details vary, but massage licenses typically require being a minimum age (usually 18 years old), having a minimum level of general education (usually a high

---

TABLE 2-3

Guide to Credentials in Massage Therapy

Type of Credential	Voluntary/ Required	Given To	Given By	Purpose
Accreditation	Voluntary	School	Nongovernment Accreditation Commission	Testify that school meets commission standards
Certificate	Voluntary	Individuals	Schools/Instructors	Proof of education completed
Continuing Education Approval	Required	Schools/Instructors	Credentialing Body	Approval of education programs for credential renewal
Diploma	Voluntary	Individuals	Schools/Instructors	Proof of education completed
National Certification	Voluntary	Individuals	Nongovernment Certification Board	Attest to competency in the profession
Occupational License	Required	Individuals	Government	Permission to practice in jurisdiction
Specialty Certification	Voluntary	Individuals	Nongovernment Organization/ Instructor	Attest to competency in specialization

school diploma), completing massage therapy education of a defined length (usually 500–1,000 clock hours), passing a designated written and/or practical test, having no criminal record, abiding by a code of conduct, and paying fees. People practicing without a license are subject to fines, and in some cases, criminal prosecution.

Alternative forms of regulation may exist in some jurisdictions. Some forms are voluntary such as certain *certification* programs. In others, those meeting certain requirements are *registered* and can call themselves massage therapists, but other practitioners are not prohibited from working.

In the United States today, 38 states plus the District of Columbia have occupational licensing or a related form of regulation for massage therapists. Licensing bills are pending in several other states. Appendix D: Massage Laws in North America on page 317 lists the massage regulating agencies in North America and their general education and exam requirements. The most current information on licensing can be found at professional organizations' websites.

A different type of license called an establishment license might also be required for a massage practice at a specific location. This is a business license to operate a commercial space where customers come for massage. Also for public protection, establishment licenses typically require revealing the business ownership, maintaining a certain level of hygiene and safety, posting services and prices, and assuring that all practitioners in the establishment have the required occupational licenses.

⟶ ORGANIZATIONS

Massage and bodywork practitioners have formed several organizations to address their needs and promote the profession. They can be categorized as general membership organizations and specialty organizations. General membership organizations welcome practitioners of different forms of massage and bodywork, and can be further categorized into professional associations and member services organizations. Specialty associations are composed of practitioners of a particular style of bodywork, such as polarity therapists, or those who work in a particular setting like the nurse massage therapists.

Professional Associations

Professional associations are nonprofit organizations run by elected leadership, whose mission is to promote their profession, to represent their members and the profession in the larger world, and to offer services to members. They set standards for the profession by developing codes of ethics and standards of practice. They typically have an IRS designation as 501(c)(6) corporations (i.e., nonprofit professional associations).

The mission of the association, its goals and plans, position statements, and services are determined by an elected board and implemented by volunteers and staff. Involvement in the work of committees, special projects, and activities of the association help develop the present and future leadership of the profession. All of the money generated by the association is reinvested in its mission.

Association services typically include providing information via official publications and website, offering professional liability insurance and group insurance plans, hosting referral services, and selling products related to the profession.

Associations raise public awareness of the profession, and conduct consumer and other surveys to collect information about the field. At annual conventions, members get together for board and committee meetings, education sessions, exhibits of the latest equipment and supplies, and networking with other members (Figure 2–3◀).

Governments consult with professional associations as representatives of the profession in developing legislation like licensing and establishment laws. They also turn to associations when seeking participants in studies and policy development. For example, professional associations participated in preparing the report of the White House Commission on Complementary and Alternative Medicine Policy (2002) (www.whccamp.hhs.gov/finalreport.html).

Organizations also look to professional associations for participation in multi-disciplinary projects. An example of this is the participation of massage organizations in the Integrated Healthcare Policy Consortium (IHPC) of the Collaboration for Healthcare Renewal Foundation (http://ihpc.info).

Some professional associations have local chapters to address the needs of members in a particular state or other local jurisdiction. Chapters provide opportunities for leadership development and networking closer to home. They are important in the United States where regulation of massage therapy occurs at the state and local levels.

The American Massage Therapy Association (AMTA), founded in 1943, is the oldest and largest professional association for massage and bodywork therapists in the United States (www.amtamassage.org). Its mission is "to develop and advance the art, science and practice of massage therapy in a caring, professional and ethical manner in order to promote the health and welfare of humanity." Its core purpose is "to promote, advance and provide innovative thinking in the field of massage therapy while facilitating, supporting and serving AMTA members." It currently has over 50,600 members in 27 countries and chapters in all 50 states.

Member Services Organizations

Member services organizations are general membership organizations whose major mission is to provide benefits like professional liability insurance, group health insurance, and publications. They also provide information of interest to their members in newsletters and on websites. These organizations may also act to protect the interests of members, for example, in matters related to licensing and legislation. They

▶ **Figure 2–3** Professional association conventions provide opportunities for continuing education and networking with other massage therapists.

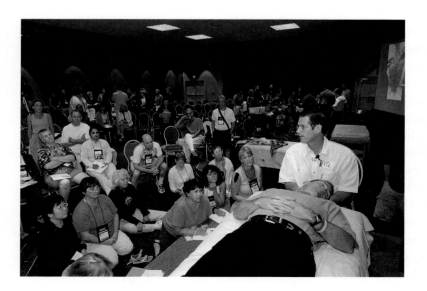

PRACTICAL APPLICATION

Explore student membership in a major professional organization. Use the organization's website and promotional materials for information.

1 Write a brief description listing the specific benefits offered with student membership.

2 Discuss with a classmate or study partner the potential value to you of joining a professional organization while still a student.

3 Answer the question: How might student membership in a major professional organization give you a head start in your career?

---

differ from professional associations in that they may be for-profit businesses, and if so, the owner sets policy and determines the direction of the organization. They typically do not hold conventions nor have elected leadership.

Associated Bodywork and Massage Professionals (ABMP), founded in 1987, is the largest member services organization for massage and bodywork practitioners in the United States, with over 50,000 members (www.abmp.com). Its goal is "to provide massage, bodywork, skin care and somatic therapies practitioners with professional services, information, and public and regulatory advocacy. ABMP is devoted to promoting ethical practices, protecting the rights of practitioners, and educating the public regarding the benefits of massage and bodywork" (www.abmp.com).

Specialty Associations

Massage therapy, like many other professions, can be divided into subgroups of practitioners with special knowledge and skills. They may focus on a particular form of massage and bodywork, a specific population of clients, or a particular setting. Specialty groups often form their own associations to address their unique needs and interests. They offer members many of the same benefits as general membership organizations. The following are examples of different types of specialty associations for massage and bodywork practitioners.

The American Organization of Bodywork Therapies of Asia (AOBTA) is a professional association founded in 1989. It represents over 1,400 practitioners of forms of bodywork based in traditional Chinese medicine developed in China, Japan, Korea, and other Asian countries (www.aobta.org). It has some state chapters.

The American Polarity Therapy Association (APTA) was founded in 1984 as an educational and charitable nonprofit organization (www.polaritytherapy.org). Its members include practitioners, teachers, and students of Polarity Therapy as developed by Randolph Stone. It promotes practitioner standards, approves education programs, sponsors education events, and publishes a newsletter and other materials.

The Rolf Institute® of Structural Integration was established in 1971 as an educational and scientific nonprofit organization (www.rolf.org). Its purpose is to promote a form of myofascial bodywork called Rolfing®, provide quality training programs in Rolfing®, certify Rolfing® practitioners, provide continuing education, and promote research and public awareness of the value of Rolfing®.

The International Association of Infant Massage (IAIM®) was formed in 1980 and incorporated in 1986 (www.iaim.net). The IAIM® mission is "to promote nurturing touch and communication through training, education, and research so that parents, caregivers, and children are loved, valued, and respected throughout the world community." The organization trains and certifies Certified Infant Massage Instructors (CIMI®) who in turn teach parents and caregivers to massage their babies.

The National Association of Nurse Massage Therapists (NANMT), established in 1987, is a nonprofit organization for nurses who are also trained in some form of massage and bodywork, and work in health care settings (www.nanmt.org). Their basic philosophy includes a respect for holistic healing, practices grounded in nursing theory, and the need to balance high-tech medicine with personalized touch-based therapies. One of their goals is to compile research related to massage in health care, and implement findings into practice.

Notice that most of the organizations described above were founded in the late 20th century, when the field of massage and bodywork experienced a period of growth and expansion. Many other specialty organizations have been formed since that time; they can be found on the Internet.

SCHOLARSHIP AND PUBLICATIONS

Scholarship in therapeutic massage and bodywork has been increasing in volume and quality over the past 25 years. Vehicles for this information have evolved from a few self-published manuals in the 1970s to a variety of well-documented and illustrated texts published by major publishing houses today.

The depth of scientific knowledge in anatomy, physiology, kinesiology, and pathology required by today's practitioners has spawned a number of books written specifically for massage and bodywork practitioners. Authors with extensive academic backgrounds in human sciences, who are also massage therapists, have provided a depth of knowledge absent in the past. The same can be said for the areas of pharmacology, psychology, and professional ethics.

As the profession of massage therapy matures, and experienced practitioners become teachers and authors, the understanding of massage therapy theory and principles deepens. In addition, massage therapists who have come from more established professions have enriched massage therapy scholarship. Nurses, physical therapists, physical and health educators, athletic trainers, psychologists, pharmacologists, and other professionals who have come into the field have helped transform massage theory and practice in a number of areas.

For example, information from other professions related to things like the therapeutic relationship, assessment skills, effects of medications, documentation, and ethics have been integrated into the massage therapy knowledge base. The result is a more developed body of knowledge for massage therapists.

A variety of publications disseminate information about massage and bodywork to practitioners and the general public. The *Massage Therapy Journal* is the official publication of the AMTA, and ABMP publishes *Massage & Bodywork*. Although intended for a general audience, *Massage* magazine also provides information about the massage and bodywork profession. *Massage Today* is a monthly publication in newspaper format that contains news about the field as well as informative articles on a variety of related subjects.

A peer-reviewed publication that reports research related to massage therapy is *The Journal of Bodywork and Movement Therapies* (www.harcourt_international .com/journals/jbmt/). Peer reviewed means that a panel of massage therapists with expertise in the subject of an article evaluates the article for accuracy, reviews any research for validity, and approves the article for publication. Although various publications have editorial review, the more rigorous process of peer review is the standard for research publications.

RESEARCH

A research base for massage therapy is developing gradually. Scientific studies about massage therapy are now conducted primarily within more established health professions and in connection with universities and hospitals. The result is an emphasis on clinical applications of massage, with less attention to applications at the top of the Wellness Massage Pyramid, such as fitness and personal growth.

Two obstacles to massage therapy research are lack of an academic infrastructure to support it and inadequate funding. Vocational schools and community colleges, where most massage therapy education takes place, do not ordinarily have the resources to conduct research. Neither do they have faculty with advanced training in experimental design and statistics to conduct the studies. The limited number of peer-reviewed research journals specifically for massage therapists means that reports of massage research are scattered among journals from other health professions.

There are, however, some developments to advance research in the profession. The Massage Therapy Foundation (formerly the AMTA Foundation) was founded in 1990 to promote massage therapy research. It funds studies and maintains a database of massage therapy research on its website (www.massagetherapyfoundation.org). The MTF published a report called the *Massage Therapy Research Agenda* in 1999. The report calls for greater research literacy among massage therapists; more funding for studies about the safety and efficacy of massage, physiological and other mechanisms of massage, massage in a wellness paradigm; and studies about the therapeutic massage profession. The MTF sponsors annual student and practitioner case report contests.

The Touch Research Institute (TRI) at the University of Miami School of Medicine was founded by director Tiffany Fields, MD, in 1992. It was the first center in the world devoted to the study of the use of touch and massage in the treatment of various ailments. Its website (www.miami.edu/touch-research.html) has information about many studies sponsored by TRI.

ETHICAL STANDARDS

Knowledge of ethics and ethical behavior are essential competencies for massage therapists. There is a growing body of literature about ethical behavior in the profession.

Ethical standards in massage therapy are reflected in the codes of ethics and standards of practice of professional organizations. The National Certification Board for Therapeutic Massage and Bodywork (NCBTMB) requires certificants to abide by their code and standards and to have continuing education in professional ethics as a condition of renewal. Professional organizations also have disciplinary procedures for censoring members not in compliance with their ethical standards. Further discussion of professional ethics can be found in Part III of this text.

ACCEPTANCE BY THE GENERAL PUBLIC

Evidence of public acceptance of massage therapy is found in the many positive articles appearing in newsstand magazines and health and fitness publications. Massage therapy is also a popular service at spas and health clubs.

Consumer surveys confirm the growing acceptance of massage therapy by the general public. In a 2003 survey, 80% of respondents viewed massage therapists as providing a stress reduction service, 69% viewed massage as a CAM therapy, and 52% saw the role of massage therapists as health care professionals. The survey showed that the general public is seeking massage therapy for stress relief, muscle soreness, and pain management. In 2003, more than 1 in 5 adults surveyed had received massage within the past 12 months (American Massage Therapy Association, 2003).

Two stereotypes that have negatively affected the level of public acceptance of massage therapy in the past are diminishing. These are the association of massage with prostitution and with quackery and medical humbug. As massage therapists achieve greater degrees of professionalism, these stereotypes will continue to decrease in the future.

RECOGNITION FROM OTHER PROFESSIONALS

There is ample evidence of the recognition of the massage therapy profession by the government and by other professionals. For example, manual therapies, including massage, were included in a report on alternative medicine to the National Institutes of Health (NIH) in 1992. The White House Commission on Complementary and Alternative Medicine Policy (WHCCAMP) cited therapeutic massage, bodywork, and somatic movement therapies as a major CAM domain in its Final Report (2002).

A majority of massage therapists (70%) in a 2005 industry survey indicated that they receive referrals from health care professionals, averaging two referrals per month. In addition, 82% of hospitals responding to a 2003 American Hospital Association survey reported massage therapy among their health care offerings. A 2002 survey of insur-

CRITICAL THINKING

Think about the effect that negative stereotypes have had on the acceptance of the massage therapy profession by the general public and by other health professionals.

1 Identify those stereotypes.

2 Write a brief explanation of why you think the stereotypes developed and why they still exist.

3 What factors related to massage therapy as an emerging profession are likely to lessen negative stereotype about massage?

CASE FOR STUDY

Jim and Explaining Massage Therapy as a Profession

Jim enrolled in a massage therapy program after high school to learn a marketable skill so he could eventually have his own business. He liked to work with his hands and was interested in health and fitness. He had received massage while recovering from a sports injury and thought he would like to be a massage therapist. He saw many career opportunities for his future in massage therapy. Jim's old high school friends could not understand the attraction of massage therapy as a career, nor did they think one had to go to school to learn something that seemed so simple.

Question:

What can Jim tell his friends to explain the profession of massage therapy to them and its growing importance as a health practice?

Things to consider:

▶ What can he say about the growing acceptance of massage by the general public and other health professionals?

▶ How can he explain the extent of his education and the skills he is learning?

▶ What can he point out about the credentials he is working toward having and the professional associations he has joined?

▶ What publications can he show them to illustrate what massage therapy is all about?

▶ How would mentioning massage therapy research help explain the profession and its place in health and healing?

What three things could Jim focus on to best explain the massage therapy profession to his friends?

1. _____

2. _____

3. _____

---

ance plans found that 74% of the HMO plans studied cover massage/relaxation therapy in some way (American Massage Therapy Association, 2005).

Representatives of the massage therapy profession have been asked to participate in a variety of professional activities. For example, an AMTA representative was appointed in 2003 to the CPT® Committee of the American Medical Association. CPT®, or Current Procedural Code, lists the codes for official reporting of medical services and procedures. Massage therapy is also represented on the Academic Consortium for Complementary and Alternative Health Care (ACCAHC).

The formal activities cited above, along with countless referrals and inclusion in integrative health care settings, attests to the growing acceptance of massage therapy and massage therapists as professionals.

Chapter Highlights

▶ Massage therapy, a modern profession with a tradition as old as time, has evolved into a wellness profession, with corresponding expectations that massage therapists be increasingly professional.

● Massage therapy is an emerging profession that has achieved some of the benchmarks of a mature profession.

▶ The body of knowledge and skills that defines the massage therapy profession is unique in many respects, while sharing some things with other professions.
  ● The uniqueness of massage therapy lies in the primacy of touch and soft tissue manipulation in its skill base, and the broad range of applications throughout the entire Wellness Massage Pyramid.
  ● The profession is rooted in the tradition of natural healing and maintains a holistic and wellness perspective.

▶ Curriculum standards for entry-level education in massage therapy range from 500–1,000 clock hours of instruction and include the knowledge and skills required for competency in the field.

▶ Accreditation is a voluntary, nongovernmental process for massage schools and programs that ensures compliance with established criteria.
  ● The U.S. Department of Education recognizes agencies that accredit massage programs and meet their standards.

▶ Continuing education beyond initial training is required for renewal of certifications, licenses, and by some general membership organizations.

▶ Four types of credentials available to massage therapists include a school diploma or certificate, national certification, specialty certification, and occupational licensing.
  ● A diploma or certificate is evidence of having completed a particular course of study.
  ● National certification is a nongovernmental voluntary credential that shows competency in the field.
  ● Specialty certification attests to education and competency in a specific form of massage and bodywork.
  ● An occupational license is a permission to practice in a certain jurisdiction, and massage therapy is regulated in 38 states and the District of Columbia in the United States and some provinces in Canada.

▶ Massage therapists have founded a number of professional organizations that include general membership organizations (i.e., professional associations and membership services organizations) and specialty associations.

▶ Scholarship in therapeutic massage and bodywork has been growing in volume and quality over the past 25 years.
  ● An increasing number of textbooks and journals have been published specifically for massage therapists.
  ● Professionals from other fields, who are also massage therapists, have enriched the scholarship in the field.
  ● Massage therapy has one peer-reviewed research journal, *The Journal of Bodywork and Movement Therapies.*

▶ The Massage Therapy Foundation, established in 1990, has developed a research agenda and provides a research database on its website (www.amtafoundation.org).

▶ Ethical standards for the profession are embodied in codes of ethics and standards of practice developed by professional associations.

▶ All of the listed accomplishments in the massage therapy profession have led to greater acceptance by the general public and recognition by other professionals.

Exam Review

Learning Outcomes

Use the learning outcomes at the beginning of the chapter and shown here as a guide to the major topics covered. Perform the task given in each outcome, and share your results with a study partner. Check off the tasks as you complete them.

- ❑ Distinguish between an occupation, a job, and a profession.
- ❑ Describe the unique knowledge base of massage therapy.
- ❑ Discuss education standards for massage therapists.
- ❑ Describe the types of credentials available to massage therapists.
- ❑ Distinguish among various kinds of professional organizations.
- ❑ Name major massage therapy organizations.
- ❑ List major publications and other sources of information about massage therapy.
- ❑ Describe the state of massage therapy research.
- ❑ Evaluate the level of acceptance of massage therapists by the general public and by other professionals.

Key Terms

To study key terms listed at the beginning of the chapter, choose one or more of the following exercises. Writing or talking about ideas helps you better remember them, and explaining them to someone else helps deepen your understanding.

1. Write a one-sentence definition of each key term. Put the term in a general category, and then distinguish it from other terms in that category. For example, "*Accreditation* is recognition awarded to institutions or education programs by a non-governmental organization that sets standards of excellence." Or, "*Certification* is a type of credential given after extensive education in a specific subject and may also include examinations, continuing education, and renewal." Try to capture the essence of each term in a concise statement.

2. Make study cards by writing the key term on one side of a 3 × 5 card, and a concise definition on the other side. Shuffle the cards and read one side, trying to recite either the explanation or word on the other side.

3. Pick out two or three terms and explain how they are related. For example, explain the relationship between *national certification* and *occupational licensing*, or between *professional associations* and *ethical standards*.

4. With a study partner, take turns explaining key terms verbally.

5. Make up sentences using one or more key terms. Variation: Read your sentences to a study partner who will ask you to explain unclear statements.

Memory Workout

The following fill-in-the-blank statements test your memory of the main concepts in this chapter.

1. As the benefits of massage therapy become better appreciated, there is a corresponding expectation that massage therapists be more _____.

2. The term *profession* is used to describe an occupation with a higher level of _____, standards, and _____ conduct.

3. Competencies define education in terms of what a practitioner can actually _____, rather than just having completed a certain number of _____ in various subjects.

4. A specific number of hours in continuing education are generally required for renewal of occupational _____, _____, and by some professional _____.

5. Credentials provide a method for employers to _____ a person's background in a given field.

6. A _____ or certificate is a statement of completion of a course of study.

7. The main purpose of occupational licensing is _____ protection and the assurance of a minimal level of _____ of practitioners.

8. Specialty associations are formed by practitioners who focus on a particular _____ of massage and bodywork, or a specific population of _____, or who work in a specific _____.

9. Two stereotypes that have negatively affected massage therapists in the past and that are diminishing today are the association of massage with _____ and _____.

10. Ethical standards in massage therapy are reflected in the _____ of _____, and standards of _____ developed by professional associations.

Test Prep

The following multiple choice questions will help to prepare you for future school and professional exams.

1. A specific position of employment is called a(n):
   a. Occupation
   b. Profession
   c. Job
   d. Calling

2. Which of the following statements about massage therapy today is *not* true?
   a. It is rooted in the tradition of natural healing.
   b. It is narrowly focused on medical applications.
   c. It maintains a wellness perspective.
   d. It is holistic at its core.

3. Recognition given to a school by a nongovernmental organization for upholding high educational standards is called:
   a. Accreditation
   b. Certification
   c. Licensing
   d. Approval

4. A detailed record of a student's performance while in school is called a:
   a. Diploma
   b. Certificate
   c. Resume
   d. Transcript

5. A credential given by a nongovernmental nonprofit organization that attests to a person's competency in a given profession is called:
   a. Specialty certification
   b. National certification
   c. Accreditation
   d. Licensing

6. In the United States, what level of government typically regulates professions like massage therapy by issuing occupational licenses?
   a. Town
   b. County
   c. State
   d. Federal

7. Nonprofit organizations run by elected leadership, whose mission is to promote their profession, to represent their members and the profession in the larger world, and to offer services to members are called:
   a. Professional associations
   b. Member services organizations
   c. Specialty associations
   d. Certification boards

8. The growing acceptance of massage therapy by the general public is confirmed in:
   a. Hospital surveys
   b. Licensing laws
   c. Consumer surveys
   d. Government reports

Video Challenge

Watch the appropriate segment of the video on your CD-ROM and then answer the following questions.

Segment 2: The Massage Therapy Profession

1. Which aspects of massage therapy as a profession are discussed in the video?

2. What credentials do the massage therapists interviewed in the video say that they have? Why do they think that their credentials are important?

3. Where does the video say that information about massage research can be found?

Comprehension Exercises

The following exercises provide questions for you to answer and tasks you can do to enhance your understanding of the material presented in this chapter.

1. Compare an established profession that you are familiar with (e.g., nurse, accountant, librarian, teacher, lawyer) with massage therapy. What characteristics of professionalism does each occupation have?

2. Who licenses massage therapists and why? What are the pros and cons of occupational licensing for massage therapists? What are the penalties for practicing without a license?

3. Why is developing a research base for massage therapy important to the profession? What are some obstacles related to massage therapy research? What organization funds massage therapy research and provides a research database on its website?

For Greater Understanding

The following exercises are designed to give you a deeper understanding of the subjects covered in this chapter. Action words are underlined to emphasize the active nature of this approach to learning.

1. Analyze the mission, services, and activities of an organization for massage therapists. Gather information using its promotional materials, publications, websites, and member interviews. Write a summary of your analysis.

2. Find the most recent massage therapy industry information reported by a professional organization. Analyze the data to see what it says about the massage therapy profession and the acceptance of massage therapy by the general public and other health professionals. What factual sources is the information based upon? Discuss the implications of the findings with the class.

3. Analyze a massage therapy publication mentioned in this chapter. Who publishes it? What types of articles and regular columns does it have? Who are the advertisers? Do you think the information is useful to massage therapists who read it regularly? Present your findings to the class.

4. Attend a state, regional, or national convention sponsored by a professional association for massage therapists. Take advantage of all of the opportunities offered at the event including education, networking, massage equipment and supplies vendors, and organizational meetings. Report to the class about your experience.

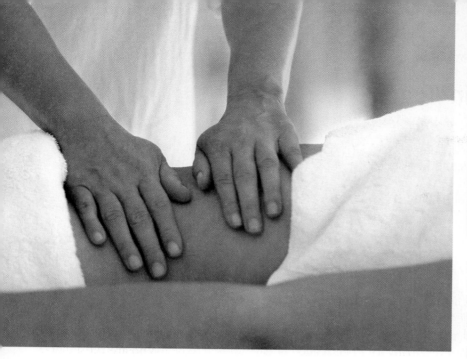

LEARNING OUTCOMES

After studying this chapter, you will have information to:

1. Trace the history of massage related to personal grooming services.

2. Describe the use of massage for athletes from ancient times to the present.

3. Explain how massage has been used over the centuries in Western medicine.

4. Identify aspects of today's massage therapy that can be traced to the natural healing philosophy.

5. Name important figures in the history of massage and describe their contributions.

6. List factors leading to the revival of massage as a popular health practice in the 1970s.

7. Describe important developments in the massage profession in recent decades.

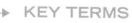

KEY TERMS

Aleiptes	Health service operator	Medical gymnast	Sobardoras
Ammashi	Massage operator	Rubbers	Trained masseuses
Bath attendant	Masseurs/Masseuses		

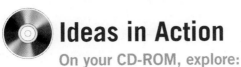

Ideas in Action

↪ HISTORY OF A VOCATION

The term *vocation* means the work a person has chosen to do for his or her livelihood, especially one for which the individual has talent or is drawn to. It comes from the Latin *vocare*, to call, and refers to the concept of having "a calling" to a particular type of work. Over the centuries, many have been called or have chosen to be massage practitioners.

Like other vocations, massage therapy has its own history. Massage practitioners of the past include servants and slaves, tribal and village healers, rubbers and masseurs, doctors and nurses, medical gymnasts, natural healers, and Swedish masseuses. Today's massage therapists are the latest in the line of countless massage practitioners that have gone before. Each generation received knowledge and skills from its predecessors and shaped the future for those who followed.

The history of massage as a vocation looks at several different aspects of the work. For example, who went into the occupation, how they were trained, what types of skills and knowledge they had, their work conditions, and their status in society. This history describes differences in various times and locations, how situations changed over the years, and what factors influenced the work of massage practitioners. It offers a better understanding of today's environment and the outlook for massage therapists in the future.

There are four major branches of the history of massage as a vocation. They roughly parallel today's work settings: personal grooming and rejuvenation, sports and fitness, health care, and natural healing. A comprehensive history of massage can be found in Calvert's *The History of Massage: An Illustrated Survey from Around the World*. A few examples from this vast history offer an appreciation for the experiences of massage practitioners in the past.

↪ PERSONAL GROOMING AND REJUVENATION

Massage has been part of personal care from time immemorial. As people groomed themselves by bathing, cleaning and cutting their hair, and trimming their nails, the pleasurable and rejuvenating effects of rubbing their skin were obvious. People in dry climates learned to rub vegetable and mineral oil on their skin to keep it moistened and healthy. This practice would have been natural for mothers caring for infants and children, those caring for the frail and elderly, and people grooming themselves and family members.

In ancient civilizations, it was often slaves or domestic servants who provided personal care services, including massage, in the private sphere or home. These servants had low social status, were uneducated, and learned their skills from fellow servants or family members.

In ancient Greece, friction and rubbing with oil was a daily practice. The ancient historian, Plutarch, reports that Alexander the Great (356–323 BCE) traveled with a personal attendant who rubbed him and prepared his bath. Other nobles of that time also "used fragrant ointment when they went to their inunction [application of skin moisturizer] and bath, and they carried about with them rubbers (triptai), and chamberlains" (Johnson, 1866, pp. 4–5).

In ancient India, royalty and nonroyalty alike enjoyed a similar practice. The Greek geographer Strabo (63 BCE–24 CE) described how Indian royalty rubbed their skin with staves or flat sticks, "and they polished their bodies smooth by ebony staves." He also mentions that the king received foreign ambassadors while being rubbed, and "there are four rubbers standing by."

In the 1800s, the British used the English word *shampooing* to describe massage practices seen in India, China, and the Middle East. The word is thought by some to come from the Sanskrit word transliterated as *tshampua*, meaning body manipulation. Shampooing was a full body experience that often involved a hot, soapy bath, followed by a form of bodywork involving percussion and friction massage, joint cracking, and applying scented oils or perfume. It was said to give "ineffable happiness and energy" and that "the Indian ladies seldom pass a day without being thus shampooed by their slaves" (Taylor, 1900, p. 40).

The ladies of Padshah Begum's Court were said to do many things throughout the day including storytelling, and "others shampoo well, and are so employed for hours every day." Johnson noted that the practice survived into the 19th century, and that "rubbing was a universal habit in India, and is almost as necessary to the native, rich or poor, as food" (Johnson, 1866, pp. 6–7).

In China in the 1800s, barbers set up shop in markets and parks offering grooming services and a type of bodywork. Patrons sat on stools while the barbers cut hair, shaved or trimmed beards, cut nails, cleaned ears, or a gave a percussive type of massage. As itinerant tradesmen, these Chinese barbers also were part street performers who played "a thousand tricks to please and amuse their customers, to whom and the surrounding audience they tell their gossiping stories" (M'Lean, c. 1914).

The blind masseurs or **ammashi** of Japan have their own unique story. In the 1800s, the government of Japan decreed that the occupation of ammashi (amma = traditional Japanese massage; shi = practitioner) be reserved for blind persons as a welfare measure. As a result, government programs for training ammashi were created, and blind amma practitioners were licensed and enjoyed public respect. (See Figure 3–1 ◀). These blind ammashi walked the streets announcing their presence: "Formerly they used to blow a small flute as they went about, and people used to call them in as they heard the sounds" (Joya, 1958). It is said that at the outbreak of World War II in the 1940s, 90% of the ammashi in all of Japan were blind, but after the war, blind ammashi were found mainly in rural districts.

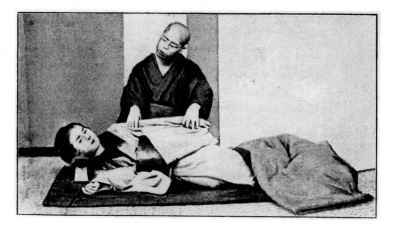

◀ **Figure 3–1** Blind Japanese masseur or ammashi, c. 1900. (From *The Art of Massage* by Kellogg, 1895.)

Public Baths

Public bathhouses are community centers for personal hygiene, grooming services, pleasure and rejuvenation, and social interaction. They are found all over the world. In the past, they were sometimes operated by the government, as in ancient Rome, but most were commercial bathhouses. Today massage continues to be an integral part of the public bath tradition in its latest form, day and destination spas.

Ancient Greece and Rome, ancient China and Japan, Medieval Europe, and the Middle East all had public baths. In times and places where individual homes did not have indoor plumbing, public baths provided bathing and grooming facilities and services, as well as community gathering places.

The Roman bath is the prototype public bath in Western civilization. These bathhouses provided by the state were built all over the Roman Empire, which extended from Asia Minor in the East to the British Isles in the west (27 BCE–476 CE). In addition to exercise courts, warm rooms (tepidarium), steam rooms (caldarium), and a cold pool (frigidarium), there were spaces for bodywork. The massage providers would have been slaves or servants to individuals, or possibly slaves or employees of the state that operated the bath.

After the fall of the Roman Empire, public baths remained popular in Medieval Europe until the 16th century when the spread of communicable diseases, and promiscuous behavior, made common bathing undesirable. A woodcut from the 16th century shows a person receiving a back rub in the corner of a public bath. (Haggard, 1932) (See Figure 3–2 ◀).

The Turkish bath, also called a *hammam*, based on the Roman prototype, became popular in the Middle East and reached Europe in the 1800s. After bathing, and perhaps a haircut and a shave, patrons received a vigorous type of bodywork from a practitioner called a *telltack*. It involved gripping and pressing the muscles, stretching, and cracking the joints (Johnson, 1866). The telltack would have learned his trade by informal apprenticeship and was unlikely to have had anything other than a practical

▶ **Figure 3–2** Massage at medieval public bath, 16th century. (From *The Lame, the Halt, and the Blind* by Haggard, 1932.)

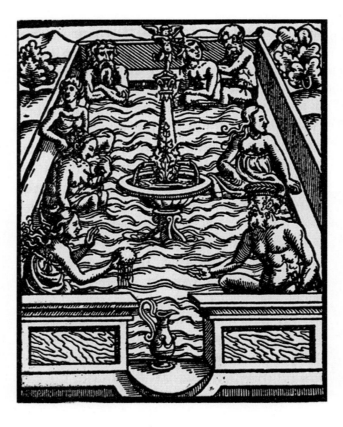

knowledge of human anatomy learned on the job. The Turkish bath was popular in the cities of Europe and North America through the first half of the 20th century and is still found in the Middle East.

The Chinese bathhouse tradition appears very similar in nature to those found elsewhere. An example can be seen in a Chinese film called *Shower* in English. The film is set in a late 20th-century Chinese bathhouse that is slated to be torn down to make way for modern buildings. Local men come to the bathhouse to take hot baths and showers, sleep on cots, listen to music, get their hair and nails trimmed, gossip, play board games, hold cricket fights, and drink tea—the Chinese version of the Turkish bath. The bathhouse owner serves as bath attendant and massage practitioner. A brief massage scene shows a patron lying on a bench and the bathhouse owner applying percussion techniques like slapping and cupping with open hands. A little later he resets a patron's shoulder that had gone out of joint (Zhang, 2000).

The occupational designation of **bath attendant** stems from ancient traditions of servants or attendants giving a rubdown, or rubbing in scented oils, after a bath. This low-skilled friction and rubbing hardly equates with the more highly skilled massage that evolved for health and healing. Nevertheless, bath attendants were misleadingly equated with massage therapists in government occupational codes until the 1980s. Bath attendants at a late 19th-century European spa are shown in Figure 3–3◀).

Salons and Spas

In the early 1900s, women went to salons or parlors for personal care services. *Beauty culture* was the term used for the art and science of grooming women's hair and nails, applying makeup or cosmetics, and other beauty treatments to enhance appearance. Massage for rejuvenation, reducing, and bust development were part of beauty culture in the early 20th century.

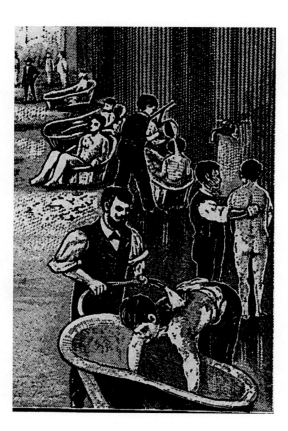

◀ **Figure 3–3** Bath attendants, c. 1890. (From *The Natural Method of Healing.* Vol. 2, Blitz Sanitorium in Germany, 1898.)

PRACTICAL APPLICATION

Find some historical objects or pictures that you could use for decoration or conversation pieces in your future office. Old massage machines, oil and liniment bottles, books, drawings, and photos can spark the interest of people who see them. Having one or more historical objects around can also offer you a special depth of connection to your chosen field.

In large urban areas in the United States, upscale salons like Elizabeth Arden and Helena Rubenstein enjoyed downtown locations, while smaller beauty salons (also known as beauty parlors and beauty shops) dotted local neighborhoods. Specialists in hair, skin, and nail grooming learned their trade in vocational schools and became licensed as beauticians or cosmetologists in most states. In their scope of practice, massage was largely limited to the head, neck and shoulders, hands and arms up to the elbow, and feet and lower leg up to the knee (Livingston & Maroni, 1945). These were superficial massage applications done during personal grooming at the salon. The first U.S. licenses for barbers and beauticians appeared around 1900.

Full body massage remained part of the beauty culture scene and was offered in salons for relaxation and rejuvenation. Swedish massage, an amalgamation of Ling's medical gymnastics (or Swedish movement cure) and Mezger's massage, became the signature massage of salons. By the 1930–40s, colleges of Swedish massage were training **masseurs** (men) and **masseuses** (women) to work in a variety of places, including personal care settings. (See Figure 3–4◀).

Graduate masseuse or graduate masseur was the title for a practitioner trained in a school, as opposed to someone who learned massage by apprenticeship or on the job, and served as a kind of credential. Careers as graduate masseuses were extolled in college catalogs. Massage students had courses in anatomy and physiology, dietet-

▶ **Figure 3–4** Swedish masseuse, c. 1935. (From *The College of Swedish Massage Catalogue*, Chicago, 1939.)

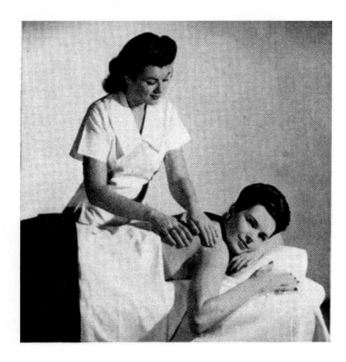

ics, hydrotherapy, light therapy, electrotherapy, and massage (College of Swedish Massage *Catalogue*, c. 1939).

Swedish masseuses were also trained in *reducing massage*, a form of massage erroneously thought to help women slim down. Swedish masseuses at reducing salons offered reducing massage, as well as nutritional advice, exercise, and steam room and steam cabinets. Many masseuses also taught exercise classes. Bust massage was advertised as developing "firmness and plumpness of the bust" (Benjamin, 2001, 2002).

Several well-respected massage programs in the 1930–40s were correspondence courses. The knowledge base was learned through the mail, followed by a week of more intensive training at the school to learn the physical skills. This arrangement, called distance learning today, was ideal for people who did not live in big cities where schools were readily available. Most people still lived in small towns prior to World War II, and transportation was difficult. These correspondence courses gave people who did not live in big cities the opportunity to receive massage training.

Massage technician or massage operator was considered a good career option in the 1930–40s for those wanting to develop a private practice—much like today. Although graduate masseurs and masseuses formed professional associations, such as the American Association of Masseurs and Masseuses established in 1943, they did not seek licensing in most states.

Over 60 years later, day spas and full service salons continue to offer personal grooming services, and some modern establishments are incorporating hydrotherapy facilities like those found in European spas. Swedish massage and other forms of massage therapy continue to be provided in these settings by graduate and, in most states, licensed massage therapists.

⤷ SPORTS AND FITNESS

From ancient Greek times, massage has been associated with sports and fitness. The Greek gymnasia were places where freeborn citizens went to train their bodies and minds. Athletes were rubbed with oil by practitioners called **aleiptes**, "whose business it was to anoint the wrestlers before and after they exercised, and took care to keep them sound and in good complexion" (Graham, 1902, p. 19). The last part of the gymnasium exercises was called *apotherapeia*, or a routine for recovery. It's purpose was ridding the body of waste products and preventing fatigue. It consisted of bathing, friction, and inunction or applying oil (Graham, 1902, p. 28).

Paidotribes in ancient Greece were like the trainers in Western sports many centuries later. They were often former athletes and served in many capacities including coach, nutritionist, masseur, physiotherapist, and hygienist. Although the paidotribes were self-taught or trained by apprenticeship, they would have been exposed to theories about diet, exercise, muscle physiology, and therapies of Greek medicine (Johnson, 1866).

Rubbers and Athletic Masseurs

When amateur sports gained popularity in the 18th–19th centuries, the rubdown after a bath was a mainstay of the care of athletes. It consisted of rubbing and friction of the limbs. It was performed by the trainers themselves, but also by specialists called **rubbers**. Rubbers were unschooled massage practitioners who might have been athletes themselves who had a knack for rubbing. They learned their skills on the job or from other rubbers. When describing the treatment for sore shins, trainer and early Olympic track coach Michael Murphy noted, "if the runner has the services of a trainer and rubber he will be properly cared for" (1914, p. 161).

As in the Greek gymnasium, athletic facilities like the YMCA and sports centers also had pools, showers, and steam rooms. The bath attendant was a familiar figure there who might also be skilled in a rubdown-style massage. In 1902, a trainer named Pollard commented that "in all cases vigorous rubbing should follow the use of water; a bath attendant who knows something about massage is invaluable, for how to rub down a man or a horse is an art" (p. 21).

Early 20th-century trainers were multitalented and helped athletes with sports skills, conditioning, motivation, and injury rehabilitation. Many had been athletes themselves, and were drawn to training, or had "good hands" and became masseurs. In professional sports like boxing, and club sports like track and field, athletic masseurs were either self-taught or apprenticed. Their knowledge of anatomy consisted of what they learned around the gym. A trainer-masseur from the early 1900s named Harry Andrews is shown in Figure 3–5 ◀.

The specialty of massage for athletes became more sophisticated in the mid-20th century. Although many trainers had learned through experience on the athletic field, others were starting to be trained in colleges and universities. The term *athletic masseur* was used to indicate a higher level of training and knowledge than that of the rubbers of the past.

In the 1930–40s, some athletic masseurs were graduates of colleges of Swedish massage. Working with athletes and professional sports teams was one of the career paths for graduate masseurs. Others were trained in physical education programs in colleges and universities, where they learned basic sciences, musculoskeletal anatomy, kinesiology, sports injuries, and other sport sciences—as well as massage applications for athletes.

Albert Baumgartner, a former trainer at the State University of Iowa, believed that "any sports trainer should be a well-qualified masseur" and that "the athletic masseur should come from the ranks of the sports teachers." He further stated that "a physical education instructor should not think himself too refined to enter the profession of the athletic masseur" (1947, p. 11).

▶**Figure 3–5** Athletic masseur, c. 1900. (From *Massage and Training* by Andrews, 1910.)

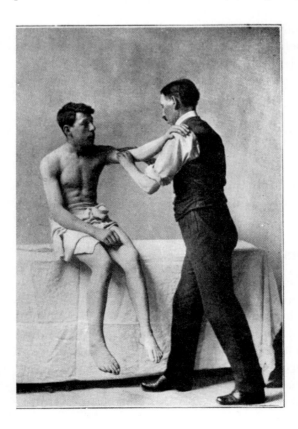

This affiliation with physical education departments in colleges eventually led to a separate profession for athletic trainers. The National Athletic Training Association (NATA) was formed in 1950. Athletic trainers soon dropped massage as used in training athletes in the past and patterned their new profession on physiotherapy, focusing almost exclusively on injuries.

For about 20 years, the old skills of the athletic masseurs were not available to college and professional athletes in the United States except where the old-school rubbers and athletic masseurs continued their work. This was not the case in many European countries, where the tradition of athletic massage remained strong.

Then in the 1970s in the United States, within the emerging profession of massage therapy, the tradition now called *sports massage* was revived. Athletes who had been turned on to massage as a training aid because of the success of European athletes sought specialists in this old art. The knowledge and skills of massage for athletes had fallen out of the realm of the modern professions of coach and athletic trainer, and so it made sense that massage specialists with an affinity for athletics would respond to the call.

Trained massage therapists, like the graduate masseurs and masseuses before them, already had knowledge of muscular anatomy and physiology, and highly developed hands-on skills. Work with athletes, or sports massage, continues to be a specialty for massage therapists.

Fitness/Health Service Operators and Expert Masseuses

In the first half of the 20th century, masseurs and masseuses worked in athletic clubs, private gymnasia, and YMCAs providing massage for health and fitness buffs. As early as 1915, a rubdown by a bath attendant was an established part of the routine at the YMCA. R. Tait McKenzie described a workout at the Y as a mixture of Swedish and German gymnastics and games, "ending with a bath and a rub down" (1915, p. 170).

Commercial health clubs for office workers and businessmen were popping up in cities across America. A December 1917 advertisement for Postl health club in Chicago featured a photo of 14 trainers and masseurs who have "adequate experience and know the laws of health through long service with us." (See Figure 3–6 ◀.) They promised to give "physical and mental health, strength, and vigor," and "steal your weak stomach and tired nerves, sending you away vibrating with glowing health and ambition."

An ad for Burke's Gymnasium from 1932 boasted "the finest and most completely equipped health institution in San Francisco." There were graded classes for ladies and their children, handball and tennis courts, and acrobatics for girls. The ladies' Turkish

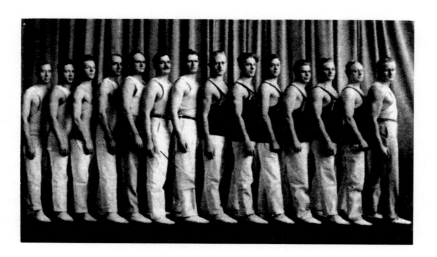

◀ **Figure 3–6** Masseurs and trainers from the Postl health club in Chicago. (From a "Physical Training for the Tired Business Man," ad in *Chicago Tribune Pictorial Weekly*, December 9, 1917.

bath, with its cabinet baths, blanket sweats, hot room, and steam room, offered a course of baths and reducing treatments. It was under the management of "expert masseuses."

By 1943, 274 YMCAs in the United States were operating health service departments that offered massage. The scope and methods of these YMCA massage operators was described by Frierwood in 1953: "The technician uses massage, baths (shower, steam, electricity cabinet), ultraviolet irradiation (artificial and natural sunlight), infrared (heat), instruction in relaxation and in some cases directed exercises. The adult members secure a relief from tensions, gain a sense of well-being, give attention to personal fitness and develop habits designed to build and maintain optimum health and physical efficiency throughout the lifespan" (p. 21).

The **health service operator** was trained in the familiar cluster of natural health and healing methods sometimes called physical therapeutics or physiotherapy. These were massage, hydrotherapy, electrotherapy, light, relaxation techniques, and exercise. The goals, however, were not medical, but focused on health, fitness, and general well-being.

Health service operators and masseurs were trained in YMCA colleges in physical education departments, as well as in colleges of Swedish massage. The Dayton YMCA in Ohio established a School of Health Service and Massage in 1937. A professional association called the Health Service Operators Society was established in 1942 "to combat the abuses of commercial bathhouses and the unethical conduct of 'cure-all' agents in the health field" (Williams, 1943, p. 30). The association was active through the 1950s.

Health clubs today have adopted the YMCA format of exercise, hydrotherapy (steam room, sauna, whirlpool), and massage. It is the same format as the ancient Greek gymnasium.

↪ HEALTH CARE

In its broadest sense, health care encompasses all of the arts and sciences of healing. Rubbing, friction, and pressing of the soft tissues have been a mainstay of health care throughout time and place. In primitive cultures, massage was performed in the treatment of a variety of ailments by shamans and traditional healers, as well as family members. It was often the domain of women.

Captain James Cook, on an expedition to Tahiti in the 1770s, gives a firsthand account of how the mother and sisters of a native named Tu used massage to treat "rheumatick pain" in his hip and leg. Cook relates, "I was desired to lay down in the midst of them, then as many as could get around me began to squeeze me with both hands from head to foot, but more especially the parts where the pain was, till they made my bones crack and a perfect Mummy of my flesh . . . . I found immediate relief from the operation. They gave me another rubbing down before I went to bed ..." (Thomas, 2003, p. 342). These women were not "professionals" in the sense of having an occupation, but performed massage as part of everyday family care skills.

On the other hand, traditional Hispanic healers called **sobardoras** are trained by apprenticeship to use massage in treating ailments of those in the community who call on their services. They also use ritual, herbal remedies, and bone-setting manipulation techniques in their work. Sobardoras are part of the healing tradition of *curanderas*, who combine folk traditions from Spain and Mexico. It is believed that curanderas inherit their power to heal, although an individual may be called to healing and given the *don*, translated as "gift." These traditional healers are professional-like in the sense that they feel called to the work, go through a long apprenticeship, and it becomes their occupation in the community (Perrone, Stockel, & Krueger, 1989).

Western Medicine

The history of modern medicine begins in ancient Greece with Hippocrates (450–377 BCE). The writings attributed to Hippocrates began a shift away from magic, ritual, and superstition in healing practices. Hippocratic writings emphasized observation, logic, diagnosis and treatment, and relationship to the patient. The Greek physician observed symptoms, related those symptoms to the internal and external environment, and prescribed therapy in accordance with nature as he understood it.

Physicians trained in the Hippocratic methods were taught rubbing and frictions: "The physician must be experienced in many things, but assuredly also in rubbing; for things that have the same name have not the same effects. For rubbing can bind a joint which is too loose, and loosen a joint that is too rigid. Hard rubbing binds; soft rubbing loosens; much rubbing causes parts to waste; moderate rubbing makes them grow" (Hippocrates, "Peri Arthron," quoted in Graham, 1902, p. 21). The implication is that practitioners must be skilled in different rubbing techniques to elicit different effects.

Those in ancient Greece who specialized in rubbing were called *triptai*. Massage and bodywork was called the *anatriptic art*. Anatriptic meant to "rub up" or toward the body's center, presumably when rubbing the arms and legs.

Ancient physicians began to identify the most effective soft tissue technique applications for various conditions. For example, Hippocrates advises "to rub the shoulder gently and smoothly" after resetting a dislocated shoulder. Celsus (25 BCE–50 CE), a Roman physician, said to stroke "the chest with a gentle hand" for a cough, and use "soft and long continued rubbing of the affected part" for a spasm. Galen (130–230 CE) advised physicians to warm the body with moderate rubbing with a linen cloth before applying oil and compressing tissues, and that "one should first rub quietly, and afterwards gradually increasing it, push the strength of the friction so far as evidently to compress the flesh but not to bruise it" (Johnson, 1866, pp. 12–19). Obviously, skilled massage applications required more knowledge and skill than mere rubbing.

The more recent tradition called *medical rubbing* began to emerge in 18th–19th century Europe. Douglas Graham's *A Treatise on Massage* (1902) devoted two chapters to the history of massage and names several physicians who used soft tissue manipulation in medical treatments during this and earlier periods. One of these was Dr. J. B. Zabludowski of Berlin, Germany, shown in Figure 3–7◀massaging the ankle, c. 1910.

Much earlier, in 1780, a well-known French professor of clinical medicine named Simon Andre Tissot wrote about massage and exercise in a book called *Gymnastique medicinale et chirurgicalein*. An English physician named William Balfour published a book on the subject in 1819. Other English physicians of the time, like surgeon Mr. Grosvenor

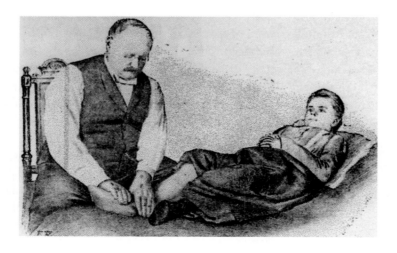

◀ **Figure 3–7** Dr. J. B. Zabludowski of Berlin, Germany, performs massage of the ankle, c. 1910. (From *Zabludowski's Technik der Massage* by Eiger, 1911.)

of Oxford, developed medical rubbing systems. In 1859, Mr. Beveridge of Edinburgh published a pamphlet called "The cure of disease by manipulation, commonly called medical rubbing."

But medical rubbing did not catch on at the time in mainstream English medicine, "and from that time to this [1866] rubbing has been left almost wholly in the hands of unprofessional persons … some of whom used simple rubbing … while others employed various kinds of liniments and ointments" (Johnson, 1866, p. 8). By the end of the 19th century, the practice of medical rubbing would evolve into a budding profession for trained masseurs and masseuses.

Trained Masseuses. About a century ago, the word *massage* replaced *medical rubbing* to describe the treatment of illness and injury with soft tissue manipulation. The French had developed soft tissue manipulation skills they called *massage*, and the term was later popularized by Johann Mezger, a physician from Amsterdam. The word *massage* stuck as the generic term for soft tissue manipulation and is used to this day. The terms *massotherapy* and *manual therapeutics*, once used to describe skilled massage, are not used anymore.

Mezger (1838–1909) developed a system of soft tissue manipulation that is the basis for today's traditional Western massage. Using French terminology, Mezger called the work massage, and its practitioners, masseurs and masseuses. He categorized massage techniques as effleurage, petrissage, friction, and tapotement; vibration was added later. The place where massage was given was called a parlor or salon. Mezger's massage became popular throughout Europe and North America.

Although a number of physicians championed massage as a treatment modality, most assigned the actual massage work to assistants. Some training schools for nurses gave general instruction in massage. Graham thought that manipulators, or massage practitioners, should have "a natural tact, talent, and liking for massage, with soft, elastic and strong hands and physical endurance sufficient to use them, together with abundance of time, patience, and skill acquired by long and intelligent experience" (1902, p. 52).

That there were many untrained massage practitioners is mentioned in textbooks from the early 1900s. Graham lamented that "it is not to be wondered at that many a shrewd, superannuated auntie, and others who are out of a job, having learned the meaning of the word massage, immediately have it printed on their card and continue their 'rubbin,' just as they have always done" (1902, pp. 51–52).

On the other hand, **trained masseuses** took courses of study in private schools and hospital programs. *A Manual for Students of Massage* written by Mary Anna Ellison (1909) outlines a typical turn-of-the-century massage curriculum. After an overview of anatomy, topics include massage techniques, how to give a general massage, vibration treatment, Schott treatment for heart disease, treatment for locomotor ataxia, Weir-Mitchell treatment for neurasthenia, and the Swedish system of medical gymnastics, which was considered a specialty.

Trained masseuses were valued by doctors who employed them. Weir Mitchell, who developed the famous Rest Cure, found many benefits from massage itself and valued observations about his patients by "practiced manipulators." He found that "their daily familiarity with every detail of the color and firmness of the tissues is often of great use to me" (Mitchell, 1877).

The level of professionalism expected of trained masseuses is evidenced by the "hints to masseuses" given by Ellison. She admonishes students to cease treatment "if you have real cause for believing that it or your personality is in any way prejudicial," and to concentrate attention on the patient (p. 138). A list of *don'ts* include: "don't discuss the doctor's methods with the patient, and don't mention the names of other patients in conversation" (pp. 143–144). Other hints are listed in Figure 3–8 ◄ and

Hints for Masseuses, c. 1909

- ❦ Don't take a case without medical permission, at least, if not supervision. Fatal results have sometimes followed massage of unsuitable cases.
- ❦ Don't discuss the doctor's methods with the patient, and don't mention the names of other patients in conversation.
- ❦ Don't talk scandal to your patients, and, on the other hand, avoid shop talk.
- ❦ Don't speak as if you were the one competent masseuse to be had.
- ❦ Don't undertake more cases than you have energy and vitality for, or both you and the patients will suffer.
- ❦ Don't accept any stimulants at a patient's house.
- ❦ Don't abuse any confidence reposed in you, or publish abroad private matters that come to your knowledge.
- ❦ Don't continue your attendance a day longer than is necessary, or if you see that massage is not providing beneficial results.
- ❦ Don't forget that you have come on business, and don't give the impression that massage is an act of condescension on your part.
- ❦ Don't neglect to study your patient's individuality, and if you can in any way rest her mind as well as her body, do so.
- ❦ Don't give the servants more trouble than you can help, whilst maintaining your position with dignity.
- ❦ Don't allow a patient to experience the discomfort of feeling your breath.
- ❦ Don't wear rings or bracelets.
- ❦ Don't sweep the patient's skin with your sleeve or any part of your dress.

◀**Figure 3–8** Hints for Masseuses (from *A Manual for Students of Massage* by Ellison, 1909).

offer good advice 100 years later, particularly Ellison's comment: "One thing I am assured of—that is, the absolute necessity for a masseuse … to keep her mind in as well-balanced condition as possible, and during her treatment to concentrate her attention (as fully as circumstances permit) on the patient and her needs, not necessarily speaking much, but having her mind full of healthfulness and hope as regards the ultimate issue of her work. She follows up *mentally*, as it were, the results she is trying to achieve *manually*." The Society of Trained Masseuses was formed in England in 1894 to raise professional standards for massage specialists working in the medical field.

CRITICAL THINKING

Analyze the "Hints to Masseuses" made in 1909 by Mary Anna Ellison listed in Figure 3–8.

1 What do the hints reveal about masseuses of 100 years ago?

2 Which ones are still applicable today?

3 What do they tell you about the historical development of ethics for massage therapists?

As mainstream health care developed in the United States through the 20th century, massage became a minor modality within the scope of other professions such as nursing and physical therapy. The occupation of masseuse and masseur never rose to the level of a separate profession within institutionalized medicine. Massage specialists were relegated to natural healing settings and deemed "alternative." That is why although massage therapy has a long tradition as a healing agent, massage is considered an alternative therapy in today's health care system.

Medical Gymnasts. A separate but related tradition of bodywork was known variously as medical gymnastics, mechanotherapy, and physical therapeutics. This was the curing of diseases through movement, that is, active and passive exercises. Although the Swede Pehr Henrik Ling (1776–1839) is the most famous individual for developing a system of medical gymnastics, others preceded him. In the 16th century, Mercurialis wrote "De Arte Gymnastica" or the science of bodily exercise, including movements for the cure of diseases. An English physician, Thomas Fuller, published "Medicina Gymnastica" in 1704, and a French physician, Clement Tissot, wrote "Gymnastique Medicinale" in 1781.

Ling's system was comprehensive and included educational gymnastics for building strong, healthy bodies, military gymnastics for hand-to-hand and small weapons combat, and medical gymnastics for treating diseases. Ling based his exercises on knowledge of anatomy and physiology as he understood them and so is credited with putting the practice on a rational or scientific basis. Physical educators, physical therapists, and massage therapists all consider Ling a "father" of their profession.

The Swedish system of medical gymnastics was considered an alternative therapy. While allopathic medicine relied on drugs and surgery as its major modalities, Ling's system was an alternative for treating a variety of chronic diseases from asthma to spinal curvature to headaches. In its heyday, before strict medical licensing, movement cure practitioners were considered primary health care providers and accepted patients for diagnosis and treatment (Roth, 1851). Many were also MDs, but there were also many lay practitioners.

One of Ling's greatest contributions was the development of **medical gymnast** as an occupation. Whereas others wrote books and taught individual students, Ling founded a school that gained international fame and trained thousands of practitioners from all over the world in his system. His school, the Royal Gymnastic Central Institute, was established in 1813 in Stockholm. It was open to men and women, and the curriculum included anatomy, physiology, pathology, hygiene, diagnosis, principles of the movement treatment, and the use of exercises for general and local development (Nissen, 1920).

Graduates of Ling's program, and spin-off programs in the United States and Europe, found employment as physical education teachers in the schools (educational gymnastics), and as medical gymnasts at Swedish movement cure institutions. In places like the Swedish Cure Institute in New York, founded by Dr. George Taylor, medical gymnasts led patients through active movements and applied passive movements or soft tissue manipulations. Medical gymnasts assisting a patient through a movement prescription are shown in Figure 3–9◀.

In the latter 19th century, medical gymnasts adopted Mezger's system of massage as a compliment to Ling's system. Later editions of textbooks originally written about the Swedish movement cure added sections on the "new" massage treatment. For example, in 1889, Hartvig Nissen wrote *A Manual of Instruction for Giving Swedish Movement and Massage Treatment*. By the late 19th century, Ling's and Mezger's systems of bodywork were so identified together that they became known in the United States as Swedish massage.

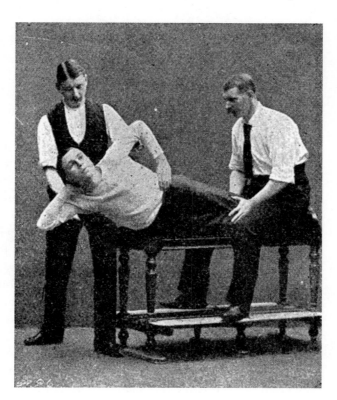

◀ **Figure 3–9** Medical gymnasts assist patient in performing movements, 1909. (From *Handbook of Medical and Orthopedic Gymnastics* by Wide, 1909.)

Many colleges that adopted the Swedish system for physical education classes also began training physical educators in the tradition of Ling. The location of these training programs within colleges influenced the direction of the development of the athletic training and physical therapy professions.

Physical therapy began to form as a separate profession around the time of World War I when practitioners, called *reconstruction aides*, were trained to help rehabilitate wounded soldiers. Many reconstruction aides were trained in departments of physical education in colleges where they learned to apply corrective exercise and massage. In fact, up until World War II, a prerequisite for many physical therapy (also called physiotherapy) programs was a degree in physical education.

Physical therapists formed their first professional association in 1921, the American Women's Physical Therapeutic Association. The name was changed in the 1940s to the American Physical Therapy Association. Today physical therapists have their own associations and training programs at the bachelor and master degree levels. Occupational licensing for physical therapists in the 1940–50s anchored the profession to mainstream medicine.

The distinction between massage therapists working in medical settings and physical therapy professionals was not crystal clear in the 1940–50s. Many physical therapists had been initially trained in colleges of Swedish massage where Ling's work was also taught. In fact, the American Association of Masseurs and Masseuses (AAMM), founded in 1943, changed its name to the American Massage & Therapy Association (AM & TA) in 1958 to reflect that some of its members identified themselves as massage practitioners and some as physical therapists.

By the 1960s, those who wanted to work in medical settings were grandfathered into physical therapy licenses. The professions of physical therapy and massage therapy were now going their separate ways. As the distinction between the professions became clearer, the "&" was dropped from the AM&TA and it became the American Massage Therapy Association (AMTA) in 1983.

→ NATURAL HEALING AND DRUGLESS DOCTORS

The natural healing movement began in the late 1800s. Natural healing practitioners rejected the allopathic methods of drugs and surgery, and instead used natural remedies to treat ailments. They were known as the *drugless doctors*. They relied on medicinal herbs, mineral waters, hydrotherapy, colonic irrigation, therapeutic massage and movement, hypnosis, meditation, and electrotherapy. They promoted healthy practices like rest, exercise, good nutrition, deep breathing of fresh air, sunbathing, singing, and laughter. Many were vegetarians. They recognized that true health is a matter of body, mind, and spirit.

Fundamental to the philosophy of natural healing is a belief in the innate healing power of nature, or "the inherent restorative power for health that resides in every organism" (Erz, c. 1924). The job of the natural healing practitioner is to facilitate that natural process and avoid "heroic" or intrusive methods. Preventing illness and promoting healthful natural living are also essential to this philosophy. The natural healing movement was a precursor to today's wellness movement and spawned the profession of naturopathic physician.

Naturopaths, the drugless healers, had begun to organize their profession in 1902 with the founding of the Naturopathic Society of America. It was reorganized as the American Naturopathic Association (ANA) in 1919. *The Naturopath*, a magazine focused on the "interests of all schools of drugless healing," and "the Art of Natural Living," also "devotes itself especially to the defense of the individual drugless practitioner persecuted by the Medical and Osteopathic Trust" (advertisement, 1925). Today, the profession of naturopathic physician is licensed in 14 of the 50 states.

Massage in the Natural Healing Tradition

Massage and the Swedish movements were important natural healing methods. Dr. P. Puderbach, director of the Brooklyn School for Massage and Physiotherapy and author of *The Massage Operator*, wrote that massage "has taken its rank as the equal of other sanative methods, and thus we see in the Massage that is applied correctly by experienced hands, a powerful means for the rejuvenation of mankind, the beautification of the human body, the alleviation of innumerable weaknesses, and the cure of many diseases that have been the curse of humanity" (Puderbach, 1925, p. 7).

Dr. Puderbach's school trained massage specialists to work in natural healing environments. Figure 3–10◀ shows an operator massaging the shoulders and using a heat lamp or radiant rays. These lamps were used to relax muscles and increase local circulation, "producing the most favorable conditions for effective massage" (Puderbach, 1925, p. 141).

Several well-known natural healing centers appeared at the turn of the century in the form of country resorts. Benedict Lust (1872–1945), a German immigrant was considered a "father" of naturopathy. Lust operated two such places called Yungborn in Butler, New Jersey, and Tangerine, Florida. Yungborn in New Jersey, established in 1896, was billed as the "original nature cure resort and recreation home" and "the parent institution of naturopathy in America." An advertisement for Yungborn lists massage, Swedish movements, and mechanotherapy as some of the many treatments available at the nature resort.

Perhaps the most famous natural healing center was the Battle Creek Sanitarium in Michigan run by J. Harvey Kellogg (1852–1943). Kellogg, who is widely known for Kellogg cereals, had a great interest in health and nutrition and was

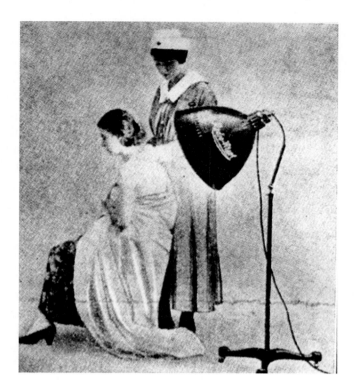

◀ **Figure 3–10** Masseuse performs massage of the shoulder under heat lamp, c. 1925. (From *The Massage Operator* by Puderbach, 1925.)

especially interested in massage. He wrote a classic on the subject titled *The Art of Massage: Its Physiological Effects and Therapeutic Applications* (1895). The manual was intended for medical and nursing students, but also became a standard text for masseurs and masseuses. Kellogg employed 10–20 masseurs and masseuses at the "San" at any one time.

Kellogg numbered the descriptions of different massage techniques and applications so that physicians could prescribe the exact methods they wanted the massage practitioner to perform on an individual patient. But the experienced masseur and masseuse were also expected to modify the application for each case and not follow the written prescription "slavishly."

Kellogg makes reference to the work of Ling in the preface to *The Art of Massage* (1895). He states that "it is rare that the most perfect results can be obtained without supplementing the treatment by massage with a judiciously conducted course of gymnastics" (p. v). He suggests that a translation of Ling's work on medical gymnastics "ought to be in the hands of every masseur" (p. vi). So just as medical gymnasts at that time were adopting massage to complement their work, masseurs and masseuses were adopting the Swedish movements as a natural complement to massage.

A popular version of natural healing was promoted by Bernarr Macfadden (1868–1955), which he called *physical culture*. Macfadden opened physical culture resorts and a Physical Culture Training School in Chicago that graduated "doctors" of hydropathy, kinesitherapy, and physcultopathy. Physcultopathists were essentially medical gymnasts trained in Macfadden's school. This is an early example of an entrepreneurial enterprise in massage therapy (Armstrong & Armstrong, 1991).

Today's massage therapy profession is a direct outgrowth of this natural healing tradition. This is evident in the affinity of massage therapists for natural healing methods, in the adoption of the wellness model to define our scope, and in our identity as an alternative or CAM therapy. Issues related to differences in philosophy and the mistrust of mainstream medicine, as well as the push for freedom of choice in medical treatment, stem from this history.

The first convention of the American Association of Masseurs and Masseuses in 1946 included a lecture on zone therapy (i.e., reflexology) by Eunice Ingham, massage and multitherapy by John Granger, an equipment demonstration by a representative of the Therm-Aire Corporation, and a talk on "cradepathy." Their first president, Clark Cottrell, said about this event "I am sure we are on the right track to the natural methods of healing" (Benjamin, 1986).

It is important to understand this connection to the natural healing tradition as the profession of massage therapy interfaces with mainstream medicine in the 21st century. This history is especially important to remember as massage therapists work to maintain their integrity while they find their place in integrative medical settings. The fundamental identity of massage therapy as a natural healing agent is a primary strength it brings to integrative health care today.

→ MASSAGE THERAPY REVIVED IN THE UNITED STATES

The 1950s were a dark time for the massage profession in the United States. Physical therapists and athletic trainers were developing their own professions and were being educated in colleges and universities. Most of the old colleges of Swedish massage were closing. Mainstream America considered natural healing the province of "health nuts" or akin to quackery, and massage was being used blatantly as a cover for prostitution. "Massage parlor" had become permanently associated with houses of ill repute.

During this time, massage was kept alive mainly by natural healers working out of their homes, in private practice, and at places like the YMCAs. Their only organized presence in the 1950s was in the American Massage & Therapy Association, formerly the American Association of Masseurs and Masseuses. In 1958 they had dropped "masseurs and masseuses" in their name partly because those terms were deemed obsolete and in disrepute. The AM&TA had a few hundred members at that time and quietly developed educational standards, a code of ethics, and a credential called the "registered massage therapist." This association would later be a force in the revival of the massage therapy profession in the 1980s.

Beginning in the 1960s and through the 1970s, there were several different happenings in American society that led to the revival of the massage profession. Two movements based in California that reintroduced massage as a valuable health practice were the Human Potential Movement and the Counterculture movement. Forms of bodywork that emerged from the Human Potential Movement included Rolfing®, the Trager® approach, and the Feldenkrais Method®. These became trademarked therapies, and practitioners continue to be trained and certified by their organizations.

A simplified form of massage was developed at the Esalen Institute in Big Sur, California. Called Esalen massage, it incorporated simple Western massage techniques and emphasized sensual aspects using scented oils, candle lighting, incense, and "new age" music. Draping of the body was optional. Its purpose was to help the giver and receiver alike get in touch with their senses. At first, Esalen massage was adopted as a tool for personal growth and learned in meditation and self-improvement centers. It was associated with the "hippie" counterculture.

Some of the hippies who performed Esalen massage recognized its potential for health and healing and wanted to do the work for their livelihood. Some of those joined the natural healers in the AM&TA, giving the organization and the profession an influx of people and new energy. Mistrust of "establishment" health care, openness to non-Western health and healing practices, ambivalence toward regulation, and awareness of the psychological and spiritual aspects of massage are some of the values that they reinforced in the field.

Other factors that contributed to a revival of massage therapy in the 1970s were an interest in Eastern philosophies and health practices, particularly from India, China, and Japan. Yogis founded ashrams in the United States that promoted ancient Indian health practices like meditation, deep breathing, vegetarianism, and massage. Trade with China was reopened in the 1970s leading to exchange of information about medical practices such as acupuncture and *tuina*. Shiatsu and amma practitioners from Japan came to the United States and trained people in their arts.

A new fitness craze called "aerobics" also emerged in the 1970s. Ordinary people began taking aerobic exercise classes and jogging and running in local fun runs and marathons. And the success of European athletes revived an interest in sports massage in the United States for massage for athletes. The wellness movement gained ground in the field of health and physical education. It urged people to take responsibility for their own well-being and emphasized a holistic approach for body, mind, and spirit.

All of these factors led to consumer demand for massage therapy and to the establishment of vocational schools to train massage practitioners. New schools of massage based on the holistic and wellness perspectives appeared in the early 1980s. The ranks of massage therapists and bodyworkers swelled, as did membership in professional associations.

MASSAGE THERAPISTS AND BODYWORKERS

In the 1970s, massage therapy was largely unregulated, entrepreneurial, and alternative. Only a few states regulated massage in the 1970s, notably Ohio, Oregon, Washington, Florida, and North Dakota.

Many who became massage therapists at that time were looking for a second career, an alternative to corporate life, and/or a more holistic approach to health care. Many were escaping what they considered soulless, overregulated professions, and were drawn to the independent, nonstandardized field of massage and bodywork.

The term *massage* was still tainted, and so the term *massage therapy* was adopted to distinguish legitimate massage from massage as a cover for prostitution. It was also accepted as the designation of choice for the field as a whole, including traditional Western massage and other forms of manual therapy. Some practitioners who had been trained in distinct forms of manipulation (e.g., Rolfing® and Polarity Therapy), and who did not wish to be associated with massage, coined the term *bodywork* to describe the larger occupational field.

Unlike physical therapists and athletic trainers, practitioners of the manipulative arts are not in agreement on one name for the profession. This ambivalence is seen in the various names of organizations like the American Massage Therapy Association (AMTA), the Associated Bodywork and Massage Professionals (ABMP), and the National Certification Board for Therapeutic Massage & Bodywork (NCBTMB). Most, however, use various combinations of *massage* and/or *bodywork* with or without references to therapy. *Somatic therapy* (i.e., body therapy) is a less used term for the field as a whole.

Regardless of what the practitioners were called, more and more consumers were looking for massage and bodywork services. And the benefits of massage touted by practitioners and their organizations were beginning to be accepted by the general public. Graduates of massage programs in the 1980s opened private practices that attracted a diverse population of clients (Figure 3–11 ◀). The momentum for massage that began in the 1970s carried over into the 1980s and beyond to the present time.

Some indication of the growth of the profession can be seen in the steady increase in the number of members in professional organizations. AMTA had 359 members in 1960; 1,051 members in 1970; 1,405 in 1980; 3,183 in 1985; and grew to over 50,000 members by 2007 (AMTA National Historian's Report, 1987). ABMP, founded in the 1980s, also has over 50,000 members today.

Professional challenges during the 20-year period 1980–2000 ranged from winning the respect of the general public to gaining acceptance as health professionals by the health care community to establishing educational and competency standards. Appropriate dress, draping standards, and the ethics of the therapeutic relationship were hashed out in professional publications and meetings.

Many of the benchmarks of professions discussed in Chapter 2: The Massage Therapy Profession on page 20, have been achieved in the last few decades. The early 1990s were particularly busy with the creation of the first National Certification Examination for Therapeutic Massage and Bodywork; the incorporation of the Massage Therapy Foundation; the founding of the Touch Research Institute at the University of Miami; and the establishment of the Office of Alternative Medicine at the U.S. National Institutes of Health. The Commission on Massage Therapy Accreditation (COMTA) received U.S. Department of Education recognition in 2002. The number of states regulating massage therapists has grown from about 6 in 1985 to 38 plus the District of Columbia in 2007, with licensing laws working their way through the legislative process in several states today.

Unified Profession

The trend in the early 21st century is toward a more unified profession of massage therapy. Although there are notable exceptions, most massage and bodywork practitioners find common ground in entry-level educational standards, licensing requirements, and national certification. They are comfortable with diversity, and just as

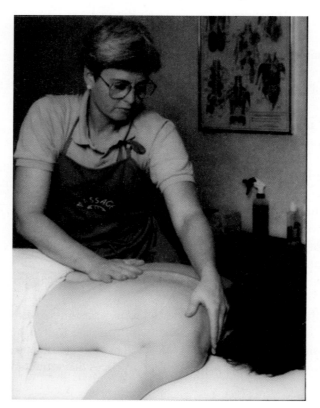

◀**Figure 3–11** Massage therapist, c. 1985. (From an ad for Wellspring Massage Therapy in Villa Park, Illinois. Author's private photo collection.)

CASE FOR STUDY

Alex and Researching Historical Background for a Legislative Issue

Alex, a massage therapist, is on the law and legislation committee of a professional organization that is preparing comments on a change in the definitions and scope of practice sections of the massage therapy licensing law. His task is to provide historical background on the issues involved.

Question:

Where would Alex look for relevant historical information that would provide broader understanding of the issues his committee is investigating?

Things to consider:

▶ History of the passage of the licensing law and amendments made over the years.

▶ Definitions and scope of practice statements in current and old versions of the licensing law in question, as well as similar laws in other states.

▶ Identification of issues that have risen over the years related to definition and scope of practice; note individuals and organizations involved.

▶ Definitions and scope of practice statements in current and old versions of licensing laws for cosmetologists, estheticians, physical therapists, and other relevant occupations.

▶ Historical relationships among professionals who use massage within their scope, e.g., cosmetologists, physical therapists, and athletic trainers; focus on similarities and differences; local issues; and organizations and people involved.

▶ Advances in the massage therapy profession throughout recent history, including advances in education and research.

Important historical information you have learned about massage laws in your geographical area:

_____

_____

_____

medical gymnasts of the 19th century embraced the new massage treatment, today's massage therapists combine different systems of soft tissue manipulation.

Many of the image problems of the past have been resolved with the creation of recognized credentials identifying legitimate massage practitioners and the adoption of codes of ethics. Some states, such as Illinois, prohibit the use of the word *massage* by anyone except licensed massage therapists.

The profession is becoming more standardized as more massage therapists enter the field through educational programs that meet accreditation and licensing requirements instead of through trademarked systems. Many techniques and approaches that were originally trademarked in the 1970–80s have been absorbed into massage therapy in generic form. For example, myofascial massage, trigger point or neuromuscular therapy, and various styles of shiatsu were originally introduced in trademarked systems, but are now integrated into many basic massage therapy programs.

There has been some discussion of splitting the field into levels or tiers, thereby distinguishing between so-called relaxation massage and medical massage. The intent of this proposal is to resolve issues related to minimum education standards. Perhaps this is a reflection of the historical tension between medical and natural healing models, and the use of massage for personal care. A better option might be to hold fast to the wellness model and embrace the whole scope of the field as outlined in the Wellness Massage Pyramid. Educational standards could be resolved by adopting entry-level standards for everyone, with additional knowledge and skills needed for those working in specialty areas or specific settings. This is an issue to resolve in the years to come.

Chapter Highlights

▶ Over the centuries, many have been called or have chosen to be massage practitioners; their stories form the history of massage as a vocation.

▶ The 4 major branches of this history are 1) massage for personal grooming and rejuvenation, 2) sports and fitness, 3) health care, and 4) natural healing.

▶ In ancient civilizations, domestic servants and slaves performed many personal care services including helping with bathing, rubdowns, and applying scented oils.

▶ In China in the 1800s, street barbers performed a type of seated massage, and in Japan at the same time, blind masseurs called ammashi traveled the streets blowing a flute to attract customers.

▶ Massage has been available in public bathhouses all over the world. The occupational designation of bath attendant stems from this ancient tradition.

▶ In the early 1900s, massage was part of personal care services called beauty culture.

- A limited use of superficial massage continues in the scope of practice of barbers and cosmetologists, who began to be licensed around 1900.
- Full body massage for rejuvenation and reducing and breast massage were performed by Swedish masseuses in the 1920–40s in beauty culture settings.
- Practitioners trained in schools were called graduate masseuses and masseurs.

▶ Massage for athletes has a long tradition.

- Massage with oil by aleiptes and paidotribes was part of the routine at the ancient Greek gymnasium.
- Bath attendants and rubbers provided massage to amateur athletes in the 18–19th centuries in Europe and North America.
- In the 20th century, athletic masseurs were trained in schools.
- By 1950, athletic trainers had developed their own profession specializing in sports injuries, and athletic massage in America largely died out.
- Sports massage was revived in the United States in the 1970s within the growing profession of massage therapy.

▶ In the early 20th century, masseurs and masseuses provided massage in health clubs in American cities.

- Health service operators and masseurs offered massage and related services in YMCAs.
- The Health Service Operators Society was established in 1942.

▶ Massage has been used for healing from time immemorial by families and tribal and community healers.

- At the beginning of Western medicine, massage was used by Greek and Roman physicians.
- Some European physicians of the 18th–19th centuries utilized soft tissue manipulation in medical treatment.
- American physicians of the early 20th century prescribed Mezger's massage to be performed on patients by assistants.
- The occupation of trained masseuse was formed as a greater level of skill and professionalism was required to work with patients.

▶ Practitioners of Ling's system of medical gymnastics applied active and passive movements to treat various chronic diseases.

- Ling founded a school in Stockholm, Sweden in 1813 to train educational and medical gymnasts.
- Medical gymnasts, also known as movement cure practitioners, were alternative medical providers in the late 19th century. They eventually adopted Mezger's massage into their work, which then became known in America as Swedish massage.

▶ By the 1950s, a separate profession of physical therapy was formed for physiotherapists working in mainstream medical settings.

- The American Women's Physical Therapeutic Association was founded in 1921.
- Swedish massage practitioners working within a natural healing framework founded the American Association of Masseurs and Masseuses in 1943, changed to the American Massage & Therapy Association in 1958, and known as the American Massage Therapy Association today.

▶ Massage was an important part of natural healing systems of the late 19th and early 20th centuries.

- Naturopaths, or drugless healers, began to organize their profession in 1902 with the founding of the Naturopathic Society of America.
- Massage operators were trained in schools to work in natural healing resorts.
- In 1895, Kellogg wrote *The Art of Massage*, which became a classic massage textbook.
- A popular version of natural healing called physical culture, with practitioners called physcultopathists, was promoted by Bernarr Macfadden.

▶ Today's massage therapists are part of the natural healing tradition as evidenced in their attraction to natural healing methods, adoption of the wellness model, identity as a CAM profession, mistrust of mainstream medicine, and champions of choice in medical treatment.

▶ An understanding of the tradition of massage within natural healing is important to massage therapists as they find their places today in integrative medical settings.

▶ The use of massage in the United States declined in the 1950s. It was revived in the 1970s through a variety of factors including the Human Potential Movement and counterculture, which spawned Esalen massage; general interest in Asian health practices; physical fitness and wellness movements; and the use of massage by elite athletes.

▶ An increased number of people seeking massage therapy, and the founding of new massage training schools, helped increase the number of massage practitioners in the 1980s.

- The 1980–90s were a period of growth and the professionalizing of massage therapy.

▶ In the early 21st century, massage therapy has become a more unified profession comfortable with diversity in approaches and moving towards generally recognized standards.

Exam Review

Learning Outcomes

Use the learning outcomes at the beginning of the chapter and shown here as a guide to the major topics covered. Perform the task given in each outcome, and share your results with a study partner. Check off the tasks as you complete them.

- ❏ Trace the history of massage related to personal grooming services.
- ❏ Describe the use of massage for athletes from ancient times to the present.
- ❏ Explain how massage has been used over the centuries in Western medicine.
- ❏ Identify aspects of today's massage therapy that can be traced to the natural healing philosophy.
- ❏ Name important figures in the history of massage and describe their contributions.
- ❏ List factors leading to the revival of massage as a popular health practice in the 1970s.
- ❏ Describe important developments in the massage profession in recent decades.

Key Terms

To study key terms listed at the beginning of the chapter, choose one or more of the following exercises. Writing or talking about ideas helps you better remember them, and explaining them to someone else helps deepen your understanding.

1. Write a one- or two-sentence description for each historical term for massage practitioner including the place, time, work setting, knowledge and skills, social status, training, and other key elements that define their work.

2. Make study cards by writing the historical term for massage practitioner on one side of a 3 × 5 card, and a concise description on the other side. Shuffle the cards and read one side, trying to recite either the description or term from the other side.

3. With a study partner, take turns explaining the historical terms verbally.

4. Take the study cards made in problem 2, turn them so that only the terms are showing, and shuffle the cards. Now place the cards in chronological order from terms used in ancient times to the present. Note when more than one term was used in a specific time period (e.g., trained masseuses and massage operators).

5. Take the study cards in problem 2, turn them so that only the terms are showing, and shuffle the cards. Sort them into work settings such as personal care, sports and fitness, health care, natural healing, and private practice.

Memory Workout

The following fill-in-the-blank statements test your memory of the main concepts in this chapter.

1. Four major branches of the history of massage as a vocation are personal _____ and _____, _____ and fitness, _____ care, _____ healing.

2. A British delegation to China in the 1790s described street _____, who offered grooming services, including a form of seated bodywork.

3. _____ masseurs of Japan walked the streets announcing their presence by playing a small flute.

4. The occupational designation of _____ _____ stems from ancient traditions of servants or other assistants giving a rubdown, or rubbing scented oils into the skin after a bath.

5. As early as 1915, a _____ by a bath attendant was an established part of the routine at the YMCA.

6. Traditional Hispanic healers called _____ specialize in massage to treat a variety of ailments.

7. In the 18th–19th centuries, the general name for soft tissue manipulation as used in medical settings was _____ _____.

8. The Society of Trained Masseuses was formed in (country) _____ in (year) _____ to raise professional standards for massage specialists working in the medical field.

9. In the 1950s, massage was being used as a cover for prostitution in the United States, and the term massage _____ had become permanently associated with houses of ill repute.

10. In the 1970s a movement in the field of health and physical education encouraged people to take responsibility for their own well-being and emphasized a holistic approach to health. This was known as the _____ movement.

Test Prep

The following multiple choice questions will help to prepare you for future school and professional exams.

1. In ancient civilizations, who typically provided personal care services like grooming and bathing in the home?
   a. Well-paid employees
   b. A class of priests and priestesses
   c. Slaves and domestic servants
   d. Older family members

2. The name used by the British to describe a practice from India that involved a hot soapy bath, followed by a form of bodywork involving percussion and friction massage, joint cracking, and applying scented oils or perfume is:
   a. Anatriptic art
   b. Shampooing
   c. Padshah's bath
   d. Ammashi

3. The prototype public bath in Western civilization and forerunner of today's day spa is the:
   a. Greek gymnasium
   b. Roman bath
   c. Mineral bath
   d. Beauty salon

4. Women massage practitioners working in beauty and reducing salons in the early 1900s were typically called:
   a. Manipulators
   b. Health service operators
   c. Swedish masseurs
   d. Swedish masseuses

5. In the 1940s, massage practitioners who worked with athletes and who were well trained in the massage field were typically called:
   a. Athletic masseurs
   b. Paidotribes
   c. Rubbers
   d. Bath attendants

6. In the United States in the late 1800s, Ling's medical gymnastics used to treat chronic diseases was known as:
   a. Physical culture
   b. Mechno-manipulation
   c. Swedish massage
   d. Swedish movement cure

7. The person who developed a system of soft tissue manipulation in the 1800s that is the basis for today's traditional Western massage is:
   a. Pehr H. Ling of Sweden
   b. Johann Mezger of Amsterdam
   c. J. Harvey Kellogg of the United States
   d. Douglas Graham of the United States

8. In the United States in the 1970s, a simplified form of massage was developed in California that incorporated simple western massage techniques and emphasized sensual aspects using scented oils, candle lighting, incense, and "new age" music. It was called:
   a. Swedish massage
   b. Esalen massage
   c. Shampooing
   d. Anatriptic art

Video Challenge

Watch the appropriate segment of the video on your CD-ROM and then answer the following questions.

Segment 3: History of Massage as a Vocation

1. Identify the various settings in which massage practitioners of the past worked, giving examples from the video.

2. Describe the dress of massage practitioners of the past as shown in the video. Explain how their dress, even though outdated today, shows a sense of professionalism.

3. Look closely at the photos of massage shown in the video. Do you notice anything that would probably be done differently today, e.g., draping or techniques? Is there anything that would be done exactly the same today?

Comprehension Exercises

The following exercises provide questions for you to answer and tasks you can do to enhance your understanding of the material presented in this chapter.

1. Name the four branches of the history of massage as a vocation. Give examples of settings today that correspond to these historical branches.

2. Briefly trace the history of sports massage, and identify the names used over the centuries for massage practitioners specializing in working with athletes.

3. What do the terms *massage parlor* and *masseuse* mean in the context of the history of massage?

For Greater Understanding

The following exercises are designed to give you a deeper understanding of the subjects covered in this chapter. Action words are underlined to emphasize the active nature of this approach to learning.

1. Imagine that you are walking around a village in ancient China, and describe the different forms of massage and bodywork that you might see there. Repeat for

the cities and towns of ancient Rome, Medieval Europe, 1880 Europe, and then 1920, 1950, and 1990 United States. <u>Note</u> that at any one time and place, massage and bodywork can be found in a number of settings and performed by practitioners with different backgrounds.

2. <u>Visit</u> a day or destination spa, and note the services on the menu. Receive a massage or other spa services if possible. <u>Compare and contrast</u> your experience to what others would have experienced in bath houses and natural healing resorts of the past. <u>Report</u> your findings to the class.

3. <u>Look</u> through magazines or newspapers from the 1890s, 1900s, 1920s or other historical time period. <u>Find</u> references to massage, drugless healing, and related topics in articles and advertisements. <u>Report</u> your findings to the class or a study partner.

4. <u>Locate</u> a historical facility in your community where massage has been available for a long time or was offered in the past (e.g., old YMCA, Turkish bath, athletic club, beauty salon, resort, mineral spring spa). <u>Look</u> for an ad for the facility from the past, especially one that mentions massage. <u>Share</u> your discovery with the class. [Variation: <u>Report</u> on a place you visited on vacation that had historical connections to massage.]

PART II

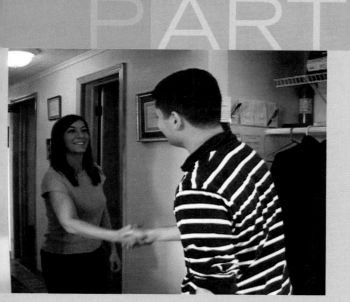

PERSONAL AND
COMMUNICATION SKILLS

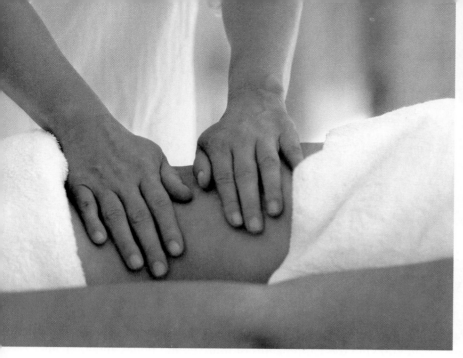

Personal Development and Professionalism

LEARNING OUTCOMES

After studying this chapter, you will have information to:

1. Appreciate the importance of personal growth for professional development.
2. Understand service as an important value for massage therapists.
3. Develop a strong work ethic.
4. Manage time effectively.
5. Project a professional image.
6. Explain the intellectual skills needed by massage therapists.
7. Improve powers of concentration.
8. Understand the role of intuition in massage therapy.
9. Develop emotional intelligence.
10. Adopt ethical standards as massage therapy students.
11. Develop fundamental physical skills.
12. Create a program of holistic self-care.

KEY TERMS

Compassion	Emotional intelligence	Professional image	Service
Concentration	Intellectual skills	Problem solving	Time management
Critical thinking	Intuition	Self-care	Work ethic

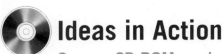

Ideas in Action

On your CD-ROM, explore:

- ▶ Professional dress, posture, and speech
- ▶ Image detractors
- ▶ Emotional intelligence
- ▶ Holistic self-care plan
- ▶ Interactive video exercises

→ PROFESSIONALISM IN MASSAGE THERAPY

As noted in Chapter 1, becoming a successful massage therapist is a journey of transformation. Part of that journey is learning to be a professional. What is professionalism? It is more than knowing the Latin names of muscles and bones and applying massage techniques skillfully. In her book, *Professionalism in Health Care* (2005), Makely said it well:

> Professionalism is a state of mind, a way of "being," "knowing," and "doing" that sets you apart from others. It gives you direction to how you look, behave, think, and act. It brings together who you are as a person, what you value, how you treat other people, what you contribute in the workplace, and how seriously you take your job .... To *be* a professional, you must *feel like* a professional. (pp. xiv–xv)

Feeling like a professional comes from the inside, but it manifests in the image you present by your appearance, behavior, and attitude. Likewise, by presenting a professional image, you cultivate feeling like a professional. When you finally become a professional, the inside and outside are totally in sync, and your professional presence is genuine.

Attitude is the sum of how a person presents him- or herself to the world—a way of acting, thinking, and feeling. To have a professional attitude is to embody all that it means to be a professional.

Becoming a professional massage therapist inevitably involves change and personal growth. Some of the key growth areas are dedication to service, developing a strong work ethic, establishing a professional image, cultivating intellectual skills, improving concentration, developing intuition, nurturing emotional intelligence, fostering ethical character, and developing physical skills. Social and communications skills are also essential, and will be discussed in detail in Chapter 5: Social and Communication Skills on page 107.

→ SERVICE

The essence of the massage therapy profession is serving others. Dedication to **service** means that we hold clients' well-being above our own desires for money, power, and worldly recognition. It means that the primary motivation for being massage therapists is to help people achieve their personal wellness goals.

Dedication to service helps keep priorities in order. It focuses attention on the well-being of clients rather than on ourselves. It guides our way and can offer a higher and more satisfying motivation than merely making money. It spurs us to be the best that we can be. It provides a moral compass for ethical decision making.

There are much easier, more prestigious, and more lucrative ways to make a living than being a massage therapist. But using massage therapy to help others live healthier, happier, and more stress-free lives provides great satisfaction to those who chose this work.

Many start on the road to becoming a massage therapist for other reasons. But those who stay and find satisfaction in their work realize that the ultimate motivation is to be of service to those who come to us for massage.

WORK ETHIC

A strong work ethic provides a firm foundation for all other aspects of professionalism. Makely defines **work ethic** as "positioning your job as a high priority in your life and making sound decisions about how you approach your work" (p. 5). It means taking your work seriously, staying focused, and applying yourself to doing a good job.

A strong work ethic is reflected in good attendance and punctuality, reliability and accountability, positive attitude and enthusiasm, and taking responsibility for doing the highest quality work of which you are capable. It starts when you are a student and carries on into your professional life. It is a trait that employers value highly and an essential characteristic for success in private practice.

Good attendance means showing up when expected or when scheduled, and punctuality means showing up on time. Punctuality also entails getting to school or work early enough so that you are settled in and ready to go when the class starts or when the client arrives. Running in late or at the last minute prevents you from preparing, centering, and focusing yourself. It shows disrespect for your classmates, teachers, and clients.

Reliability is a related trait that means people can depend on you to do what you say you are going to do, when you say you will do it. If you are reliable, people will have trust and confidence in you. Accountability means that you accept responsibility for your actions, and do not make excuses for repeated mistakes. You apologize sincerely for and correct mistakes that you have made.

A positive attitude and enthusiasm are revealed in how you speak about your work and the energy you put into it. The word *enthusiasm* comes from the Greek language and means possessed or inspired by the gods. If you have enthusiasm, you exhibit keen interest and eagerness. You value your work and look forward to studying, practicing, and learning more about it.

With a strong work ethic, you take responsibility for doing your highest quality work every time. Regardless of whatever else is going on in your life, you strive for quality in your work. You exhibit competence in applying the knowledge and skills of your profession for the good of your clients.

TIME MANAGEMENT

Time management involves planning a workable schedule. It is a matter of priorities, which means making time for what matters most and letting go of the rest. A common mistake of students is to try to fit school into an already crowded schedule. Being rushed or late, eating on the run, cramming for classes and exams, and suffering from sleep deprivation are symptoms of poor time management. You have to *make* time for what you value most.

So the first step in time management is to identify goals and priorities for the time under consideration. That could be for a week, a month, or a year. It might be defined by your life at the moment, such as the time you are in school or for the semester. If priorities are not clear, it is difficult to make good choices about the use of time.

Students who start with school as a top priority are more likely to produce a time management plan that leads to success.

Plotting out a weekly schedule is the next step toward getting your use of time under control. The time management chart in Figure 4–1 ◀ is an example of planning adequate time for regular activities.

A time management plan for students includes the following: work, school (classes and homework/practice), commuting, regular appointments and meetings, family time, sleeping, eating, rest/relaxation, and recreation. A good rule of thumb is to plan 60–75% of your time, and leave 25–40% for unplanned or spontaneous activities. Working while attending school tends to decrease "spontaneous" time, but may be manageable for a short period.

A good time management tip is to identify *time wasters* and eliminate them from your life. A time waster would be something that does not contribute to your high-priority goals. Delayed gratification and learning to say "no" to yourself, with sights on a higher goal, are important signs of emotional maturity.

Reserve your prime time for high-priority tasks. For example, plan to study when you are most awake and full of energy. Also figure in adequate travel time between scheduled events. For example, list 7:30 AM—leave for school, as well as 8:30 AM—anatomy class begins.

Plan enough time for homework and practicing massage skills. For each hour of lecture class allot 2–3 hours of study time. Practice massage as required in your program for at least 4–6 hours per week outside of class time. Practice is not only for doing your homework and honing your massage skills, but also for building the strength and stamina to make a living as a massage therapist after graduation. By graduation, you should be comfortably performing the number of hours of massage (class + practice time) that you are aiming for in your practice startup.

Get in the habit of using a daily or weekly planner to keep track of regular and special appointments, events, and deadlines. Check your schedule at the beginning of each month, week, and day for an overview of the time period. Refer to your planner when making appointments so that you don't double schedule a time period.

▶ **Figure 4–1** Sample time management planning chart for a massage student.

Time Period September – December (Fall Semester)			Class Time: 24 hrs		Study/Practice Time: 20 hrs		
Time	**Monday**	**Tuesday**	**Wednesday**	**Thursday**	**Friday**	**Saturday**	**Sunday**
5:00 am	sleep	sleep	sleep	sleep	sleep	sleep	sleep
6:00	sleep	sleep	sleep	sleep	sleep	sleep	sleep
7:00	up & eat	up & eat	up & eat	up & eat	up & eat	up & eat	sleep
8:00	travel	travel	travel	travel	travel	travel	up & eat
9:00	class	class	class	class	work	work	recreation
10:00	class	class	class	class	work	work	recreation
11:00	class	class	class	class	work	work	recreation
12 noon	lunch	lunch	lunch	lunch	work	work	lunch
1:00 pm	class	class	class	clinic	lunch	lunch	study/practice
2:00	class	class	class	clinic	work	study/practice	study/practice
3:00	class	class	class	clinic	work	study/practice	study/practice
4:00	travel	travel	travel	travel	work	study/practice	study/practice
5:00	dinner	dinner	dinner	dinner	work	study/practice	dinner
6:00	work	study/practice	work	read/study	dinner	dinner	read/study
7:00	work	study/practice	work	read/study	recreation	recreation	read/study
8:00	work	study/practice	work	read/study	recreation	recreation	recreation
9:00	read/study	study/practice	read/study	read/study	recreation	recreation	recreation
10:00	relax/meditation	relax/meditation	relax/meditation	relax/meditation	recreation	recreation	relax/meditation
11:00	sleep	sleep	sleep	sleep	sleep	sleep	sleep

PRACTICAL APPLICATION

Analyze your own work ethic as reflected in your behavior so far in massage school and your attitude towards class work and homework. Concentrate on attendance, punctuality, behavior in class, and getting assignments in on time, as well as good attitude and enthusiasm.

1 Do you see areas for improvement?

2 Can you pick out three things you can start doing today that show a commitment to your massage training and enthusiasm for massage therapy?

3 How will that help you in your career as a massage therapist?

Good time management while at school will naturally spill over into postgraduate employment and private practices. Build good habits in school that will serve you well afterward.

PROFESSIONAL IMAGE

Your appearance reflects your inner state of professionalism. A **professional image** makes a favorable impression on your clients and identifies you as someone they can have confidence in and trust. Your appearance should be clean, neat, modest, and appropriate for the setting in which you work. Establishing a professional presence involves attention to dress, grooming, posture, and language.

Dress

The way you dress sets the tone of your relationship with clients—respectful, non-sexual, and trusting. It also helps set boundaries by saying to the client that this is a professional relationship. Remember that as a professional massage therapist you are not dressing to impress your friends or attract a romantic date. Your appearance reflects your professionalism (Figure 4–2 ◀).

Many massage therapists adopt a uniform look by wearing loose pants and polo shirt, hospital scrubs, sports clothes, or martial arts outfit. A spa might have a required uniform like a smock with the company logo. With a little thought and creativity, you can find work clothes that are attractive, practical, and express who you are as a professional.

Some guidelines for professional dress are:

▶ Have work clothes that are separate from your everyday clothes.
▶ Choose clothes that are conservative and modest.
▶ Choose clothes that can be cleaned easily.
▶ Wear clothes that allow the freedom of movement you need for your work.
▶ Wear clothes appropriate for your work setting and in compliance with your employer's dress code.
▶ Wear closed-toe shoes, or other coverings that enclose the feet (e.g., socks with sandals).
▶ Keep clothes clean, neat, and odor-free.

▶ **Figure 4–2** Your appearance reflects your professionalism.

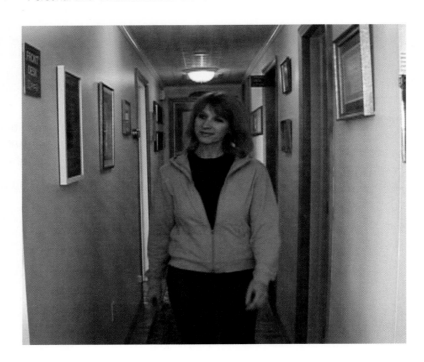

Some generally accepted *don'ts* for professional dress are:

- ▶ Don't wear tops that show cleavage or breast tissue (e.g., low-cut tops or sleeveless shirts with large armholes).
- ▶ Don't wear tops with large or long sleeves that may touch the client.
- ▶ Don't wear pants that are tight or provocative (e.g., show the navel).
- ▶ Don't wear short shorts or short skirts.
- ▶ Don't wear denim jeans, either long or short.
- ▶ Don't wear sandals without socks or go barefoot.
- ▶ Don't wear t-shirts with advertising or sayings that may be offensive.
- ▶ Don't wear jewelry that is likely to touch the client (e.g., dangling necklaces and rings). Rings can also be unsanitary if dirt and skin cells collect around and underneath them.
- ▶ Don't wear clothing that suggests a social setting rather than a professional setting.

An employer may have a mandatory dress code. Ask about it in your job interview so you are clear about what is expected. Most dress codes identify acceptable and unacceptable attire and indicate whether a uniform is required. They specify rules about jewelry and body decoration like tattoos and piercings.

Grooming

Grooming is an important part of appearance that includes nails, hair, and skin. Your hands, the instruments of massage, should receive special attention. Keep fingernails clean and short, that is, below the line of the fingertips. If you hold up the palm of your hand and look at the fingers, the fingernails should not be visible. Keep cuticles neat and trimmed.

Rough spots on the hands can be softened and cracks prevented with the application of healing lotions and creams. Since you will be washing your hands frequently, it is important to use soap with lotion added and to dry your hands thoroughly to prevent chapping. Chapped hands with cracked skin provide an entry point for germs and can feel rough on the client's body.

Use face makeup conservatively. Applying makeup to enhance appearance in a professional setting is appropriate. Being "made-up" to make a trendy statement or as you might for a date or social event is not appropriate.

Body piercings and tattoos may be all right if within the norms acceptable to your employer and clients. Cover any tattoo that you think might be offensive to clients. Consider removing potentially offensive tattoos that you might have had done before your professional life as a massage therapist.

Wash your hair regularly using unscented or lightly scented products. Adopt a hairstyle that prevents the hair from falling forward when bent over, or from touching the client in any way. Men with facial hair should keep it clean and trimmed.

Body odor can be a problem in a profession such as massage that involves physical activity and close contact with clients. Always use an underarm deodorant. Those who do not shave under the arms should be aware that hair retains sweat, and that unpleasant odor develops faster there than on shaved areas. If necessary, wash under the arms during the day, and change your shirt after a few massage sessions.

Breath odor is another potential trouble spot. If you like to eat spicy foods or smoke, adopt strategies to eliminate the resulting odor. Breath mints can be effective for normal instances of "stale breath." Smokers must also consider the smell of smoke on their hands, clothes, and hair. Nonsmokers are more sensitive to cigarette and cigar smoke, so they can often smell odors that smokers cannot. Remember that when working around your client's head and face, they will be very aware of the smell of your hands. Here is a summary of guidelines for good grooming:

▶ Keep nails trimmed and manicured below the tips of the fingers.
▶ Keep hair clean and in a style that prevents it from touching the client.
▶ Keep skin on hands healthy and soft.
▶ Wear conservative face makeup.
▶ Take precautions to prevent offensive body odor.
▶ Take precautions to prevent offensive breath odor.
▶ Keep areas around body-piercing jewelry clean.

Posture

Good posture is not only healthy, it also enhances your professional presence. Keep your back and neck in good alignment, head up, and muscles relaxed. Good posture should feel balanced and uplifting. Avoid slouching, leaning, tilting, and other poor postural habits. By correcting poor postural habits, you set a good example for clients. Chapter 6: Goal-Oriented Planning on page 149 outlines the elements of good sitting and standing posture in greater detail.

Speech

Speech also projects professionalism. Communications with clients are friendly and caring, but never too personal or casual. The way that you talk to friends and family might not be appropriate in a professional setting.

Avoid street slang and use good grammar. Call adult females "women" and adult males "men." Do not use terms of familiarity such as "sweetie," "dear," "doll," or "dude" when talking to clients.

Also avoid overly formal language and use of technical terms that clients might not understand. It is not appropriate to "show off" by using anatomical terms unfamiliar to the general public. For example, the term *thigh* will do just as well as *femur*

CRITICAL THINKING

Visit three different places where massage therapists work, and evaluate the level of professionalism you see there.

1. Report your findings to the class or study group, noting specific details of dress, grooming, posture, speech, and image detractors on which you base your evaluation.

2. Compare what you see in different settings and notice whether there is more than one way to look and be professional.

3. Determine which elements you find essential to presenting a professional image and those that are a matter of choice.

in most cases. Using anatomical terms when educating the client about what you are doing is acceptable if done in moderation and the client is able to understand what you are saying. Communication skills are discussed in greater detail in Chapter 5: Social and Communication Skills on page 108.

Image Detractors

Needless to say, annoying habits detract from a professional image. Avoid nervous habits like finger tapping, nail biting, knuckle cracking, leg bouncing, and hair twirling. Other detractors include wearing noisy jewelry, chewing gum, smoking, eating, or drinking in a client's presence.

→ INTELLECTUAL SKILLS

Massage therapy is performed with the head, heart, and hands. **Intellectual skills** or thinking skills play an important part in being a professional massage therapist. From learning about the human body to planning massage sessions to making ethical decisions, the ability to use your head is essential.

Intellectual or cognitive skills can be thought of as having six levels (Bloom, 1956). The first level is knowledge of terms, concepts, principles, facts, and methods. At this level the massage therapist can recall or remember things like the names of bones or different massage techniques. The second level is comprehension, in which he or she can reorganize, paraphrase, or explain the material beyond mere recall. For example, the therapist can describe in his or her own words how a synovial joint works, or why a specific massage technique has a certain effect.

The third level is application, in which knowledge is used in real-life situations. For example, when giving a massage for stress reduction, the massage therapist uses principles learned previously, for example, using long, flowing strokes and avoiding stimulating techniques like tapotement. The fourth level is analysis, or breaking down a communication or situation into its parts and identifying specific elements, relationships among parts, patterns, and overall organization. Analysis is an important skill in assessing a problem a client is having or in considering an ethical question.

The fifth level is synthesis, or putting together pieces to create a whole, or arrive at a solution. For example, after an analysis of a problem presented by a client, a massage therapist takes all that he or she knows about massage therapy and creates a session plan to achieve certain goals. The sixth level is evaluation, for example, judging

TABLE 4–1

Six Levels of Intellectual Skills

Level	Intellectual Skill	Description
1	Knowledge	Recall or remember terms, concepts, principles, facts, and methods
2	Comprehension	Reorganize, paraphrase, or explain the material beyond mere recall
3	Application	Use information in real-life situations
4	Analysis	Break down a communication or situation into its parts, and identify specific elements, relationships among parts, patterns, and overall organization
5	Synthesis	Put together the pieces to create a whole, or a solution
6	Evaluation	Form a judgment; determine the worth, value, or quality

to what extent a certain massage application was successful in achieving session goals. These last three levels (analysis, synthesis, and evaluation) are the foundations of goal-oriented session planning, explained in Chapter 6: Goal-Oriented Planning on page 136. The six levels of intellectual skills are summarized in Table 4–1 ◀.

Higher Level Thinking

There will be many situations in your career that call for higher level thinking. Two types of higher level thinking useful to massage therapists are critical thinking and problem solving. Related to those are applications like planning sessions for clients and making ethical choices. Higher level thinking involves all six levels of intellectual skills described above.

Critical thinking helps you get at the truth and avoid being deceived. Levine, a childhood learning specialist, noted that "Non-critical thinkers accept far too much at face value. They may be more concrete and have trouble looking beneath the surface, analyzing and evaluating that which is more than meets the eye" (Levine, 2002, p. 203). Noncritical thinkers tend to be naive and gullible. Levine cautions though about going too far and becoming cynical, doubting everything and trusting nothing. Asking pertinent questions to discover the truth is a sign of healthy skepticism.

Critical thinking weighs reasons to believe against reasons to doubt. It looks for objective evidence, confirmation of claims, errors, distortions, false information, and exaggerations. It looks beneath the surface for authenticity and honesty. It takes into consideration the thinker's own prejudices and beliefs, which is an exercise in self-reflection.

Critical thinking is bolstered by communicating the thought process to another person. In explaining their thinking, people clarify their ideas and test their logic and conclusions. Listening to others can add information, opinions, and provide valuable insights from another perspective.

An example of critical thinking about a product being sold involves a series of questions. For example, what are the claims about this product? Is there any objective evidence for the claims? How good is that evidence? Who is presenting the claims, and do they have a personal stake (e.g., monetary interest) in the situation? What do others say about this product? What is the basis for their thinking? Have I used the product, and do the claims ring true given my experience? Is there anything that might influence my perception of the product; for example, knowledge of similar products or attractive packaging? Do I have likes or dislikes, prejudices or beliefs that might influence my evaluation? What is the level of risk involved in believing or not believing the claims? And if I decide to buy the product, how will I benefit from it, and do I really need it?

Critical thinking is important to massage therapists in situations like spending money on equipment and supplies, and deciding whether to believe a claim made for massage or other healing practice. It is useful in choosing continuing education in a particular form of massage therapy, and for evaluating a contract for a business partnership. Important issues in the profession call for critical thinking, like whether to support a certain provision in a licensing law or a position taken by a professional association. Critical thinking is a good habit for a mature professional.

Problem solving in its various forms is a systematic approach to finding a solution to a problem using critical thinking skills. The starting point for problem solving is some issue, question, or dilemma for which there are response options. Time and effort are taken to gather the information needed to make an informed choice or formulate a solution. Gathering information involves listing the facts, soliciting opinions, understanding the history of the situation, and recalling similar situations. Decisions made in similar circumstances, and their results, are important to note. Information gathered is then analyzed and evaluated, and finally a choice or decision is made.

A significant aspect of problem solving is self-reflection as found in critical thinking. Things that may color your thinking such as fears, prejudices, habits, past experiences, and feelings are taken into consideration in a conscious way. This is not to negate them, but to put them into the equation with other information. Self-reflection promotes greater objectivity.

Evaluation involves weighing the pros and cons of choices for action, or clarifying the priority of values involved. The conclusion or final choice of action is based on some criteria like highest values (ethical decisions), legal considerations, good business principles, or meeting client goals (goal-oriented session planning).

Systematic problem solving leads to better decisions because the process helps avoid common pitfalls like jumping to conclusions, narrow thinking, and lack of clarity about reasons for choices. It allows thoughtful consideration of complex situations. Higher level thinking skills are summarized in Table 4–2◀.

The basic elements of problem solving are found in its specific applications. For example, goal-oriented session planning described in Chapter 6: Goal-Oriented Planning on page 136, and ethical decision making described in Chapter 8: Foundations of Ethics on page 190 are variations on the basic process of problem solving.

↳ CONCENTRATION

Concentration is the ability to sustain attention on something for a period of time. *Attention span* is the length of time a person can concentrate before becoming distracted. Concentration is a mental skill that can be developed with practice.

The ability to concentrate is important to massage therapists for several reasons. For students, it makes learning easier and attending classes more productive. You can hear what the teacher is saying in class, pay attention to details, and make connections between facts and concepts. You can attain a greater depth of understanding.

Massage therapists are more present while talking to clients and during massage sessions if they focus their attention. An aware client can feel when the massage therapist's mind is wandering, much the same way you can tell if someone in front of you is not listening to what you are saying. A wandering mind interferes with the essential connection or presence with a client.

TABLE 4-2
Higher Level Thinking Skills Used in Massage Therapy

Critical Thinking	▶ Process for discovering the truth and avoiding deception
	▶ Weigh reasons to believe against reasons to doubt
	▶ Look for objective evidence, confirmation of claims, errors, distortions, false information, and exaggerations
	▶ Look beneath the surface for authenticity and honesty
	▶ Take into consideration the thinker's own prejudices and beliefs, which is an exercise in self-reflection
Problem Solving	▶ Systematic approach to finding a solution to a problem using critical thinking skills
	▶ Starting point is an issue, question, or dilemma for which there are choices for responding
	▶ Information needed to make an informed choice or formulate a solution is gathered
	▶ List the facts, solicit opinions, understand the history of the situation, and recall similar situations
	▶ Information gathered is analyzed and evaluated, and finally a choice or decision is made
	▶ Solution based on some criteria like highest values (ethical decisions), legal considerations, good business principles, or meeting client goals (goal-oriented session planning)

Details also tend to get lost if the mind is jumping from one thing to another. For example, it takes time to absorb sensations from your hands and interpret them as you apply massage techniques. If your mind is not present, even if your hands are working, a lot of information will be lost.

Letting the mind wander in activities like daydreaming, ruminating about the past, worrying, or looking forward to a future event is a barrier to good concentration. Being easily distracted by sights and sounds in the environment shortens the attention span. The mind goes off somewhere and is not paying attention to the task at hand.

Attention is also important in performing massage because it focuses our energy. Heckler explains that "*energy follows attention* means that feeling, sensation, and aliveness increase and become more vivid at the place where we direct our attention" (1997, p. 98).

Improving Concentration

Concentration can be improved through minimizing attention disruptors, single-tasking, creating a more distraction-free environment, and practicing focusing the mind through meditation techniques.

Stressful situations, lack of sleep, illness, and overuse of stimulants like caffeine can temporarily disrupt the ability to concentrate. Conversely, relaxation techniques, getting enough sleep, taking care of health problems, and proper nutrition improve the ability to concentrate. Recreation activities and light entertainment can offer a break from work, helping to calm and focus the mind. As mentioned previously, massage itself is known to improve mental alertness and focused attention.

Single-tasking, or doing one thing at a time, is a prerequisite for concentration. Its antithesis, *multitasking*, or doing more than one thing at a time, is a modern stress producer. Watching television while trying to study, reading e-mail while on the phone, and planning a grocery list in your mind while doing massage are examples of multitasking. The quality of one or both activities suffers as a result of split attention. Single-tasking is a practice in concentration.

Simple, uncluttered space minimizes visual distracters. Silence, "white noise," or quiet background music also help concentration. Students can cut down distracters by sitting in the front of the classroom and eliminating behavior like eating and drinking, doodling, and talking during class time. Electronic devices are perhaps the biggest distracters of modern times. During periods of concentration, turn off all electronic devices such as cell phones, pagers, and personal digital assistants. Being constantly interrupted breaks concentration.

Massage therapists create distraction-free environments for themselves and their clients. Dim lights, soft music, and minimal talking allow concentration on the massage itself.

Meditation

Meditation techniques are designed to quiet the mind and enhance the ability to pay focused attention. Meditation has been described as "the natural process of becoming familiar with an object by repeatedly placing our minds upon it" (Mipham, 2003, p. 24). This is the essence of modern meditation techniques—choosing something like a word or object to place attention on, and when the mind wanders, bringing it back to the object of attention. It is that simple—and that difficult—since the mind likes to wander.

Learning focused attention is like trying to teach a puppy to sit and stay. You place the puppy into a sitting position and tell him to stay. He stays for a few seconds, then sees something interesting and wanders off. You gently bring him back to the same spot, sit him down, and tell him to stay. This routine is repeated again and again, and gradually his ability to stay improves. Similarly, a person's ability to concentrate improves with meditation practice.

A good posture for practicing meditation is seated in a comfortable chair or cross-legged on a cushion. Keep the back upright and in alignment, and let the hands rest on the knees. If in a chair, feet are flat on the floor. Meditation can be practiced with the eyes closed or open slightly (soft eyes) looking 6–10 feet ahead. Good meditation posture is demonstrated in Figure 4–3 ◀.

The surroundings should be quiet and free of distractions. Although meditation can be practiced at any time, many find the early morning or late evening more conducive for calming the mind. Set aside 10–30 minutes daily for best results. Consistency is important for developing concentration ability over time.

A simple form of meditation is called *peaceful abiding*. The object of attention in peaceful abiding is the breath. "In peaceful abiding, we ground our mind in the present moment. We place our mind on the breath and keep it there" (Mipham, 2003, p. 24). By having a focal or reference point like the breath, we can better detect when concentration is broken, and bring it back as we practice focused attention. The end result is a clear, focused, uncluttered mind.

Another form of meditation is called *quiet sitting*. This is the practice of taking time to calm your mind, collect your thoughts, and center yourself. It is taking a break from the distractions of life and sitting quietly for a moment. The idea is to

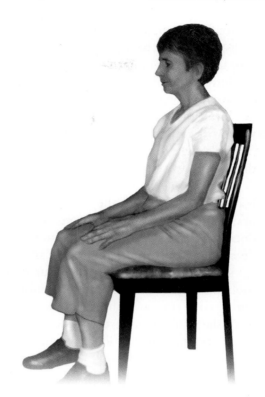

◂ **Figure 4–3** A good posture for practicing meditation is seated in a chair with the back upright and in alignment, the hands resting on the knees, feet flat on the floor, with soft eyes looking 6–10 feet ahead.

find a comfortable place to sit, close your eyes, and calm your breathing and your thoughts. Keep your thoughts centered on this quiet moment, and let go of unnecessary thinking. After a few moments, resume activity keeping the calmness you have created (Simpkins & Simpkins, 2000).

In *active meditation,* an activity like walking, knitting, or even doing the dishes can be used as a practice for focusing the mind. The point here is to focus on thoughts relevant to what you are doing, and let go of unrelated thoughts. If your mind drifts into other thoughts, gently bring it back to the task at hand. By raising awareness of when the mind is wandering and learning to bring it back to the object of attention, you are increasing your ability to concentrate.

Athletes work to improve their powers of concentration for better sports performance. Zen practices like kyudo (archery), flower arranging, and tea ceremony are ancient forms of active meditation. Eventually, massage itself becomes an active meditation in the sense that you are concentrating on what you are doing without distraction.

Many massage therapists do a variation on quiet sitting before beginning a massage session. They take a few moments to stand outside the door to the massage room and collect and focus their thoughts. This prepares them to be present and to give the massage session focused attention.

⟶ INTUITION

Intuition is defined as "a direct perception of the truth, independent of any rational process … [it] lets us see and respond to our environment without calling rational problem-solving into play. There is an organic knowing at work" (McCormick and McCormick, 1997, p. 99).

Intuition is related to *instinct*, which McCormick and McCormick call "the hardware of intuition." Our instincts help guide us through complex situations without having to stop and think everything through (1997, p. 99). Instincts come in handy when we are faced with unfamiliar situations, don't have all the facts, or have to act quickly. "Trust your instincts" is good advice when safety is involved. The terms *common sense* and *horse sense* have this same connotation (i.e., knowing through an inner voice).

Intuition is like a sixth sense. People with developed intuition can sense things, or have hunches about things they cannot rationally explain.

Intuition has its place in the practice of massage therapy. Massage therapists who work intuitively are not thinking through every move they make. Their hands "know" where to go and what to do. These are called *intelligent hands*, as if the hands themselves were doing the work disconnected from the brain.

Of course, just because the brain is not consciously thinking doesn't mean it is not involved. All of the stored knowledge and experience are available in the brain and working on an unconscious level as skills are performed. If something doesn't seem right according to intuition, the thinking brain becomes engaged to do rational problem solving as the situation requires.

A case can be made for the value of adding intuition to the massage therapist's tool chest of knowledge and skills. Intuition is developed by quieting the mind and letting go of conscious thinking. When a student is first learning massage techniques, he or she thinks about every move, but after a while and with practice, the mind can loosen its grip and intuition be given more rein. Such a massage is felt by the receiver as smooth and effortless.

↪ EMOTIONAL INTELLIGENCE

Emotional intelligence is the "heart" in the familiar triumvirate—head, heart, and hands. Emotional skills work hand-in-hand with intellectual and physical skills for full maturity as a massage therapy professional.

Neuroscientists are exploring the complex connections between the limbic structures of the brain, which are the seat of emotions, and the neocortex or thinking brain. It turns out that rather than being totally independent, these two "minds" interact continuously. The head and heart work together for best results:

> In a sense we have two brains, two minds—and two different kinds of intelligence: rational and emotional. How we do in life is determined by both.... Indeed, intellect cannot work its best without emotional intelligence.... The new paradigm urges us to harmonize head and heart. (Goleman, 1995, pp. 28–29)

Emotional intelligence is defined by a set of skills related to five domains: (1) knowing one's emotions, (2) managing emotions, (3) motivating oneself, (4) recognizing emotions in others, and (5) handling relationships (Goleman, 1995, pp. 43–44). Emotional skills are important in laying the foundation for success; for example, maintaining a positive outlook, building healthy relationships with clients, dealing with conflict, and making good decisions. They are essential for success in school and building thriving practices afterward.

Like mental IQ, everyone is born with brain circuitry that provides a starting point for emotional intelligence. And like thinking skills, emotional skills are first learned in childhood and developed throughout a lifetime.

Self-Awareness

The keystone of emotional intelligence is self-awareness; that is, recognizing a feeling as it happens and its accompanying emotion or impulse to act. Understanding the difference between a feeling and an emotion is a good starting point for self-awareness.

Although these are often equated, there is a subtle difference between *feelings* and *emotions*. The verb *feel* comes from an old English word related to sensation and perception, while *emotion* comes from an old French word related to movement and behavior. "Emotions are the outward expressions we use to either display or disguise an underlying feeling, matching or masking our inner state" (McCormick & McCormick, 1997, p. 84). People described as *emotional* freely display their feelings outwardly.

There is no agreement about which emotions are primary. However, some common emotions and their variations can be identified: enjoyment (happiness, joy, amusement, sensual pleasure, satisfaction); love (friendliness, kindness, devotion, adoration, infatuation, selfless love or *agape*); surprise (shock, astonishment, amazement, wonder); anger (outrage, resentment, annoyance, irritability, hatred, violence); sadness (grief, sorrow, loneliness, self-pity, depression); fear (anxiety, nervousness, dread, fright, phobia, panic); disgust (contempt, disdain, scorn, aversion, revulsion); shame (guilt, embarrassment, remorse, humiliation, regret, contrition). Figure 4–4 depicts the broad range of emotions of which humans are capable.

Temperament is a term for a person's basic disposition, or tendency toward certain moods or emotions. A developmental psychologist at Harvard identified at least four temperamental types: timid, bold, upbeat, and melancholy. He studied how temperament is shaped by "hardwiring" in the brain and how early experiences modify these tendencies (Kagan, Snidman, Arcus, & Reznick, 1998).

Extremes of temperament can be a negative factor in being a massage therapist. For example, being excessively shy or sad can interfere with developing a practice. Being excessively bold can result in poor judgment about behavior toward clients. Recognizing our basic temperament and learning to improve aspects that interfere with our life and work is part of developing emotional intelligence. An added incentive to become more self-aware is that the more we understand ourselves, the more we'll understand and have empathy for clients.

Naming our moods and emotions is an empowering step. Naming requires the ability to pause and look at emotion from the thinking brain. Humans have a unique capability of self-reflection that allows us to look at ourselves with some outside perspective. This provides the separation necessary to recognize the difference between emotions and our reactions to them. Naming emotions lays the foundation for identifying their causes and learning to manage them.

Managing Emotions

Once there is self-awareness, managing emotions becomes possible. Managing emotions involves learning to handle emotions so they are healthy expressions of our feelings and appropriate for the setting. This means recognizing them and responding in ways that benefit self and others. A balance must be achieved between suppressing emotions and letting them get out of control. As Goleman observes, "When

Enjoyment	Love	Compassion	Surprise	Sadness	Fear	Disgust	Shame	Anger
Happiness	Friendliness	Empathy	Shock	Grief	Anxiety	Contempt	Guilt	Outrage
Joy	Kindness	Sympathy	Astonishment	Sorrow	Nervousness	Distain	Embarrassment	Resentment
Amusement	Devotion	Pity	Amazement	Loneliness	Dread	Scorn	Remorse	Annoyance
Sensual Pleasure	Adoration		Wonder	Self-Pity	Fright	Aversion	Humiliation	Irritability
	Infatuation				Phobia	Revulsion	Regret	Hatred
Satisfaction	Selfless Love				Panic		Contrition	

▶ **Figure 4–4** The broad range of human emotions.

emotions are too muted they create dullness and distance; when out of control, too extreme and persistent, they become pathological, as in immobilizing depression, overwhelming anxiety, raging anger, manic agitation" (1995, p. 56).

Two examples of managing emotions related to being a massage therapist are dealing with annoyance with a client and continuing to work while feeling sad about a recent loss. In the first instance, being direct with the client about the cause of annoyance (e.g., habitual lateness) is appropriate, whereas allowing feelings of anger to fester is not. In the second instance, something simple like having fresh flowers in the room may cheer you up, while ruminating about your situation would not help.

A basic aspect of managing emotions is controlling impulses. Emotion is by definition an impulse to action. Being overcome with emotion can short-circuit the rational brain, leading to actions regretted later. Anger management is an example of learning impulse control. Strategies include walking away, counting to 10, and taking a cooling-off period. Chronic anxiety may be managed by learning relaxation and mind-calming techniques.

Delayed gratification is also possible when a person has impulse control. That means resisting an impulse today for a greater reward at a later date. The ability to delay gratification is a sign of maturity and makes many things possible, such as staying with an exercise routine, studying for classes, saving money for a new massage table, or responding ethically to a client.

Motivating Yourself

Two useful skills for self-motivation are nurturing an optimistic outlook and learning to get into the flow of peak performance. Taking responsibility for cultivating these abilities is part of emotional intelligence.

Optimism is a known contributor to success in school, sports, and even healing. Being optimistic means expecting that things will turn out all right in the end, despite setbacks and difficulties. An optimistic attitude helps a person persevere when the going gets rough. Being pessimistic, or expecting failure, leads to giving up when there are bumps in the road.

Optimism may be part of inborn temperament; however, a positive outlook can be nurtured. It is related to what psychologists call *self-efficacy*, the belief that you have the skills to meet the challenges you will face. A sense of self-efficacy can be nurtured by teachers who present challenges within students' current abilities and build on those abilities by making the challenges progressively more advanced. Once a person knows this principle, he or she can work on developing a sense of self-efficacy, and therefore, a sense of optimism.

Flow, or being *in the zone,* refers to a state of complete harmony during peak performance. There is a fluidity, sense of ease, and mastery that makes the performance a joyful experience. Performers get lost in the action as they become totally absorbed in what they are doing. Flow has an emotional component because, "in flow, the emotions are not just contained and channeled, but positive, energized, and aligned with the task at hand" (Goleman, 1995, p. 90).

Flow is a state that can be accessed. It involves quieting and focusing the mind on the task at hand and experiencing the sheer joy of the activity. It occurs most easily when the activity is challenging, but not too hard. Flow is thwarted by worry, boredom, or too much thinking.

Flow can be experienced in learning something new, practicing a skill, or during a challenge such as a test. Mihaly Csikszentmihalyi noted that "the best moments usually occur when a person's body or mind is stretched to its limits in a voluntary effort to accomplish something difficult and worthwhile … for each person there are thousands of opportunities, challenges to expand ourselves" (Goleman, 1995, pp. 91–92).

Recognizing Emotions in Others

Empathy, or recognizing emotions in others, is an important skill for massage therapists. It is essential for good communications with clients and developing effective therapeutic relationships. It is the basis for creating rapport and is the root of caring.

The ability to read someone else's emotions is based primarily on nonverbal cues. It means noticing things like tone of voice, facial expression, and gestures, and then matching emotions accurately to what is observed. Reading emotions can be very subtle; that is, interpreting *how* things are said, not just the words that are said. For example, a person with empathy can detect underlying sadness, anger, or anxiety in a client's words or actions. Empathy is emotional attunement with others.

Empathy does not mean taking on someone else's pain as your own. It differs from *sympathy*, which is defined as a relationship in which whatever affects one person correspondingly affects the other, and *pity*, which is feeling sorrow for someone else's misfortune. Sympathy and pity result from a lack of emotional boundaries with others and can lead to burnout for practitioners in the caring professions.

Compassion takes empathy one step further. **Compassion** is the "deep awareness of the suffering of another coupled with the wish to relieve it" (*American Heritage Dictionary*, 2000). Compassion combines empathy with a dedication to serve others. Compassion within the context of the massage therapy profession means the wish to relieve the suffering of others with the work of our hands.

Handling Relationships

The fifth domain of emotional intelligence is handling interpersonal relationships. The fundamental relationship between a massage therapist and client is called the *therapeutic relationship*. Elements of a healthy therapeutic relationship include clarity about the nature of the relationship, understanding of individual roles within the relationship, and establishing clear boundaries related to roles.

For the massage therapist, it means taking responsibility for the relationship and being honest, trustworthy, and ethical. For the client, it involves confidence in the therapist's abilities, trust and respect for the therapist, and satisfaction with the service provided. The massage therapist takes the lead in resolving conflict, responding to a client's anxiety or anger, and keeping good professional boundaries.

Examples of situations calling for skill in interpersonal relationships include resolving a misunderstanding about a cancellation policy, counseling a client with a body odor problem, or showing concern for a grieving client. Massage therapists might also have to respond to clients who use offensive language, come for massage under the influence of alcohol, or make romantic or sexual advances.

Interpersonal relationship situations will be discussed in greater detail in Chapter 5: Social and Communication Skills on page 108.

ETHICS FOR THE MASSAGE STUDENT

Ethics is the study of the nature of moral behavior, of right and wrong. It examines choices for behavior and uses a decision-making process to determine the degree of morality of certain actions.

Ethics have a positive aspect related to *what to do*, and a negative aspect related to *what not to do*. Common values upon which ethical choices are made include honesty, integrity, compassion, quality care, respect for persons, privacy and confidentiality, abiding by laws, keeping professional ethical standards, and doing no harm.

Professional ethics refers to common ethical situations that arise within a specific occupation like massage therapy. Codes of ethical behavior and standards of practice are developed by professional associations as the collective standard for the profession. Part IV of this book is devoted to ethics for massage therapists.

Massage therapy students have their own unique circumstances that require ethical consideration. Some are the same for all students, but others are unique to massage therapy students. The standards for massage students listed below are a good start to learning professional ethics as massage therapists. Ethical principles regarding relationships in school are discussed in more detail in Chapter 9: Therapeutic Relationship and Ethics on page 200.

Standards for massage students include:

Professionalism

1. Dress professionally for school.
2. Practice good hygiene.
3. Bring equipment and supplies needed for class.
4. Avoid offensive language and behavior with classmates.
5. Come to class on time and sober.

Class Work

6. Meet or exceed attendance requirements.
7. Put your best efforts into class, homework, and tests.
8. Devote adequate time to study and practice.
9. Present your own work in class, homework, and on tests (do not plagiarize or cheat).

Relationship with Classmates

10. Respect all classmates regardless of gender, ethnic background, religious tradition, sexual orientation, disability, or other distinguishing characteristic.
11. Respect the powerful effects of a relationship based on touch.
12. Refrain from a sexual relationship with a classmate until after graduation.
13. Take precautions to prevent the spread of disease in school.
14. Keep personal information about classmates confidential.
15. Practice informed consent with classmates.

Professional Boundaries

16. Change clothes modestly during hands-on classes.
17. Practice proper draping in class.
18. Keep good professional boundaries when practicing on family and friends.
19. Never engage in sexual behavior in the context of practicing massage therapy.

Relationship with the School

20. Treat your teachers and school administrators with respect.
21. Abide by school policies.
22. Represent your school professionally at public events.
23. Take care of school equipment and use it safely.

⟶ PHYSICAL SKILLS

Massage is performed with the whole body, not just the hands and arms. Being a massage therapist requires a certain level of body awareness, touch skills, physical fitness, and good body mechanics. Self-care practices related to the physical body not only develop the physical conditioning necessary to do massage, but also help prevent repetitive strain injuries that can cut a career in massage therapy short.

Body Awareness

Body awareness is the ability to sense where your body is in space while at rest and in motion and to coordinate movement with mind. It entails an integration of body and mind so that a person exists as an embodied being.

People who lack body awareness have difficulty following instructions for good body mechanics and for performing techniques because they are not "in their bodies." There is a disconnect between body and mind, as expressed in this quote from James Joyce: "Mr. Duffy lived a short distance from his body."

Body awareness is one of the beneficial effects of receiving massage and bodywork, and it is a wellness goal for clients. Body awareness is essential for learning massage techniques and for skillful implementation of massage sessions. Athletes and dancers, artists and craftsmen, musicians, and others who use their bodies in their work and leisure pursuits develop good body awareness over time. It is an awareness that can be developed through movement exercises. It can only be learned by doing and paying attention.

Being centered and grounded are two basic concepts related to body awareness important to massage therapists. Center has a physical and psychological dimension and refers to a focal point or point of organization from which being and movement occur. Its opposite is being scattered, off balance, and moving from the periphery. Being centered refers to finding your center and staying there while you move about.

Center of gravity is a biomechanical concept meaning "the point about which a body's weight is equally balanced in all directions" (Hall, 1991, p. 371). Think of the point at which your body is balanced from top to bottom, front to back, and left to right. Your exact center of gravity depends on your body shape, and how tall you are. The center of gravity for most women is in the hip region and higher toward the chest for most men.

A similar concept of center is found in Eastern practices. In Chinese, the center is called the *tan t'ien* (pronounced *dan tyen*) located about 1.5 inches below the navel and one-third of the way from front to back (Chuckrow, 1998). In Japanese, it is called *hara*. The hara is not only a place of physical centering, but a point of organization on many levels. Heckler states that "center is a state of unity in which effective action, emotional balance, mental alertness, and spiritual vision are in a harmonious balance. When we are centered our actions are coherent with what we care about" (1997, p. 96). You can begin to find this centered state by learning to move from the physical center.

The tai chi stance and walk are simple exercises that give you a sense of moving from the center. They can also be the foundation of learning good body mechanics for applying massage therapy. Figures 4–5◀ and 4–6◀ describe these useful exercises for developing good body awareness.

Ground refers to the firmness of the earth. The act of grounding refers to establishing a connection or being rooted to the earth through the legs and feet. The meaning can be extended to having a stable base and connection to a foundation

▶ **Figure 4–5** Tai chi stance with front foot pointing straight ahead and back foot at a 45° angle, heels in line, and feet shoulder-width apart. Shift weight back and forth feeling the movement from the hara or center.

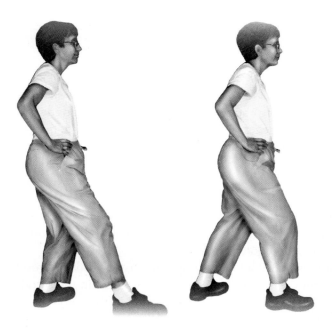

whether standing or sitting. This idea becomes important as you learn to move from and use the power of your legs in applying massage techniques. The energy of the movement comes up from the ground through the legs, into the center, and then into the upper body. This concept will be explored further in the section on good body mechanics.

Skilled Touch

Since touch is the basis of massage, skilled touch is essential for success as a massage therapist. Skilled touch has four dimensions important to massage therapists: (1) contact, (2) qualities, (3) communication, and (4) palpation.

Contact refers to the sense presence of the massage therapist's hands on the client's body. When contact is good the client feels a full, confident, deliberate, and warm connection to the massage therapist (Figure 4–7 ◀). Poor contact can feel tentative, hesitant, unsure, fearful, or nervous.

▶ **Figure 4–6** Tai chi walk along straight line. From tai chi stance, shift weight to the back leg and turn the front foot 45° degrees outward. Then shift weight to front leg while bringing the back leg to the front along the straight line; the new front leg receives the weight. Shift weight back and repeat the walk. Keeping hands on the hips helps you feel the movement from the center.

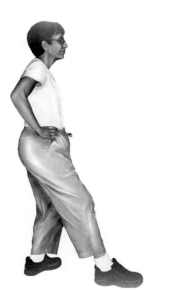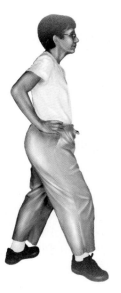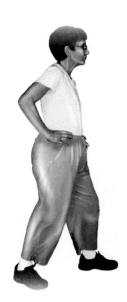

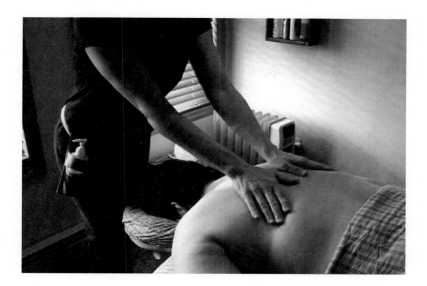

◀ **Figure 4–7** Good contact feels full, confident, and deliberate, and establishes a warm connection between massage therapist and client.

Qualities of touch are related to contact and vary from soft and gentle to hard and rough. Human beings are capable of many nuances in quality of touch, and massage therapists become more conscious of how they are touching their clients and what is an appropriate quality to use in a given situation. For example, athletes often prefer a firmer, deeper, and more vigorous massage, while a person who is ill requires a gentler touch.

Communication through touch is achieved by the contact and different qualities of touch applied during massage, or before or after the session when greeting or saying good-bye to a client. Be conscious of what you might be communicating when you touch your clients. Caring and openness are examples of what can be communicated through touch. Touch during massage should be caring, but never personal, sexual, or aggressive.

Respect for your clients' boundaries is a significant aspect of skilled touch. Know what is off limits for everyone (e.g., touching genitals), and for each individual client (e.g., ticklish feet or an old injury site). Obtaining informed consent for permission to touch is an important communication skill discussed in Chapter 9: Therapeutic Relationship and Ethics on page 209.

Palpation is sensing information about the client through touch and by the feel of tissues and movement at joints. Palpatory literacy involves the ability to locate specific anatomical structures and detect normal and abnormal conditions. The nature and importance of palpation skills in goal-oriented planning is discussed further in Chapter 6: Goal-Oriented Planning on page 146.

Body and Hand Mechanics

Body mechanics refers to the alignment and use of the body while performing massage. Good body mechanics minimize shoulder, neck, and back problems, as well as injuries to the arms and hands.

Standing. Good body mechanics start with the table at the proper height for you. A table too high or too low makes good body mechanics difficult. To determine a good table height, stand facing the table with your hands at your sides. Adjust the table legs so that your knuckles touch the tabletop (Figure 4–8 ◀). Become aware of the alignment of your back and neck when performing massage with the table at this height. Further adjust the table height as needed to keep good alignment.

▶ **Figure 4–8** Adjust the table legs so that your knuckles touch the table top when you are standing and your arms are hanging down.

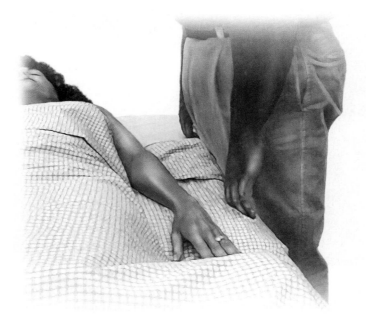

When facing the head or foot of the table, use a forward-leaning stance. The front leg is bent more than the rear leg, and the back and neck are in vertical alignment. Avoid bending over the client or hunching the shoulders. Bend the knees to lower your body. Apply pressure by leaning into the technique as your weight shifts from back leg to forward leg. This is why grounding is so important, because the energy for the technique comes up from the ground then goes through the legs. Generate power from your center or hara. Good body mechanics in the forward-leaning stance is demonstrated in Figure 4–9◀.

When facing the table directly, a side-to-side or horse stance allows for good body mechanics. Bending the knees and shifting the weight are also important in this stance. See Figure 4–10◀.

Sitting. Sitting on a chair or stool when massaging the receiver's head, hands, and feet can help reduce strain on the body. Sit near the edge of the seat with your feet flat on the floor and upper body in good vertical alignment. Adjust the height of the chair to allow good alignment (neutral position) of the wrists. Feet are grounded to

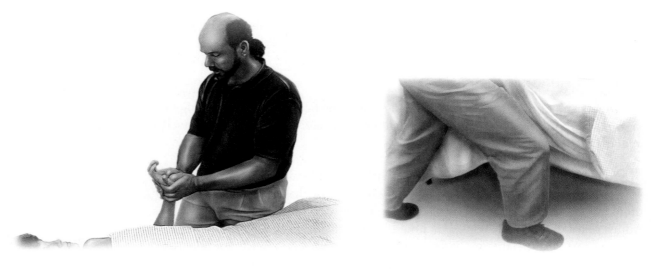

▲ **Figure 4–9** Good body mechanics when facing the head of the table; legs in forward-leaning stance with feet grounded, upper body in good alignment.

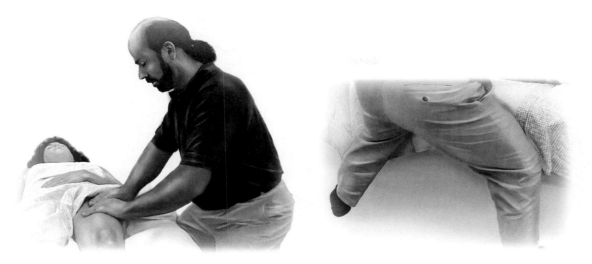

▲ **Figure 4–10** Good body mechanics when facing the table directly; legs in horse stance with feet grounded, upper body in good alignment.

the floor, and seat is grounded to the chair (Figure 4–11◀). Use the sitting position only for working areas with smaller muscles or for energy bodywork.

Hands. Good hand mechanics minimize strain on the fingers, thumb, and wrist joints. The thumb is especially vulnerable to misuse during high-pressure techniques like trigger point work or shiatsu. Stacking the joints is a protective principle in which joints are lined up so that the line of force is through the bones and not across the joint. Figure 4–12A◀ shows correct thumb alignment for applying direct pressure. Avoid applying pressure with the thumb abducted since this puts strain on the thumb joint, as shown in Figure 4–12B.

It is best to keep the wrists in a neutral position (neither flexed nor hyperextended) as much as possible. When applying compression techniques, avoid hyperextending the wrist. If reinforcing one hand with the other during compression techniques, place one hand directly over the metacarpals and not over the bent wrist. Correct and incorrect positions for compression are demonstrated in Figure 4–13◀.

Consider the use of the elbow for heavily muscled areas, or a hand tool such as a T-bar to apply direct pressure to a small area. The forearm may also be used to apply broad sliding strokes to the thighs or back (Figure 4–14◀).

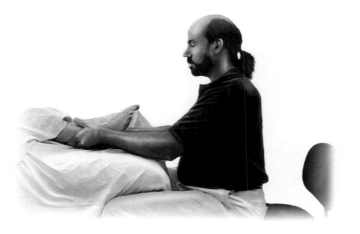

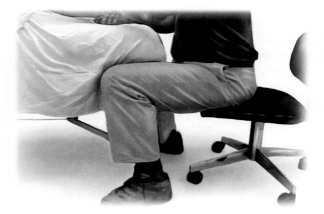

▲ **Figure 4–11** Good body mechanics while performing massage from seated position; sit near edge of chair with feet flat on floor, upper body in good alignment.

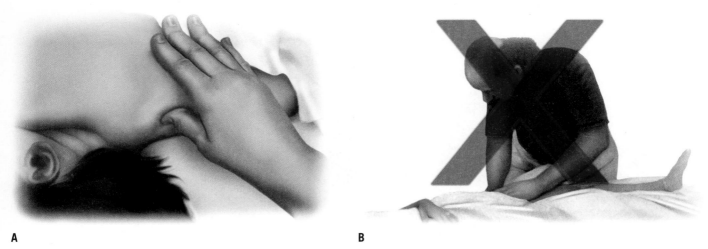

A   **B**

▶ **Figure 4–12 A.** Correct hand mechanics with thumb aligned with wrist while applying direct pressure; **B.** Incorrect hand mechanics with thumb abducted while applying direct pressure.

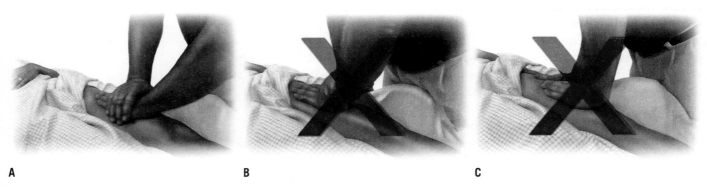

A   **B**   **C**

▶ **Figure 4–13 A.** Correct hand and wrist position for compression techniques; **B.** Incorrect hand position for compression techniques putting pressure on the wrist with the top hand; **C.** Incorrect hand position for compression techniques hyperextending the wrist.

▶ **Figure 4–14** Use of the forearm to apply broad effleurage to the hamstrings.

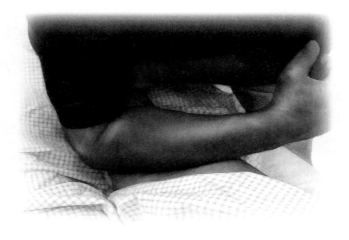

→ PHYSICAL FITNESS

In addition to being good role models for their clients, having a good level of physical fitness allows massage therapists to work without undue stress and strain. Learning the fundamentals of fitness is also good for better understanding the health of clients. Basic fitness includes cardiovascular function, strength, flexibility, and body composition.

Testing by a fitness professional using the latest methods will give the most accurate results. However, the simple tests described below offer a general fitness profile and demonstrate the concepts involved. Elements of a physical fitness profile are shown in Figure 4–15◀.

Cardiovascular Fitness

A basic cardiovascular (CV) fitness profile includes resting heart rate, blood pressure, and cardiovascular endurance. Measurements of these three aspects of CV fitness give an indication of how efficient and strong the heart is, and the level of stress on the blood vessels and the system as a whole.

Take your resting heart rate (RHR) either at the wrist below the base of the thumb, or on the anterior neck (carotid artery). For the most accurate reading of RHR, sit still for a few minutes and then find your pulse with your index and middle fingers, not the thumb. Count the number of beats for 1 minute (or number of beats per 15 seconds × 4). Normal resting heart rate is 60–80 beats per minute.

▶ **Figure 4–15** Physical fitness profile form.

Name _____ Date _____

♥ **Cardiovascular Fitness**

Resting Heart Rate (RHR) _____

Blood Pressure (BP) _____ / _____

Cardiovascular Endurance	poor	fair	good	excellent

⊤ **Muscular Strength/Endurance**

Abdominal/Sit-Ups	poor	fair	good	excellent
Upper Body/Push-Ups	poor	fair	good	excellent

() **Flexibility**

Sit and Reach	poor	fair	good	excellent

△ **Body Composition**

Body Mass Index (BMI)	underweight (less than 19)	healthy (19-24.5)	overweight (25-29.9)	obese (30+)

Waist Measurement (inches) _____

(women 32.5 – 37 inches; men 35 – 40 inches) **

*Fitness test results tables can be found in books like *Fitness for Dummies* by S. Schlosberg and L. Neporent (Wiley Publishing).

**Waist measurement as an indication of healthy body composition is discussed in *You on a diet: The owner's manual for waist management* by M. F. Riozen and M.C. Oz (Free Press).

Blood pressure (BP) is measured with a device called a sphygmomanometer or blood pressure machine. Blood pressure readings have two numbers (e.g., 120/80). The first or top number is the *diastolic pressure*, that is, the pressure of the blood on the vessels when the heart contracts. The second number is the *systolic pressure*, that is, the pressure on the blood vessels between beats. Anyone with BP over 140/90 is considered hypertensive and should see a doctor about it. High blood pressure puts stress on blood vessels and can lead to stroke and other serious health problems.

Cardiovascular endurance refers to the heart's capacity to keep up with a certain workload, and its ability to recover afterward. A simple test to demonstrate this concept is the 3-minute step test. This test is performed by stepping on and off a 12-inch-high bench or step for 3 minutes and then immediately checking your heart rate (HR) (Figure 4–16◀). Check the HR again at 1-minute intervals to see when it starts to drop back to the RHR. The lower the HR after the exercise, and the faster the recovery, the better the CV endurance is.

Good CV endurance increases the capacity to work longer without fatigue and offers protection against heart disease. Cardiovascular endurance is improved by participating in an exercise like walking, running, or cycling for at least 30 minutes 5 days per week. The activity should be vigorous enough to get the heart rate elevated and the body sweating, but not so high that you cannot carry on a conversation. The better the CV endurance, the more effort it will take to feel like you're working.

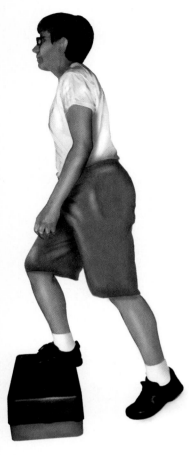

▶ **Figure 4–16** Step test for cardiovascular endurance.

Muscular Strength and Endurance

Overall muscular strength and endurance is developed naturally as the time spent performing massage gradually increases. However, by increasing muscular fitness beyond what is needed to apply massage techniques, less of the muscles' total capacity is used up when working, so there is less stress and fatigue at the end of the day.

Muscular strength refers to a muscle's ability to move a maximum amount of resistance once, while *muscular endurance* indicates the capacity to move against resistance for a number of repetitions over time. Strength and endurance are related since the stronger a muscle is the less hard it has to work to complete a task. Simple tests for muscular endurance include the number of push-ups or squats you can do, or the number of sit-ups in 1 minute (Figure 4–17◀). These tests taken together evaluate the major muscle groups of the body.

In addition to strength in large muscle groups, massage therapists benefit from having exceptional strength in the shoulders, arms, wrists, and hands. Resistance exercises for the upper body can help build strength in these important areas. Use of resistance bands offers a convenient way to increase strength in muscles used most in massage.

▶ **Figure 4–17** One-minute sit-up test for abdominal muscle strength and endurance.

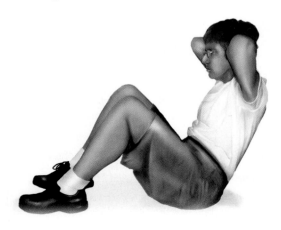

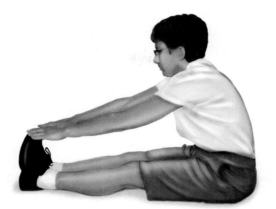

▶ **Figure 4–18** Sit-and-reach test for overall flexibility.

Flexibility

Flexibility is the "ability to flex" or the possible range of movement at joints. Range of motion at each joint can be measured precisely with an instrument called a goniometer, which works like a protractor used in geometry.

A simple test for overall body flexibility is the sit-and-reach test, which is really a test of lower back, hamstring, and shoulder flexibility. Sit with the bottoms of your feet flat against a stair or low box. With no warm-up tries, reach forward as far as you can toward your toes and hold the position (Figure 4–18◀). Note how far you reach, that is how far short of your toes or past your toes your fingers extend. For good flexibility, you should be able to reach past your toes.

Flexibility is maintained by regular stretching. Getting into the habit of stretching everyday and between client appointments can protect you from tight, shortened muscles. A regular stretching routine should include stretches for the legs and hips, arms and shoulders, and wrists and hands. Figures 4–19A–F◀ show a variety of stretching techniques for massage therapists to address the shoulders, arms, and hands.

Body Composition

Body composition refers to your body-fat percentage; that is, how much of your body is composed of fat tissue in comparison to other tissues (muscle, bones, organs, etc.). It is a general indication of health and a signal for health risk factors. Tests like skin-fold calipers, underwater weighing, bioelectrical impedance analysis (BIA), and other methods have been developed to measure body composition with varying levels of accuracy.

The BMI (body mass index) is a method that compares your height and weight to arrive at an index number to determine your weight status. Some BMI calculations also factor in chest and waist measurements. BMI is not as accurate a measurement as the more technical methods mentioned above, but offers a general indication of healthy body composition and is used here for demonstration purposes.

A simple BMI calculation is: weight ÷ (height in inches × height in inches) × 705. BMI categories are underweight (less than 18.5), healthy (18.5–24.9), overweight (25–29.9), and obese (30 or greater) (National Heart, Lung, and Blood Institute). Visit the National Heart, Lung, and Blood Institute website (www.nhlbisupport. com/bmi/bmicalc. htm) for a quick calculation of your BMI.

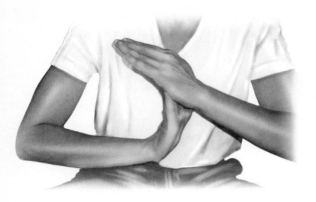

▲ **Figure 4–19A** Palm stretch by hyperextending the fingers.

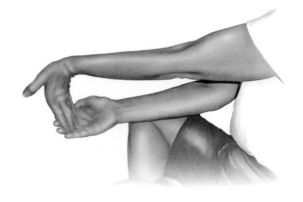

▲ **Figure 4–19B** Forearm and palm stretch by hyperextending the wrist.

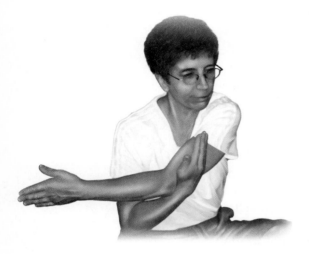

▲ **Figure 4–19C** Shoulder stretch by horizontal flexion of arm.

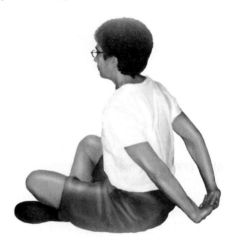

▲ **Figure 4–19D** Shoulder and pectoral muscles stretch by reaching behind.

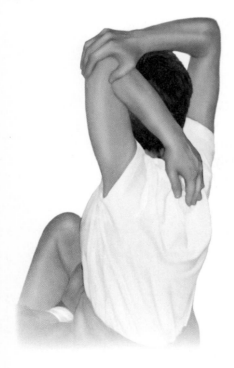

▲ **Figure 4–19E** Triceps and side stretch with arm overhead.

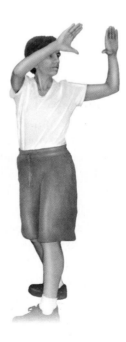

▲ **Figure 4–19F** Shoulder and torso stretch by twisting and looking behind.

CASE FOR STUDY

Robin and Getting into Shape for Massage

Robin started massage school about two months ago and is now noticing that she has difficulty getting through technique classes without feeling extremely tired and sore. She always thought of herself as being in good shape, but now realizes that doing physical work like massage might require a higher fitness level. She knows that to be successful in school and in a massage practice afterwards, she must get into better physical condition.

Question:

What can Robin do to get into better physical condition for doing massage?

Things to consider:

▶ Current physical fitness profile
▶ Areas (e.g., muscles, joints) that feel stressed after practicing massage
▶ Current types and level of exercise (e.g., CV, strength, flexibility)
▶ Quality of body mechanics while practicing massage techniques

▶ Related health practices:
  ● Amount of sleep each night
  ● Eating habits
  ● 3R's (rest, relaxation, recreation)
▶ Areas for improvement
▶ Possibilities for fitness activities

Now put yourself in Robin's place. What three things can you do to improve your physical fitness for performing massage?

1. _____

2. _____

3. _____

Body type and shape are determined by heredity, and affect body composition. But genetic predisposition can be managed with a program of good nutrition and exercise.

BODY–MIND PRACTICES

Some physical exercises do not fit neatly into the strength, flexibility, and cardio fitness categories described above. Yet they are useful for improving various aspects of physical fitness with the added benefit of developing coordination, body awareness, and concentration. And they are performed in a way that promotes relaxation. These can be thought of as body–mind practices or "any type of exercise that requires a conscious effort to link how [what] you are feeling to what your body is doing" (Schlosberg, 2005, p. 14).

Body–mind practices popular today include yoga, tai chi, qi gong, and Pilates. Although the first three practices stem from larger systems of philosophy and health practices in India and China, they can be found today adapted and simplified for Westerners. It is not necessary to know or accept the entire philosophical context to benefit from the exercises themselves.

Yoga is an ancient practice from India that concentrates on holding various postures thought to balance energy as understood in Ayurveda, and which improve bodily strength, flexibility, and body awareness. Yoga also includes meditation and breathing exercises.

Tai chi [ti-*chi*], an ancient practice from China originally based on martial arts, involves movements that promote balance, coordination, control, and strength. The movements are performed alone or in movement routines called forms. The quality of movement in the popular Yang style is slow and flowing. Tai chi stances and loco-motion, weight transfer, and quality of movement are ideal for learning good body mechanics for performing massage.

The Chinese also developed exercises to stimulate the flow of life energy or Qi (also *chi*). *Qi gong* [chi-*gong*] literally means *energy exercises* and focuses on the mind, posture, breathing, and movement. Qi gong is a very useful supplement to Asian bodywork therapy since it has the same goal; that is, to improve the flow of Qi in the body's energy channels (Chuen, 1991).

Pilates [pih-*lah*-teez] is a modern system of exercise developed by Joseph Pilates, who created the movements to treat injured dancers. Pilates emphasizes the body's core; that is, the abdominal muscles, upper and lower back, and hips and thighs. The exercises focus on using good alignment and strengthening muscles used for good pos-ture (Figure 4–20◀). Pilates is eclectic, borrowing from yoga, ballet, and standard strengthening exercises. It's uniqueness and benefit lies in its concentration on core muscles, good posture, and correct form. It increases body awareness and control as it promotes good body mechanics.

There are many styles or spin-offs of these systems of exercise. Doing a little home-work and critical thinking about them will help you choose one or a combination of practices appropriate for your wellness goals.

▶ **Figure 4–20** Pilates exercises strengthen the body's core muscles.

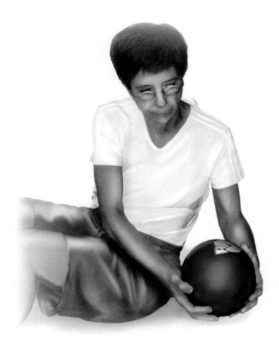

STRESS-CONTROL STRATEGIES

Massage therapists appreciate the major role that stress can play in undermining health and fitness. Students are under special circumstances that increase the stress in their lives, and therefore need stress-control strategies to help maintain good health. Good stress-control habits developed while in school can continue throughout your life.

Consequences of stress overload for students include problems like inability to pay attention in class (distraction), poor attendance and lateness, test anxiety, and chronic emotional upset. Stress-control plans include strategies like good time management, adequate rest and relaxation, and anxiety reduction techniques including massage.

Poor time management is perhaps the biggest stress producer for students. Developing a good time management plan as described earlier in this chapter is the cornerstone of a stress-control strategy.

Adequate rest, relaxation, and recreation are essential stress-control strategies. Getting 7–9 hours of sleep per night and having at least 30 minutes of "downtime" or quiet time per day are good goals. Recreation (think of *re-creation*) activities offer a break from work and revive the spirit. Schedule the three Rs of stress control into your time management plan.

Massage therapists, who are looked to as experts in stress reduction, accumulate a number of different methods to promote relaxation. These include relaxation audiotapes or CDs, physical practices like yoga and tai chi, meditation and quiet sitting, and massage itself. The more students practice relaxation techniques, the better able and more credible they will be when helping clients who come to them to reduce the stress in their lives.

HOLISTIC SELF-CARE PLAN

It can be a challenge to balance family and friends plus work and school while training to become a massage therapist. It takes a comprehensive, realistic plan. **Self-care** is a term used by massage therapists to describe how they take care of their own well-being while they fulfill their career goals and are of service to clients.

A holistic self-care plan includes those activities that support your development as a massage therapist and minimize factors that lead to illness and injury. It means having a plan for physical, mental, and emotional health and fitness, and avoiding undue stress and burnout. Even though self-care plans are as unique as the individuals involved, they have some common elements.

Self-care plans include healthy nutrition, physical fitness, rejuvenation, and stress management. Good body mechanics while performing massage is essential to prevent injury and increase longevity as a massage therapist. Quiet sitting or some other form of meditation helps maintain mental alertness and emotional calm. Taking time for recovery, rest, and relaxation prevents burnout. Good time management is the foundation of putting it all together and making it happen.

Keeping a journal or logbook, especially while putting a self-care plan into place, can help track progress and identify aspects that need to be strengthened. Figure 4–21 ◀ is an example of a page from a journal for tracking a holistic self-care plan.

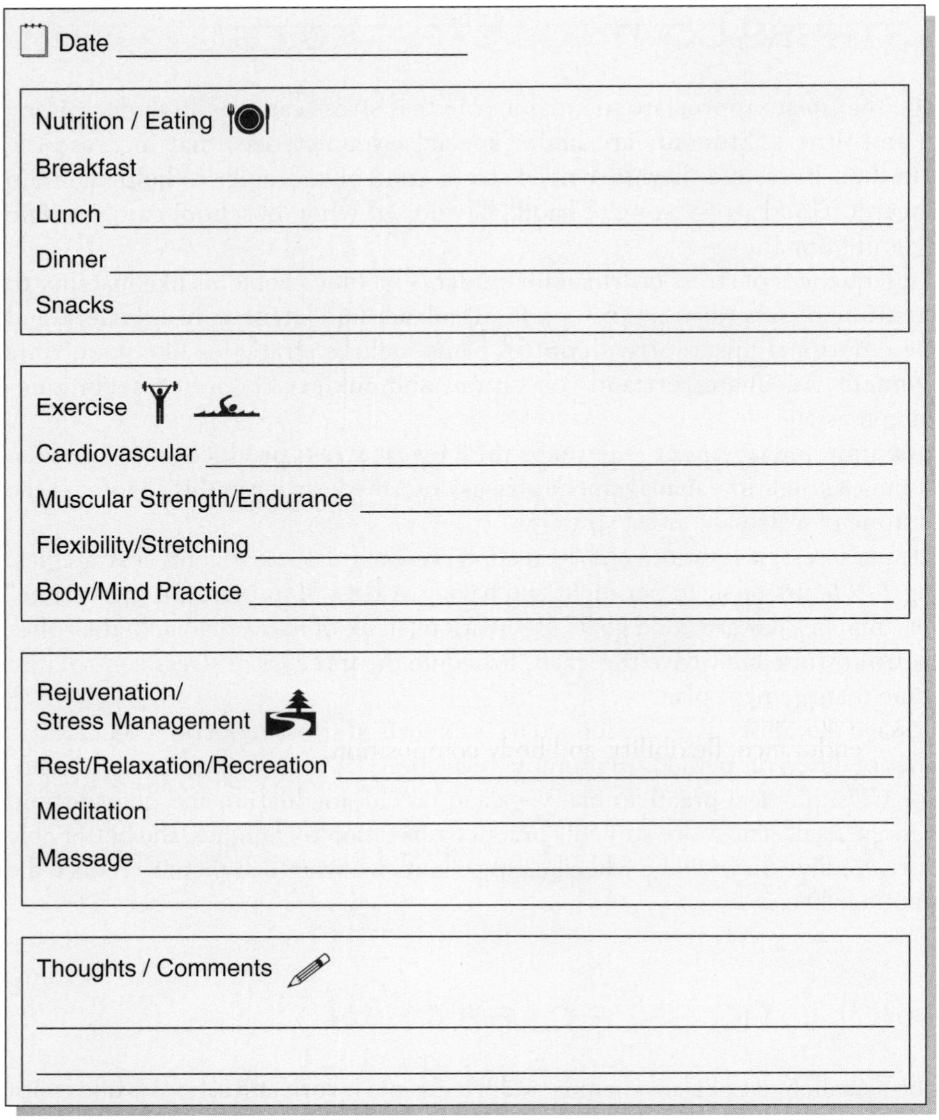

▶ **Figure 4–21** Sample daily log for holistic self-care plan.

🗒 Date _____

Nutrition / Eating 🍽

Breakfast _____

Lunch _____

Dinner _____

Snacks _____

Exercise 🏋 🏊

Cardiovascular _____

Muscular Strength/Endurance _____

Flexibility/Stretching _____

Body/Mind Practice _____

Rejuvenation/
Stress Management 🌲

Rest/Relaxation/Recreation _____

Meditation _____

Massage _____

Thoughts / Comments ✏

_____

_____

Chapter Highlights

- ▶ The journey to becoming a professional massage therapist involves personal growth and change.
- ▶ To have a professional attitude is to embody a professional way of acting, thinking, and feeling.
- ▶ Dedication to service means that the client's well-being is held above the massage therapist's own desire for money, power, and worldly recognition. This provides a moral compass for ethical decision making and motivation to be the best that you can be.
- ▶ Having a good work ethic means giving work a high priority in your life and is reflected in good attendance, punctuality, reliability, accountability, positive attitude, and enthusiasm.
- ▶ Good time management provides a practical plan for scheduling priorities and eliminating time wasters.
- ▶ Projecting a professional image means dress that is modest, clean, and allows freedom of movement, and good personal grooming, posture, and speech.

▶ Intellectual skills needed by massage therapists span the range from knowledge to comprehension, application, analysis, synthesis, and evaluation. Higher level thinking skills include critical thinking and systematic problem solving.

▶ The ability to concentrate makes studying more productive and performing massage better focused.

● Concentration is improved through minimizing attention disruptors, single-tasking, creating a more distraction free environment, and learning to focus the mind with meditation techniques.

▶ Intuition is direct perception of the truth without using rational problem solving and is useful for performing smooth, effortless massage.

▶ Emotional intelligence is defined by self-awareness, managing emotions, self-motivation, recognizing emotions in others, and handling relationships.

● Emotional intelligence is essential for developing healthy and ethical therapeutic relationships with clients.

▶ Standards for massage students lay the foundation for professional standards after graduation and include the areas of professionalism, class work, relationship with classmates, professional boundaries, and relationship with the school.

▶ Being a massage therapist requires certain physical skills including good body awareness, skilled touch, and body and hand mechanics.

● Physical fitness includes cardiovascular health, muscular strength and endurance, flexibility, and body composition.

● Mind-body practices like yoga and tai chi develop coordination, body awareness, and concentration.

▶ Self-care is taking care of your own well-being while fulfilling family, work, and school responsibilities.

● A holistic self-care plan encompasses the many aspects of well-being including the physical, mental, emotional, and social.

● Stress-control strategies like good time management, adequate rest, and relaxation techniques help prevent overload and burnout.

● Keeping a log or journal tracks progress and is motivating.

Exam Review

Learning Outcomes

Use the learning outcomes at the beginning of the chapter and shown here as a guide to the major topics covered. Perform the task given in each outcome, and share your results with a study partner. Check off the tasks as you complete them.

❑ Appreciate the importance of personal growth for professional development.
❑ Understand *service* as an important value for massage therapists.
❑ Develop a strong work ethic.
❑ Manage time effectively.
❑ Project a professional image.
❑ Explain intellectual skills needed by massage therapists.
❑ Improve powers of concentration.
❑ Understand the role of intuition in massage therapy.

❑ Develop emotional intelligence.
❑ Adopt ethical standards as massage therapy students.
❑ Develop fundamental physical skills.
❑ Create a program of holistic self-care.

Key Terms

To study the key terms listed at the beginning of the chapter, choose one or more of the following exercises. Writing or talking about ideas helps you better remember them, and explaining them to someone else helps deepen your understanding.

1. Write a one-sentence definition of each key term. Put the term in a general category, and then distinguish it from other terms in that category. For example, "*Intuition* is a direct perception of the truth, independent of any rational process." Or, "*Intellectual skills* are thinking or cognitive abilities." Try to capture the essence of each concept in a term statement.

2. Make study cards by writing the key term on one side of a 3 × 5 card, and a concise definition on the other side. Shuffle the cards and read one side, trying to recite either the explanation or term on the other side.

3. Pick out two or three terms and explain how they are related.

4. With a study partner, take turns explaining key terms verbally.

5. Make up sentences using one or more key terms. Variation: Read your sentences to a study partner who will ask you to explain unclear statements.

Memory Workout

The following fill-in-the-blank statements test your memory of the main concepts in this chapter.

1. Dedication to service offers a higher and more satisfying _____ than merely making money, and provides a moral _____ for ethical decision making.

2. Reliability means that people can _____ on you to do what you say, and if you are reliable people will have _____ in you.

3. Use a daily or weekly _____ to keep track of appointments.

4. Have work clothes that are _____ from your everyday clothes.

5. Communications with clients should be friendly and _____, but never too personal or _____.

6. Problem solving is a _____ approach to finding a solution.

7. A good meditation posture is sitting in a chair with your back upright and in _____, and hands resting on the _____. Eyes are either closed or softly looking _____ feet ahead.

8. Intuition is a direct perception of the _____, independent of any _____ process.

9. Recognizing a feeling in oneself and its accompanying impulse to act as it happens is called _____.

10. Establishing a connection to the earth through the legs and feet is called being _____.

11. Good body mechanics start with the table at the proper _____ for you.

12. A basic cardiovascular fitness profile includes _____ heart rate, _____ pressure, and cardiovascular _____.

13. Body–mind exercises like yoga and tai chi help improve _____, body _____, and _____.

14. The three R's of stress-control strategy are _____, _____, and _____.

Test Prep

The following multiple choice questions will help to prepare you for future school and professional exams.

1. Taking your work seriously, staying focused, and applying yourself to getting the job done right is known as having a good:
   a. Service orientation
   b. Punctuality
   c. Work ethic
   d. Sense of ethics

2. Planning a workable schedule for good time management is a matter of:
   a. Setting priorities
   b. Instant gratification
   c. Finding time wasters
   d. Luck

3. Which of the following is considered professional dress?
   a. Short shorts
   b. Denim jeans
   c. Closed-toe shoes
   d. Dangling jewelry

4. Nervous habits like finger tapping, nail biting, knuckle cracking, leg bouncing, and hair twirling can be:
   a. Stress reducers
   b. Image detractors
   c. Image enhancers
   d. Grooming problems

5. Using knowledge in real life situations is an example of intellectual skill at the following level:
   a. Comprehension
   b. Application
   c. Analysis
   d. Synthesis

6. What type of higher level thinking weighs reasons to believe something against reasons to doubt it?
   a. Logical thinking
   b. Problem-solving
   c. Clinical reasoning
   d. Critical thinking

7. Which of the following does *not* improve the ability to concentrate?
   a. Single-tasking
   b. Multitasking
   c. Meditation
   d. Distraction-free environment

8. A deep awareness of the suffering of others coupled with a desire to relieve it is called:
   a. Empathy
   b. Sympathy
   c. Compassion
   d. Appreciation

9. The ability to sense where your body is in space while at rest and in motion, and to coordinate movement with mind is called:

   a. Body awareness   c. Grounding

   b. Physical fitness   d. Centering

10. When applying massage techniques with good hand mechanics, what position are the wrists in?

   a. Extended   c. Flexed

   b. Hyper-extended   d. Neutral

Video Challenge

Watch the appropraite segment of the video on your CD-ROM and then answer the following questions.

Segment 4: Personal Development and Professionalism

Segment 4a: Personal Development: Professionalism

1. What do the massage therapists interviewed in the video say about clothes and projecting a professional image?

2. What advice do the massage therapists give about greeting clients?

3. Which of the image detractors discussed in the video do you recognize in yourself? Make a commitment to minimize detractors to improve your professional image.

Segment 4b: Personal Development: Emotional Intelligence

1. Identify ways that the massage therapists interviewed in the video show a high level of emotional intelligence. How is that important to a successful massage therapy practice?

2. What do the facial expressions of the massage therapists in the video convey to their clients? What similarities do you see in the massage therapists' expressions? Do you see any differences?

3. What do the massage therapists interviewed in the video say about establishing good relationships with their clients?

Segment 4c: Personal Development: Self-Care Plan

1. What methods of developing physical fitness are shown in the video? How do they compare with your physical fitness activities?

2. What do the massage therapists interviewed in the video say about the importance of stress control in their lives and careers? What are their stress control strategies?

3. What aspects of time management are mentioned in the video? How can you improve time management in your life?

Comprehension Exercises

The following exercises provide questions for you to answer and tasks you can do to enhance your understanding of the material presented in this chapter.

1. What are some important elements of a good work ethic? Why is this important for success in school and as a future massage therapist?

2. Name the five domains of emotional intelligence, and give two examples of how emotional intelligence could be important for a massage therapist.

3. Explain why having good body and hand mechanics is important for massage therapists.

For Greater Understanding

The following exercises are designed to give you a deeper understanding of the subjects covered in this chapter. Action words are underlined to emphasize the active nature of this approach to learning.

1. <u>Volunteer</u> a few hours a week for at least 4 consecutive weeks at a place that serves a special population, such as the elderly, disabled, homeless, caregivers, or children with special needs. <u>Write</u> in a journal about your experiences, especially how you feel about the value of service—its satisfactions and its challenges.

2. <u>Fill out</u> a time management chart for the rest of this semester or the next. <u>Discuss</u> your plan with a study group or classmate, and <u>evaluate</u> it according to the priorities you set for yourself. <u>Note</u> how well it supports your success in the massage school program.

3. <u>Imagine</u> the massage practice you will create after graduation. <u>Describe</u> what you will wear and your grooming plans. <u>Choose</u> one day when all students come to class dressed as they would for working with real clients. <u>Evaluate</u> each other's choices, and <u>suggest</u> improvements if appropriate.

4. <u>Choose</u> a situation related to massage therapy for an exercise in critical thinking and problem-solving; for example, whether you should buy a certain a product (e.g., type of oil, table, or massage tool); or take a certain elective class; or spend time and money on a particular certification program; or support a proposed licensing provision (e.g., hours of continuing education for license renewal). <u>Analyze</u> the situation listing pertinent questions, <u>evaluate</u> the situation, and <u>decide</u> on a course of action. What influenced your final decision?

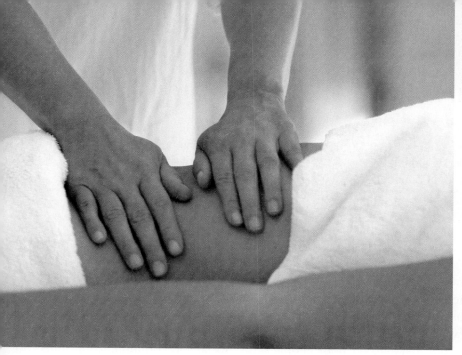

Social and Communication Skills

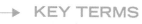 ## LEARNING OUTCOMES

After studying this chapter, you will have information to:

1. Practice basic courtesy and good manners.
2. Greet clients appropriately and with confidence.
3. Use body language to enhance communication.
4. Be a good listener.
5. Resolve conflicts peacefully and positively.
6. Set professional boundaries with clients.
7. Frame useful interview questions.
8. Make effective presentations.
9. Write clear business correspondence.
10. Use the telephone in a professional manner.

KEY TERMS

Body language	**Courtesy**	**Listening**	**Social skills**
Communication skills	**Interview skills**	**Professional boundaries**	**Verbal communication**
Conflict resolution			

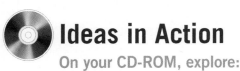

Ideas in Action

On your CD-ROM, explore:

▶ Greeting clients
▶ First impressions
▶ Professional boundaries

▶ The intake interview
▶ Interactive video exercises

RELATIONSHIPS

Massage therapy practices are built and maintained upon a foundation of good relationships. These include relationships with clients, other health professionals, and people encountered in a place of employment or while managing a private practice. Massage therapy is a person-to-person profession, and even the most skillful massage techniques cannot make up for poor people skills. Social and communication skills are inseparable and essential abilities for massage therapists.

Social skills encompass behaviors between people that promote harmony, understanding, and connection, while peacefully solving problems like disagreements, misunderstandings, and reconciliation after harm done. The primary goal of social skills is building good relationships. The social skills described in this chapter are specific to massage therapists and the situations they encounter daily.

Communication skills are the means of information exchange between people, and include verbal (i.e., speech and writing) and nonverbal (i.e., body language and facial expression) methods. Touch is also a powerful tool of communication. Good communication avoids misunderstanding, confusion, and lack of clarity that can produce social friction. Social and communication skills are polished through awareness, learning, experience, and practice.

COURTESY AND GOOD MANNERS

Courtesy and good manners are behaviors that are expected in social situations, such as saying "please" and "thank you," listening when someone is speaking to you, and introducing newcomers to a group. Courteous behavior shows respect for others and exhibits thoughtfulness about their feelings, comfort, and safety. It is essential for client satisfaction and good customer service.

The unwritten rules of good manners vary in different societies and in different situations, and change over time. Today, good manners include turning off audible signals on cell phones and other electronic devices in places where silence is appreciated, such as theaters, classrooms, and massage rooms. Good manners also include not having personal conversations on the phone and not eating when clients are present.

Good manners in school show respect for teachers, classmates, and yourself. They are often more conspicuous by their absence. Disturbing class by talking when the teacher is talking, eating during class, letting a cell phone ring, fidgeting, and leaving a mess where you were working are examples of bad manners in school.

Courteous, respectful language goes along with good manners. Use of offensive slang, crude sayings, and angry or demeaning words are especially out of place in school and professional settings.

While good manners open the door to good professional relationships, bad manners can slam the door shut. People have certain expectations about how they will be treated, and showing disrespect can evoke feelings of anger, disappointment, or annoyance. Having good manners is a sign of emotional intelligence and thoughtfulness.

Because what is considered good manners varies by culture and changes over time, professionals working in diverse environments become very aware of their behavior toward others. Business is particularly sensitive to this as it expands into a global marketplace. Professionals remain aware and flexible, adapting to times and circumstances to support building good relationships.

Courtesy and good manners can become second nature, but awareness and practice are prerequisites. Many of the social and communication skills described in this chapter are considered good manners and are expected of trained professionals.

→ GREETING AND FIRST IMPRESSIONS

It is a truism that you only get one chance to make a first impression. When you greet clients, potential employers, and others for the first time, they get an immediate impression of your professionalism.

> Whenever we walk into a room, our clothing, manners, and mannerisms are on display. Others assess our self-confidence and our ability to present ourselves based on 60 seconds of information. Each of us has our own signature of professional presence—an indelible statement that we make the instant we show up. (Bixler and Duggan, 2001, p. 7)

Because massage therapy is based on touch and close contact, it is especially important to establish good rapport right away, as well as confidence, trust, and a certain comfort level. In addition to projecting a professional image (through dress, grooming, posture, and speech) as described in Chapter 4: Personal Development and Professionalism on page 73, the manner of greeting is also part of a first impression.

Greeting a First-Time Client

The elements of greeting a client are to make eye contact, say the person's name, introduce yourself, shake hands, and give further directions. In the therapeutic relationship, the massage therapist is in charge, so it is her or his responsibility to take the initiative in greeting and helping the client feel comfortable.

Ten minutes before a client is expected, check your dress and grooming and office space to make sure it projects a professional image. Tidy up yourself and the space to look clean and well organized. Review the available client information. If possible, greet the client in a reception area.

When the client arrives, stand up, make friendly eye contact, and smile. Really look at the person to gauge his or her state of being and comfort level. Are they happy or sad, in pain, nervous, shy, or tired? Your assessment of the client for planning the massage session starts now. Then say the client's name to continue to make a connection, and introduce yourself.

When meeting a client for the first time, acknowledge the person by name and then introduce yourself. Say, for example, "Hello Dennis, my name is Debra and I will be your massage therapist today." You would have learned the client's name from checking the appointment book.

Finally, when you are confident that it will be well accepted, shake hands and invite the client to sit down (Figure 5–1 ◀). All this takes place in a matter of seconds.

The handshake is the first time you touch your client so it is especially important in establishing good rapport. Try not to reach over a barrier, like a desk or counter, when you shake hands.

▶ **Figure 5–1** Greet a first-time client with a firm handshake.

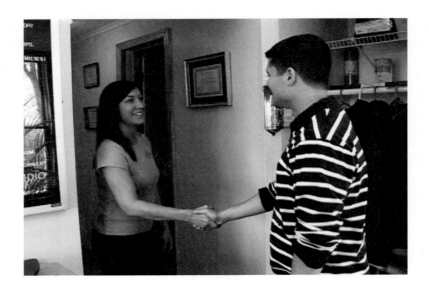

Extend your hand to the client first. Meet the client's grip palm to palm with good quality contact as you would during the massage. Squeeze firmly, but not too hard, for about 3 seconds and then release the hand. A general rule is to meet the other person's force, and squeeze more gently if the person is weak or injured.

Avoid the "bone crusher," "limp noodle," and "two-finger wiggle" handshake styles. Variations of the handshake include the "handshake sandwich" with your two hands around the client's one hand, which may be perceived as overpowering or patronizing; and the handshake with the left hand on the other person's forearm or shoulder, which is more intimate. Do not use these variations, or perhaps use them only later in the relationship as a comforting gesture in special circumstances. If a person is missing the right hand, or has a prosthetic arm, extend your left hand instead. The handshake should not feel rushed, but also should not linger too long, suggesting familiarity.

Hugs are a gesture used frequently in American society and may be appropriate in certain situations. However, when establishing professional boundaries, the handshake is a clearer statement of the business nature of the relationship and is safer for first-time clients. Use your judgment about hugs before or after subsequent appointments. Do not feel that you must hug a client to appear friendly or caring. Hug only if you have clear professional boundaries with a particular client, if you want to express particular affection for some specific reason, if it is acceptable to the client, and if it fits your personality. Remember that hugs may seem invasive to certain clients.

There are cultural differences in what is considered acceptable for greetings. For example, in some Asian and Middle Eastern countries, direct eye contact shows disrespect. Or touching at any time outside of the massage may seem too intimate. These are judgment calls that will become more accurate with more awareness and experience.

After the handshake, a client needs direction about what to do next. It could be, "Please sit down while we go over your goals for the session," or "Let's take a moment to go over your health history," or whatever you would like the client to do next. Be clear in your direction when pointing to a chair, or leading the client to the massage room. Clients receiving massage for the first time will need more guidance and assurance.

INTRODUCTIONS

Making introductions is a basic social skill used during the regular business day and at meetings or conferences. Introductions help people feel comfortable and welcome, as well as transmit useful social information. They are an essential networking tool.

The "golden rule" of introductions is to mention the name of the most honored person first. Other considerations are rank, gender, and age. If people are of equal rank, the woman's name is mentioned first. In a professional practice, the client is always the most honored person, but in other situations, determining the most honored is a judgment call.

The first person's name is followed by a phrase like, "I'd like you to meet [second person's name]," or simply, "This is [second person's name]." If possible, follow up the second person's name with a comment containing information about one or the other person. Ideally the comment would be something to further identify a person, or acknowledge his or her relationship to the situation. Say, for example, "John is a massage therapist at the Marian Hospital Integrative Health Care Center," or "Deidre works with me at the Rejuvenation Spa in Centerville," or "Kristin is going to the workshop on sports massage next month." This opens the door to further conversation and a sense of connection.

Here are some examples of brief introductions:

"Mary, I'd like you to meet Bill. Bill has a massage therapy practice in Milwaukee specializing in orthopedic massage. Mary is in from Minneapolis."

"Dr. Hernandez, this is Jerry Black, a massage therapist. Jerry has a question about a possible contraindication for one of his clients. Would you mind talking to him about it?"

"Dylan Smith, I'd like you to meet Reuben Jones. You two have something in common as fellow reflexologists."

Name tags that are worn prominently and can be read clearly are valuable social devices. Wear yours so that others can readily identify you, call you by name, and introduce you to other people more easily. If you work in a clinic or spa with other employees, a name tag identifies you to clients. Name tags worn at conferences facilitate networking.

There are times when introductions are not necessary. For example, if other massage therapists or clients are in the reception area, you would not be expected to introduce everyone to everyone else as you would in a social situation. Your business is with your client, and no other introductions are expected.

VERBAL COMMUNICATION

Speech or **verbal communication** is the primary medium of delivery on telephone calls and for important tasks like greeting and interviewing clients, explaining policies and procedures, networking with other health professionals, and giving presentations. The delivery of the spoken word in verbal communication is usually more important than the content. It is estimated that in a spoken message, body language accounts for 55% of the communication, voice for 38%, and the words for 7% (Cole, 2002, p. 95).

A good general rule is to speak with moderate speed in a calm, steady, strong voice. Vary the energy, rhythm, and inflection to make the delivery more interesting. Articulate clearly and avoid mumbling. Try to modulate accents unfamiliar to listeners.

Talk more slowly to people who have a different native language than the one you are speaking. Learn a few key words in the language of your regular clients; for example, words for *hello*, *pressure*, *pain*, *turn over*, and *good-bye*. If speaking a language that is not your own, be more conscious of using your voice quality, hand gestures, and body language to clarify your meaning.

When speaking to persons with hearing challenges, face them directly so they can read your lips. Speak slowly with good articulation, but do not exaggerate your words. You may increase the volume on your speech a little, but do not shout, especially to a person wearing a hearing aid. Learn some sign language if you work in a situation where you have regular clients who are hearing-impaired.

Voice quality is also important. Lower-pitched voices sound more confident and competent. Avoid seeming harsh or being overly loud or soft. Be aware that your tone of voice can type you, for example, a whining, nasal voice sounds like a complainer; a high-pitched, quavering voice sounds nervous; a breathy, slow voice sounds seductive. To add volume and richness to your voice, breathe deeply and relax your neck muscles and vocal cords. Your voice should come from the diaphragm rather than the throat (Cole, 2002).

Poor speech habits include using sounds like "uh" as space fillers, constantly clearing the throat, pausing too long between words, and speaking too fast. Ending sentences with a high inflection, as in asking a question, sounds uncertain and unconfident.

When speaking to clients, body language should project a friendly, open, and relaxed attitude. Avoid crossed arms, staring too intently, and frowning. A warm smile helps put people at ease.

Speech is a product of experience and habit and can be improved with practice. Become aware of your speech and develop speaking habits that enhance your verbal communications with clients and other social contacts.

↳ BODY LANGUAGE

Body language speaks volumes. Your posture, how close you stand to others, hand gestures, eye contact, and facial expression communicate your mood, interest, and even respect for a person you are talking to. As a massage therapist, knowing some of the common meanings of body language can help you project the meaning that you want and also understand others better.

Good upright, aligned posture commands respect and confidence. On the other hand, slouching, tilting, looking around, and drooping of the head can communicate disinterest, evasion, or boredom.

The comfortable distance between two people who are talking varies somewhat with culture. Be aware of your own comfort level and how it might differ from a client's preferred distance. Moving closer can indicate an interest in the subject, friendliness, or just difficulty hearing. Moving uncomfortably close is a type of physical boundary crossing.

Arms crossed in front of the body convey a sense of protection or distancing, while arms uncrossed and relaxed convey openness. Legs crossed can project the same sense as crossed arms. Hands on the hips signal impatience or anger. Fidgeting or habits like tapping a pencil or doodling project boredom, nervousness, or distraction.

Hand gestures are particularly communicative. In some cultures people seem to "talk with their hands" as they accentuate the meaning of their words with gestures. Putting a hand over the heart area or placing a hand lightly on another person's arm expresses sympathy and is a way of "reaching out" or making a connection. On the other hand, putting a hand out in front with palm facing the other person implies "stop" or "wait a minute." A common gesture to avoid is finger pointing, which seems accusatory and scolding.

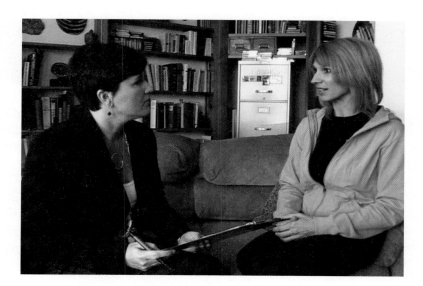

◀ **Figure 5–2** Relaxed posture and a friendly smile communicate an open and welcoming attitude toward clients.

Eye contact is extremely important. Looking at someone when you are speaking or being spoken to makes an essential connection. Knowing when to break eye contact is also important. Staring, looking too intently or too long, can be uncomfortable to a recipient. Break eye contact every so often and then come back. Looking away or around the room when someone is speaking to you is taken as a sign of disrespect or dismissal.

The eyes can also communicate things like friendliness, concern, annoyance, anger, pleasure, confusion, questioning, flirting, and seduction. Eyes communicate best along with other aspects of facial expression. The massage therapist in Figure 5–2 ◀ displays openness to the client through body language and a friendly smile. Having an expression that is hard to decipher, the so-called "poker face," might be useful in some circumstances, but tends to make people distrustful and uncomfortable.

The smile is perhaps the most universally recognizable sign of friendliness. A warm smile when greeting someone is welcoming. But beware—a genuine smile is hard to fake.

Remember that body language is only one piece of the communication puzzle. It is part of the whole communication package, along with facial expression, voice quality, words, and the general situation. People's personal habits (e.g., they might always fold their arms) must also be taken into consideration. The better you know someone, the easier it is to "read" him or her. Piece all the parts together to understand the full meaning being projected.

↪ LISTENING

Listening involves taking in and trying to understand what someone else is communicating to you. "I hear you" is a familiar expression that means "I understand (or empathize with) what you just said."

Listening is an essential communication skill for building relationships, discussing important issues, planning massage sessions, solving problems, resolving conflicts, and negotiating contracts. It also plays a big part in learning and critical thinking. Listening allows you to gather information, understand others better, and take in new ideas. Being a good listener begins with the intention to hear what others are really saying and overcoming poor listening habits.

Poor listening habits include letting the mind wander and formulating replies while others are speaking. Other bad habits are interrupting speakers, tuning out

PRACTICAL APPLICATION

Situations in which the words, voice quality, and body language are not in sync can lead to miscommunication. When this happens, one or both parties may feel uncomfortable, misunderstand what is being communicated, or even look for a way to end the conversation. This awkward, out-of-sync interaction is the kind of communication you want to avoid having with your massage clients.

With a study partner, role play situations in which what is intended to be communicated does not match the voice quality, inflection, or body language used. For example, try greeting a client with arms folded and frowning. Next, try playing a client who claims to feel fine and have no pain, while the body language clearly portrays discomfort, pain, or unease. Then correct the out-of-sync elements to communicate your message clearly. Switch roles with your partner a few times and be creative.

For a variation, try role playing using different types of eye contact. Include not looking at the other person, staring too long without a break, or looking around the room. Switch roles.

1. What can you learn about a client from voice quality and body language? Can you learn even more than his or her words alone convey?

2. What messages might you inadvertently communicate to a client through your body language? How might you ensure that your communication is clear?

3. What degree of eye contact is the most comfortable? What does your study partner communicate by having little or no eye contact with you when you are conversing?

---

different points of view, jumping to conclusions, finishing people's sentences for them, and talking while others are speaking. People also tend to hear what they want to hear and tune out what they don't want to deal with. Do not try to talk over environmental noise like street sounds or music playing in the background. Background noise interferes with hearing someone else's words.

Really listening involves focusing on what a speaker is saying (the words), feeling, and meaning. Know that people sometimes have trouble expressing in words what they mean. The Chinese character for *listen* consists of four characters: the heart, the mind, the ears, and the eyes (Cole, 2002).

When "listening" for feelings, pay attention to how the words are said, that is, inflection and voice quality. Watch body language and facial expressions as well. Listening for feelings is important for developing *empathy*, that is, recognizing emotions in others, as discussed in the section on emotional intelligence beginning on page 82 in Chapter 4: Personal Development and Professionalism.

Listening for the context is also important for understanding what someone is really trying to say. Getting the full picture helps you respond appropriately. Listen for what is not being said, and ask questions to "fill in the blanks." Summarize what you think you heard and check out your accuracy. This is an important interviewing skill, as discussed later in this chapter.

Affirmative Listening

Affirmative listening involves letting the speaker know that you are paying attention. This is accomplished by occasional verbal cues and body language. These affirming cues by the listener include nodding, saying "uh-huh" or "I see" or "yes," and repeating a word or key phrase or idea. Body language like leaning slightly forward toward the speaker and orienting your body to face the speaker also indicates attention. Eye contact is also important (Cole, 2002).

Affirmative listening allows others to say all that they have to say without interruption. However, active listening is good for promoting true understanding of someone's ideas and feelings and is an important communication skill for massage therapists.

Active Listening

Active listeners become more engaged in the communication process by reflecting back to the speaker what they think was said. This is not done by parroting the words exactly, but by paraphrasing or restating the words to clarify their meaning. Booher comments on the values of reflective listening: "By paraphrasing their views, you give talkers a chance to reflect on what they just said, to make sure that's what they mean, maybe even to change what they think or feel after hearing it again" (1994, p. 151).

These lead-in phrases are useful for active listening:

"You seem to be saying …"
"If I understand you correctly, you're saying …"
"Let me see if I get where you're coming from. You think that …"
"Am I hearing this right? You think …"
"Help me sort this out. You feel that …"

Notice that some lead-ins refer to the factual meaning of what was said and some are geared toward the feelings behind the words. They are statements, not questions. By paraphrasing, you are neither agreeing nor disagreeing with what was said. You are just checking out the meaning.

Cole offers five guidelines for reflective (active) listening (1994, pp. 158–159):

1. When several points are made, summarize the one that you want to focus on. This will help you keep the conversation pointed in the direction you want to take.
2. When several emotions are expressed, reflect the final one, as this is usually the most accurate.
3. Keep your reflective listening restatement short in order to keep the focus on the speaker.
4. Only reflect what's there—don't start guessing.
5. Wait out thoughtful silences.

Active listening is useful for drawing out information, understanding new ideas, being clear about statements, and clarifying your understanding. It can also be used in conflict situations to defuse emotion (yours or the speaker's), allow the speaker to express the emotions underlying his or her words, and show empathy. Cole suggests not using reflective listening if you don't like or respect the speaker. This avoids the possibility of unintentionally displaying your negative feelings. Also, do not use reflective listening as a substitute for stating your own thoughts and feelings on a subject.

⟶ CONFLICT RESOLUTION

Conflicts can arise in any relationship. Conflicts occur when personalities or styles clash, or when people trying to work together have different goals or expectations. Differences of perception, belief, opinion, values, or understanding of facts can cause strife and disharmony. Conflicts often manifest as arguments, disappointment, anger, annoyance, or frustration. They involve two or more people at odds with one another.

Conflict resolution means resolving conflicts amicably and begins with a conscious desire to do so. It involves setting aside competitiveness and the need to win, and focusing on goals rather than obstacles. Five basic approaches to dealing with conflict are collaboration, force, avoidance, accommodation, and compromise. The approach that is most appropriate for a given situation depends on the importance of two factors: (1) concern for others versus concern for your own needs and desires, and (2) importance of the relationship (Cole, 1994). Figure 5–3 ◀ explains when each approach is most appropriate.

Collaboration, or taking the time to find a solution together, is the way to go when building a long-term relationship, when goals are too important for compromise, or when you need to work together for the greater good.

Force, or demanding that your way be followed, is only acceptable in an emergency, when the stakes are high and the relationship nonessential, or when a higher principle is at stake and you have the power to enforce your will.

Avoidance, or not acknowledging a conflict, is risky because unresolved conflicts seem to grow worse rather than go away. Avoidance may be all right if it is a temporary situation and the issue is minor.

Accommodation, or letting the other person have his or her way, is best when keeping harmony in the relationship is most important, when the issue is more important to the other person than to you, when you cannot win, or when you realize that you are wrong.

Compromise, or both people adjusting their original positions, works best when a quick resolution is the goal, when the problem is temporary, or when a complete solution is impossible after much negotiation (Cole, 1994).

Minor conflicts occur all the time in therapeutic relationships with clients. Because the relationship is of such high importance, accommodation and collaboration are the usual modes of resolution, followed in order by compromise, avoidance, and force. Force should rarely be used and only in cases of emergency.

An example of a mid-level conflict is a client who misses an appointment once and does not want to pay the cancellation fee. If keeping the client is important, then accommodation may be the answer; that is, waiving the fee for this time. Avoidance, or not bringing the issue up, is a bad idea because it does not call attention to the policy, and the client may think that it is unimportant. If the client misses again, then the stakes are higher and you might want to insist on charging the cancellation fee.

Another example is a conflict with a fellow massage therapist who shares a massage room with you at a clinic. She always leaves the massage room messy, and you have to come along afterward and clean up before your client arrives. Given that the relationship and your needs are both important, as well as the principle of the situation, your best choice is an attempt at collaboration. That would involve confronting the

▶ **Figure 5–3** Choosing the best conflict resolution approach.

Method of Conflict Resolution	Relationship Importance	Need or Desire to Win
Collaborate	Very High	Equal
Accommodate	Very High	Low
Compromise	High	Moderate
Avoid	Low	Low
Force	Low	High

Special Situations	
When building long-term relationships:	Collaborate
When you need others support to reach goals:	Collaborate
When harmony is more important than the issue:	Accommodate
When you realize you are wrong:	Accommodate
When you cannot win:	Accommodate
When time is short:	Compromise
When an issue has low importance:	Compromise
When the conflict is a one-time thing:	Avoid
When the conflict is trivial:	Avoid
When you need to act fast in an emergency:	Force
When the issue is ethical or legal:	Force

other person with the facts as you see them and asking her to be more conscientious about cleaning up. You may be surprised to find out that she thought other workers at the spa or clinic were supposed to clean up, or maybe she has to rush out to another job and forgets about cleaning up. Collaboration involves listening and coming to agreement on a solution.

Major conflicts are uncommon but do happen occasionally. There may also be unethical situations like a client who wants to date you, or expects treatment outside of your scope of practice, or asks for sexual favors. For this type of conflict, insistence on ethical behavior is the only way to go.

Tips for successful conflict resolution include being respectful in language and demeanor, keeping a positive attitude, and looking for the win–win situation. Focus on finding a way for everyone to save face, staying open to options, being a good listener, and finding common goals. Resolution barriers are needing to win, taking things personally, letting hostility fester, and giving orders. Phrases like "you must," "you should," and "you have to" are sure to rankle the other person. Remember that conflicts are inevitable among people working together, and approach conflict resolution as an opportunity to practice your social skills rather than as a chore to be avoided.

↳ PROFESSIONAL BOUNDARIES

Boundaries communicate limits or borders that define personal and professional space. They are the fences we place around ourselves to preserve our integrity as individuals. Good boundaries allow two individuals to meet with integrity and without violation of the other's space, but close enough to make connection.

CASE FOR STUDY

Elise and a Conflict in Appointment Times

Elise has a steady client who recently changed jobs and is now on a different schedule. The times he prefers for massage appointments are now outside of Elise's regular hours. She sees clients from 10:00AM–4:00PM on Tuesday–Saturday. Elise would like to keep the client, but needs to resolve this conflict in their schedules.

Question:
Can Elise find a satisfactory appointment time for this steady client?

Things to consider:

▶ How important is it for Elise to continue with this client?
▶ How much outside of her regular hours would the new appointment time have to be?
▶ Does he have time for appointments outside of his "preferred" times?
▶ How flexible is he willing to be?
▶ How firm do her work hours need to be?

▶ Does she have family or other obligations that limit her availability?
▶ How willing is each person to compromise? Accommodate the other? Collaborate to find a solution?
▶ Is there a point at which dissolving the relationship is the only option?

Write examples of different scenarios for resolving this conflict.

1. **Accommodation:** _____

   _____

2. **Compromise:** _____

   _____

3. **Collaboration:** _____

   _____

Professional boundaries clarify the nature of the therapeutic relationship and the roles of both massage therapist and client. Such boundaries communicate to the client that the relationship is professional not personal, and define ethical behavior for both parties. It is the responsibility of massage therapists to establish and maintain professional boundaries in their practices through their communications with clients.

> Boundaries are the heart of how we protect ourselves and our clients. A boundary is like a protective circle drawn around ourselves and our clients; it defines what goes on within that circle and the ways practitioners will and will not treat each other. (McIntosh, 1999, p. 25)

There are five types of boundaries according to Benjamin and Sohnen-Moe (2003): physical, emotional, intellectual, sexual, and energetic. Setting appropriate professional boundaries in these five areas is a matter of ethics as well as social propriety.

How far we sit or stand from each other sets physical boundaries for personal space. Invading people's space by getting too close to them can make them nervous and uncomfortable. Clothes also serve as physical boundaries, as does draping during a massage session. Physical boundaries limit where and when it is appropriate to touch a client and vice versa, as in the discussion presented earlier of whether or not to hug a client. Leaving the room when clients are dressing and undressing gives them personal space and preserves their boundaries.

The physical space for massage, that is, office and massage room, should be free of personal property such as family photos or collections of objects. If practicing in a home, segregate the reception area, bathroom, and massage room from personal and family space as much as possible, especially from bedrooms.

Emotional boundaries limit disclosure about feelings. Since massage therapists are not professionals in psychology, too much emotional disclosure on the client's part may cross the line of a massage therapist's scope of practice. Emotional disclosure by the massage therapist may turn the tables in the therapeutic relationship by seeming to call for help from the client.

Intellectual boundaries demand respect for other people's beliefs and restrict forcing our beliefs and opinions on others. For example, some massage therapists who are health conscious may try to indoctrinate their clients regarding their eating habits, such as their belief in vegetarianism. This is not only an intellectual boundary violation, but also a scope-of-practice problem.

Critical thinking is a form of setting intellectual boundaries by questioning what we hear from others and protecting ourselves from propaganda and indoctrination. Massage therapists may also encourage critical thinking in their clients as a means of empowerment.

Sexual boundaries in a professional relationship are absolute. They protect both massage therapists and clients. Sexual boundary violations by massage therapists are unethical and illegal.

Energetic boundaries are less obvious; for example, not letting a client's bad mood or "negative energy" affect your state of being. Clients who seek massage are frequently stressed out and carry a lot of nervous energy. Helping clients disperse this energy without permeating the massage therapist's boundaries is an important self-care consideration.

Professional boundaries are also defined by routine office procedures and policies. These include policies for clients arriving late for sessions, not showing up for appointments, standards of hygiene, and payment due dates. Communicating policies clearly reduces misunderstanding and increases satisfaction when expectations are met.

Keeping good professional boundaries is a key factor in maintaining ethical massage therapy practices. Common boundary violations will be discussed further on page 204 in Chapter 9: Therapeutic Relationship and Ethics.

CRITICAL THINKING

We have many professional relationships in our lives, e.g., doctors, dentists, lawyers, teachers, school administrators, and more. We also have relationships with service providers like hair stylists, personal trainers, and car mechanics.

Choose one such person in your life and analyze your relationship with him or her. Write a short essay answering the following questions:

1 What is your role and the other person's role in the relationship?

2 What boundaries can you identify in the relationship?

3 How were those boundaries established? Are they implicit or explicit?

4 How do the established boundaries enhance the relationship? Do you think there are adequate boundaries,

or would you feel more comfortable if the boundaries were clearer?

Now, consider your relationship with practice clients. Write out a plan for establishing professional boundaries with them. Include physical, emotional, intellectual, sexual, and energetic boundaries. Continue your essay by answering the following questions:

1 What professional boundaries will you establish as a student of massage with your practice clients?

2 What are some polite but clear methods you can employ to communicate those boundaries effectively?

3 Explain why such boundaries are important to practice now while you are still in training to be a massage therapist.

→ INTERVIEW SKILLS

Interview skills include a variety of methods for eliciting useful information from clients. Interview skills are important from the time you screen potential clients on the phone, to intake interviews with new clients, to taking health histories and conducting pre- and post-session interviews.

The listening skills presented earlier are essential to interviews, but so are different methods for framing client answers. Some basic client interview methods are asking open-ended and multiple-choice questions, and using rating scales and body charts. Chapter 6: Goal-Oriented Planning on page 145 discusses client intake interviews in more detail.

Open-Ended Questions

Open-ended questions steer clients to specific topics, but leave space for them to answer in their own words. Rather than dictating the form of response, the massage therapist listens to what the client has to say in answer to a simple question. Responses to open-ended questions often give clues for further questions. Examples of general open-ended questions used in pre-session interviews are:

▶ How are you feeling today?
▶ How has your shoulder been feeling since the last massage?
▶ How were your legs during the marathon last weekend?
▶ Has your stress level related to that work situation calmed down?
▶ Were you able to rearrange your workstation so you aren't straining your neck so much?
▶ What are your goals for the massage today?

Multiple-Choice Questions

Multiple-choice questions give clients a choice of descriptors, which helps them to be more specific and helps you to better assess the situation they are trying to describe. It gives them choices that they might not have thought of themselves, but that have meaning to you. Some useful descriptors for common complaints are:

- ▶ Is the sensation you feel numbness, tingling, or pain?
- ▶ Would you describe your pain as sharp, diffuse, dull, aching, or throbbing?
- ▶ Would you describe the pain as mild, moderate, or severe?
- ▶ Would you describe movement at your shoulder as free, fluid, stiff, or restricted?
- ▶ Are your headaches seldom, occasional, frequent, or almost constant?

Rating Scales

Rating scales offer a rough measurement of things from the client's subjective view. Ratings use numbers to measure the degree or level of the client's experience of some factor related to their goals. Ratings give an indication of the client's experience of his or her condition and can be used to measure progress or regression from the client's perspective.

A scale from 1 to 10 is familiar to most clients, with 1 indicating the best scenario and 10 indicating the worst scenario for the item being rated. Below are examples of rating stress level, pain, and function.

- ▶ On a scale of 1 to 10—1 being pleasantly relaxed and 10 being totally stressed—how would you rate your level of stress today?
- ▶ On a scale of 1 to 10—1 being pain free and 10 being extreme pain—how would you rate how your back feels today?
- ▶ On a scale from 1 to 10—1 being easy and 10 being extremely limited— how would you rate your ability to walk up stairs today?

Body Charts

Body charts are diagrams of the human figure (e.g., front, back, and side views) that are marked by the client to locate problem areas and indicate the nature of a complaint. They offer the client a visual and kinesthetic (as opposed to verbal) way to give subjective information. Body charts can be used in the initial interview, as well as before individual massage sessions.

Clients mark with a pen the exact spots of concern on an outline of a body. Symbols can also be used to locate painful areas, recent injuries, or bruises. Symbols can also be used for different feelings in the area, for example, tension, numbness, tingling, and pain.

The use of a body chart as described above is different from the body chart filled in as part of the massage therapist's written SOAP notes (see page 170 in Chapter 7: Documentation and SOAP Notes). Documentation should clearly indicate whether the client or the massage therapist is the source of information on the chart.

Interview Guidelines

In addition to framing relevant questions, conducting good interviews includes knowing how to create an openness to response, when to lead the questioning, what to avoid, and when to stop.

Clients feel more open to giving responses if they understand the reason for your questions. Explain why you are asking questions in the interview. For example, while setting up an appointment for a first-time client, say something like: "I'm going to ask you a few questions to see if massage therapy would help you reach your goals, and if so, to plan your first session." Before taking a health history, explain: "I need a little more information about your health and any medications you are taking to plan the massage session."

Use body language that encourages answering. For example, look directly at the client and listen for the answer, rather than shuffling papers or looking around the room.

Give clients time to respond if you want thoughtful and accurate answers to questions. Do not rush the clients' answers, and pause for 5–10 seconds before repeating the question or asking further questions. Remember that silence gives clients the space they need to respond.

Some clients may need more direction, especially if you are relying on open-ended questions. Switch to multiple-choice questions, rating scales, or body charts for clients who have trouble expressing themselves verbally.

Ways to take more of a lead in questioning include asking for clarification of a statement, keeping clients on the topic if they are digressing, and helping them to get to the point. Ask clients to clarify conflicting statements. Ask for a final statement of agreement in important matters like billing policies, informed consent, or goals of a massage session. For example, say, "Do we agree on those two primary goals for this session?"

Avoid creating an atmosphere where clients feel like they're being interrogated; for example, by not smiling, or asking rapid-fire questions, or questioning their answers. Avoid being judgmental or dismissing their answers as unimportant. Do not deny their experiences.

Avoid questions not directly relevant to their massage therapy sessions. For example, it would be inappropriate to have a person coming to you for a relaxation massage go through an extensive medical history interview.

A good rule of thumb is to make interviews just long enough to get the essential information for planning a safe and effective massage session—no longer. Clients are coming for massage, which is a hands-on experience. Unnecessary questions take away from that valuable session time. A summary of interview guidelines appears in Figure 5–4 ◀.

◀ **Figure 5–4** Summary of interview guidelines.

Interview Guidelines

When conducting client interviews, follow these guidelines:
1. Create an inviting and open atmosphere.
2. Explain to the client *why* you are asking questions.
3. Look directly at the client when asking a question.
4. Give clients time to think and speak.
5. Use affirmative listening for encouragement.
6. Use active listening to clarify what was said.
7. Lead back a client who is digressing.
8. Ask for clarification of conflicting statements.
9. Use open-ended questions to hear the client's own words.
10. Use multiple-choice, rating, or body charts to frame answers.
11. Ask only relevant questions.
12. Stop when you know enough.

Avoid:
1. Creating an atmosphere of interrogation
2. Asking rapid-fire questions
3. Speaking too fast
4. Being judgmental
5. Dismissing answers
6. Denying the client's experience
7. Posing unnecessary questions

↪ PRESENTATIONS

Massage therapists make presentations in a variety of informal and formal ways. One-to-one, informal presentations include explaining policies and procedures to new clients, and showing clients self-massage techniques to use at home. More formal presentations may include talking to local community groups about the benefits of massage, or to a governing body in favor of or opposing legislation that affects massage therapists. Explaining, demonstrating, and persuading are useful communication skills in these situations.

Since presentations are essentially teaching opportunities, the audience receiving the presentation can be thought of as a group of learners. Include as many facets of learning as you can; for example, auditory, visual, and kinesthetic elements.

The first rule in making presentations is to know your goals. Why are you making the presentation? What do you expect to gain from it? Second is to know the audience and their expectations. Knowing the audience includes understanding their level of knowledge and experience with what you are presenting. Knowing their expectations helps you plan your presentation to meet their goals as well as yours. Then organize and plan what you want to say.

Explanations are verbal descriptions telling the what, how, and/or why of something. For routine tasks like explaining policies and procedures to new clients, develop a loose script with an opening statement, points to emphasize, and an ending such as "Do you have any questions?" Use props like a copy of the policies that you can read together. Give yourself a time limit and stick to it.

It might be useful to explain to clients why you are using particular techniques to address their goals for massage sessions. For example, you might explain that "Given that our goal today is to reduce your post-exercise soreness, I'll be doing a lot more stroking, kneading, and stretching to improve circulation and elongate those tight muscles. I'll be paying more attention to your legs since that's where you're feeling the soreness most." Do not explain more than clients need to know, and gear the explanations to their current knowledge of the human body and experience with massage. Anatomy charts and models are handy props for reinforcing verbal explanations of what is happening in the body during massage.

Demonstrations involve showing an audience how something is done or how something works by actually performing the action while giving a verbal description or explanation. Demonstrations enhance learning by giving the audience the opportunity to watch actions that would take many words to describe. A demonstration is worth 10,000 words. For example, demonstrating self-massage or stretching techniques to clients is more effective than verbal explanations alone. Performing massage techniques while explaining the effects of massage adds a valuable component when making a presentation to a community group or other health professionals.

When doing a demonstration, keep things simple. Avoid the urge to expound on everything you know about a topic or things that you find interesting. Tell your audience what you will show and why it is important to them, followed by a step-by-step explanation as you perform the actual demonstration. Allow for questions from the audience either during or after the demonstration.

The room setup is particularly important for demonstrations because the audience needs to see what you are doing. Be aware of how far away the audience members are from you and their angle of viewing. For larger groups, having a video camera that can project the demonstration onto a screen is useful.

The art of persuasion comes into play when you are trying to convince an audience to behave a certain way, take a specific course of action, agree on a particular solution to a problem, or accept a certain fact or belief. For example, you might persuade a client to allow you to massage a tight area even though it will be uncomfortable at first, or persuade legislators to vote for a massage licensing bill, or convince an audience that getting massage regularly is a good idea.

The first concern in persuasion is establishing credibility, trust, and confidence in you, the persuader. Informing the audience of your training and experience is useful, as is presenting a confident and professional appearance.

An organized presentation of ideas is next. The four steps in a persuasive presentation are (1) get the audience's attention; (2) present the conclusion, action, or decision that you are looking for and its key benefits; (3) build your case in detail; and (4) call for a specific action or decision (Booher, 1994). To build your case, establish a need or goal, and then show how your plan can meet it. Anticipate objections, and answer them in your presentation. Clear thinking is persuasive in itself. Avoid being too pushy or demanding. Invite others to your way of thinking.

A word of caution is in order here. Persuading clients to accept a certain approach to their therapeutic goals or to allow you to perform specific techniques when they would really rather not is more coercion than persuasion and is considered unethical. In Chapter 9: Therapeutic Relationship and Ethics on page 209, the idea of *informed consent* is explained as a way of giving clients choices while presenting your case.

All presentations should end with an opportunity for the audience to ask questions for clarification. For a client, you might say, "Was that clear? Do you have any questions?" For a formal presentation you might invite questions during the talk, or leave time for a short question-and-answer period at the end.

WRITTEN CORRESPONDENCE

As much as the way you dress and speak, written correspondence is a statement of who you are and a reflection of your level of professionalism. There is a greater likelihood that you will be listened to and understood, and your goals achieved, if your written correspondence is well formatted, grammatically correct, neat, and clearly stated.

Memos, e-mails, and business letters are the most common types of written correspondence for massage therapists. These forms of communication demand basic writing skills like correct spelling, punctuation, and grammar. Simple sentence construction and clear organization of thought are hallmarks of good business correspondence. Brevity is a virtue in written documents.

Memo

Memos are informal notes used to communicate information in short form to clients, coworkers, and colleagues. They dispense with some of the formalities of the business letter, but can retain a professional look by being printed on business stationery. All of the elements of a memo are important, especially the date, which is often overlooked. The block format makes skimming the memo content easier for the recipient.

Memos are appropriate for short notes, unofficial business, and other informal correspondence. Note that memos are still business correspondence and should project a professional image using professional language. The memo format and an example are found in Figure 5–5 ◄.

MEMO

Date

To
From
Subject

Main message (1–3 sentences)
Closing (1–2 sentences)

Signature/Initials

Example

MEMO

October 22, 2007

To: Jose Rodriquez
From: Timothy Kim, Massage Therapist
Re: Presentation at Rotary Club Meeting

Hello Jose—This is a note to confirm that I will give a 30-minute presentation on the benefits of massage at the Rotary Club luncheon on November 15, 2007, at 12:00 noon at the Bebop Café in Brenton. I understand that you will have a microphone and overhead projector available for my use.
Thank you again for the invitation to speak to the club.

Jim

E-Mail

E-mail is essentially an electronic memo. The e-mail format varies with the computer program used, but usually contains all of the elements of a standard memo. E-mail is becoming the preferred method of correspondence in both personal and professional settings. Delivery is fast, inexpensive, and e-mail is easy to respond to. However, there are some pitfalls to watch out for when using e-mail for business purposes.

First is your e-mail address. Have separate personal and professional e-mail addresses if possible. Use a professional-sounding address name like your own formal name or the name of your practice (e.g., jonesmassagetherapy@email.com). Avoid abbreviations and trendy e-mail jargon. Leave out "emoticons" for more professional correspondence; for example, smiley face :) sad face :(or perplexed :/. Remember that using all capital letters is like SHOUTING at the recipient—don't do it.

State your message concisely and clearly. People are being overwhelmed by the volume of e-mails they receive, and the messages you send are more likely to be read if they are short. Always put an informative title in the subject line. Use a phone call, paper memo, or letter if the message is lengthy. Memos and letters can be faxed if fast delivery is desirable.

Business Letter

Formal business letters are used for official correspondence with government agencies, insurance companies, vendors, employers, and clients. When corresponding for the first time with other health professionals, use the business letter format. They are also preferred for legal matters. The formal business letter format and the use of official stationery lends a more serious tone to a document.

Business letters have more identification and introductory information than memos and usually longer paragraphs. There are several different acceptable formats, and it is advisable to choose one to use for your practice and stick to it (Hahn, 2003). The basic business letter format in Figure 5–6◀ uses a modified block style, that is, aligned with the left-hand margin.

◀ **Figure 5–6** Business letter format and example.

Business/Practice Name
Address/P. O. Box
City, State, Zip Code
Phone/E-Mail

Date: Month-Day-Year

Recipient Name
Address/ P. O. Box
City, State, Zip Code

Dear [Title] First name, middle initial, last name:

Introductory paragraph

Middle paragraph

Closing paragraph

Sincerely,
Signature

Printed name, title

Anita Davis, Licensed Massage Therapist
1234 Box Street
Everytown, CA. 44444
(123) 456-7890 / adavis@email.com

June 14, 2007

Mineral Water Spa
567 South Street
Watertown, CA. 44445

Dear Ms. Edie Giacomo:

Thank you for the opportunity of interviewing for the position of full-time massage therapist at the Mineral Water Spa last Wednesday. I enjoyed seeing your facility and meeting other spa staff members. I was impressed by the level of professionalism and care for guests that I saw there.

I have enclosed the additional information you requested. This includes a copy of my license to practice massage therapy, my massage school transcript, and a list of my continuing education for the past five years.

Please let me know if you need anything else for your review of my credentials. I would welcome the opportunity to be a massage therapist at the Mineral Water Spa.

Sincerely,
Anita Davis

Anita Davis, Licensed Massage Therapist

For greater speed of delivery, business letters can be sent via overnight delivery services. They can also be sent as attachments to e-mails, with the actual paper letter sent at the same time via regular mail. For legal matters, consider sending letters "certified" mail for a record that they have been received, or use a carrier like UPS that has a tracking service.

Written Correspondence Guidelines

Remember that business correspondence has a different function than social correspondence and is more formal. Some general guidelines for written correspondence related to a massage therapy practice are:

▶ Choose the appropriate format for the correspondence (memo, e-mail, or letter).
▶ Use official printed stationery for memos and letters.
▶ Type business correspondence; memos may be written or printed legibly.
▶ Use correct grammar, punctuation, and spelling.
▶ Keep sentences simple, and organization logical.
▶ Use a more formal tone, and avoid slang and jargon.
▶ Do not put anything in writing that you would not like to see in a court of law.
▶ Keep a file of all of your written correspondence in chronological order.

TELEPHONE USE

Telephones and answering machines are essential communication tools for massage therapy practices. Clients usually call via telephone for their first appointments, so it is important to have good phone skills. Use the good speech habits as described earlier in this chapter.

Chances are that in private practice, a prospective client's first encounter with you will be via an answering machine. Script your answering machine message to be clear and concise. For example: "Hello. You have reached Green Fields Massage Therapy. I am unable to take your call at this time. Please leave a short message including your name and phone number, and I will return your call as soon as possible. Please wait for the beep to record your message." Re-record your message until you are satisfied that it sounds open, inviting, and professional.

When answering your phone, visualize a prospective client at the other end. In other words, be friendly and relaxed (Figure 5–7◀). If you feel hurried or stressed,

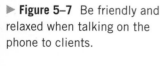
▶ **Figure 5–7** Be friendly and relaxed when talking on the phone to clients.

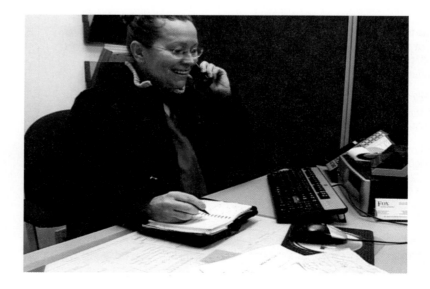

pause and take a deep breath to calm yourself before you answer. Identify yourself right away. For example: "Hello. This is Thomas Alter of Green Fields Massage Therapy. How may I help you?"

Here are some other tips for telephone use:

▶ Have a phone line dedicated to your practice.

▶ Do not make client calls on a cell phone while driving or in public places.

▶ Do not accept other incoming calls (e.g., call-waiting) when on the phone for business.

▶ Turn off ringers and cell phones when in a massage session.

▶ Do not interrupt a massage session to answer a phone call.

▶ Avoid distractions or multitasking while on the phone.

▶ Smile while on the phone. It can project a friendly impression.

Return calls promptly within 24 hours, if possible. If you will be unavailable to return calls for more than a day, change your message to alert callers when you will return their calls. This shows that you are reachable and reliable.

Chapter Highlights

▶ Good social and communication skills are essential for success as a massage therapist.

  ● Social skills promote harmony and connection between people, and resolve disagreements and misunderstandings.

  ● Verbal and non-verbal communication skills facilitate the exchange of information and are polished through awareness, learning, experience, and practice.

▶ Courtesy and good manners are the foundation of customer service.

  ● What is considered good manners varies by culture and can change over time.

▶ First impressions are important to establish rapport with new clients.

▶ Greeting clients involves making eye contact, saying the person's name, introducing yourself, shaking hands, and giving further directions.

  ● The handshake is the first time you touch your client so it is important to have good, firm contact.

  ● Use good judgment in hugging clients to maintain professional boundaries and avoid violating the client's comfort level.

▶ Introductions help people feel comfortable and welcome, as well as transmit useful social information.

  ● In introducing two people, say the most honored person's name first.

▶ Verbal communication is improved through practice.

  ● Speak in a calm, steady, strong voice; vary energy, rhythm, and inflection to make delivery interesting; articulate clearly and avoid mumbling.

▶ Body language speaks volumes.

  ● Use good upright, aligned posture and avoid slouching, tilting, and a drooping head.

- Use welcoming and friendly posture and gestures; communicate with your eyes and smile.

▶ Being a good listener begins with the intention to hear what others are really saying and to overcome poor listening habits.

- Focus on what the speaker is saying (words), feeling, and meaning. Avoid letting the mind wander and formulating replies while others are speaking.

▶ Affirmative listening lets the speaker know that you are paying attention through verbal cues and body language.

▶ In active listening, you reflect back to the speaker in your own words what you think he or she said.

▶ Five basic approaches to conflict resolution are (1) collaboration, (2) accommodation, (3) compromise, (4) avoidance, and (5) force.

- Choose the best approach to any specific conflict, taking into consideration the priority of your own needs versus the other person's needs and the importance of the relationship. Try for a win-win resolution.

▶ Professional boundaries clarify the nature of the therapeutic relationship, and the roles of both massage therapist and client.

▶ Five types of professional boundaries are (1) physical, (2) emotional, (3) intellectual, (4) sexual, and (5) energetic.

- Keeping good professional boundaries is a key factor in maintaining ethical massage therapy practices.

▶ Interview skills are used to elicit useful information from clients.

▶ Client interview methods include asking open-ended and multiple-choice questions and using rating scales and body charts.

- Conducting good interviews also includes knowing how to create openness to response, when to lead the questioning, what to avoid, and when to stop.

▶ Massage therapists make presentations in a variety of informal and formal ways to both individuals and groups.

- Know your goals and your audience, and then organize and plan what you want to say.
- Explanations are verbal descriptions telling the what, how and/or why of something.
- Use loose scripts and props for routine explanations to clients.

▶ Demonstrations involve showing an audience how something is done or how something works by performing the action while giving a verbal description.

- Keep descriptions clear and simple, and be sure the audience can see the demonstration well.

▶ In making persuasive presentations, first establish your credibility, then get the audience's attention, present your point and build your case for it, and call for action.

- Always provide an opportunity for listeners to ask questions.

▶ Written correspondence reflects your level of professionalism.

- Use correct spelling, punctuation and grammar, as well as simple sentence construction and brevity.

- Memos and business letters are written in a more formal tone on printed stationery using the correct format.
- E-mail is an electronic memo and follows the rules of any other business correspondence.
- Keep a file of all written correspondence in chronological order.

▶ Telephones and answering machines are essential communication tools.

- Use a clear and concise answering machine message, and return calls within 24 hours.
- Turn off ringers and cell phones when in a massage session.
- Avoid distractions and multi-tasking while on the phone.

Exam Review

Learning Outcomes

Use the learning outcomes at the beginning of the chapter and shown here to identify social and communications skills you need to develop further. Rate each social or communications skill listed in the outcomes on a scale from 1 to 5 according to your current level of expertise: 5 (excellent), 4 (very good), 3 (good), 2 (poor), and 1 (very poor). Reread the chapter sections on skills you rated 1 or 2, and perform related exercises below until you can rate all skills at least 3, or good.

Rating	Learning Outcome (Skill)
☐	Practice basic courtesy and good manners.
☐	Greet clients appropriately and with confidence.
☐	Use body language to enhance communication.
☐	Be a good listener.
☐	Resolve conflicts peacefully and positively.
☐	Set professional boundaries with clients.
☐	Frame useful interview questions.
☐	Make effective presentations.
☐	Write clear business correspondence.
☐	Use the telephone in a professional manner.

Key Terms

To study key terms listed at the beginning of the chapter, choose one or more of the following exercises. Writing or talking about ideas helps you better remember them, and explaining them to someone else helps deepen your understanding.

1. Write a one-sentence definition of each key term. Put the term in a general category, and then distinguish it from other terms in that category. For example, "*Interview skills* are communication skills used to elicit useful information from clients." Or, "*Professional boundaries* set limits on behavior, and clarify the distinct roles of the massage therapist and the client." Try to capture the essence of each term in a concise statement.

2. Make study cards by writing the key term on one side of a 3 × 5 card and a concise definition on the other side. Shuffle the cards and read one side, trying to recite either the explanation or word on the other side.

3. Pick out two or three terms and explain how they are related. For example, explain how courtesy, professional boundaries, and body language are related.

4. With a study partner, take turns explaining key terms verbally.

5. Make up sentences using one or more key terms. Variation: Read your sentences to a study partner who will ask you to explain unclear statements.

Memory Workout

The following fill-in-the-blank statements test your memory of the main concepts in this chapter.

1. Good social skills promote _____, _____, and _____ between people.

2. A general rule when shaking hands is to _____ the other person's force, and squeeze more gently if they are weak or _____.

3. Wearing name tags at professional conferences facilitates _____.

4. The _____ of the spoken word is usually more important than _____.

5. Good upright, aligned posture commands _____ and _____.

6. Poor listening habits include letting the mind _____, and formulating _____ while others are speaking.

7. Boundaries communicate _____ or _____ that define personal and professional space.

8. Sexual boundary violations by massage therapists are _____ and _____.

9. Rating scales offer a rough measurement of things from the client's _____ view.

10. Clients feel more open to giving responses during interviews if they understand the _____ for your questions.

11. Presentations are essentially _____ opportunities.

12. Business correspondence has a different function than _____ correspondence, and is more _____.

Test Prep

The following multiple choice questions will help to prepare you for future school and professional exams.

1. Which of the following directions for greeting a first time client is *not* correct?
   a. Make eye contact
   b. Offer your hand to shake
   c. Wait for the client to speak before introducing yourself
   d. Smile

2. When introducing two people, whose name is said first?
   a. The oldest
   b. The youngest
   c. The most honored
   d. The woman's

3. In terms of body language, arms crossed in front of the body can convey a sense of:
   a. Protection and distancing
   b. Welcome and openness
   c. Confidence and trust
   d. Friendliness and invitation

4. The type of listening that lets a speaker know that you are paying attention is:
   a. Attentive listening
   b. Distracted listening
   c. Active listening
   d. Affirmative listening

5. What type of conflict resolution is most appropriate when building long-term relationships, or when you need to work together with someone for the greater good?
   a. Force
   b. Collaboration
   c. Accommodation
   d. Compromise

6. Which type of professional boundary demands respect for other people's beliefs and restricts forcing our beliefs and opinions on others?
   a. Physical
   b. Emotional
   c. Intellectual
   d. Energetic

7. Which type of interview question steers clients to specific topics, but leaves space for them to answer in their own words?
   a. Open-ended question
   b. Multiple-choice question
   c. Rating scale
   d. Body chart

8. The first rule in making presentations is to know:
   a. How much time you have
   b. Your goals
   c. Your audience
   d. The room set-up

9. The most appropriate form of written correspondence for official business is:
   a. A memo
   b. An e-mail
   c. A brief note
   d. A business letter

10. Which of the following statements about phone use in your private practice is *not* good advice?
    a. Try to return phone calls within 24 hours
    b. Keep phone ringers on low volume during massage sessions
    c. Do not interrupt a massage session to answer the phone
    d. Do not interrupt a phone call with a client to answer another call, for example, with call-waiting

Video Challenge

Watch the appropriate segment of the video on your CD-ROM and then answer the following questions.

Segment 5: Social and Communication Skills

1. Review the scenes in the video in which massage therapists are greeting clients. Identify ways that professionalism, competence, and confidence are communicated.

2. What do the massage therapists interviewed in the video say about talking too much and listening to clients?

3. What principles of good communication do you see in video scenes showing client interviews? How do the massage therapists create a sense of openness to encourage client response?

Comprehension Exercises

The following exercises provide questions for you to answer and tasks you can do to enhance your understanding of the material presented in this chapter.

1. What is meant by *people skills*? Why are they important to massage therapists?

2. In addition to words, what are you listening for when talking to clients? What is the difference between affirmative and active listening?

3. What are professional boundaries? Give some examples of physical, emotional, and intellectual boundaries with clients.

For Greater Understanding

The following exercises are designed to give you a deeper understanding of the subjects covered in this chapter. Action words are underlined to emphasize the active nature of this approach to learning.

1. Create and practice a routine for greeting regular clients to make them feel welcome, comfortable, and confident in you. Take into consideration your body language, voice quality, and words. Have a study partner help you develop this professional "persona." (Variation: Videotape your greeting and analyze it with classmates. Modify it as needed to project what you want.)

2. Practice affirmative and active listening with a partner. Listen to how his or her day went yesterday, and at first simply nod and give affirmative signals that you are listening. Then practice active listening by reflecting back what you thought the person said for clarification.

3. Recall a conflict that you had recently with a friend, family member, or coworker, and explain how the conflict was resolved, identifying which of the five basic approaches you used. Would you judge the solution to be a good one? Why or why not? How might you have resolved it in a better way?

4. Conduct health history interviews with classmates, family, or friends using a health history form in Appendix F: Intake and Health History Forms on page 330. Use open-ended questions, multiple-choice, rating scales, and body charts to collect information. Evaluate your performance and modify it the next time for better delivery.

PART III

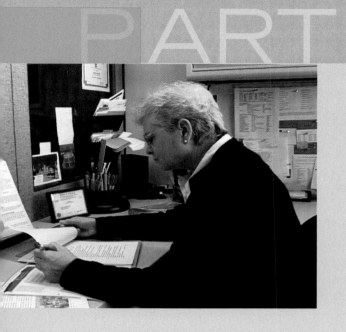

PLANNING AND DOCUMENTATION

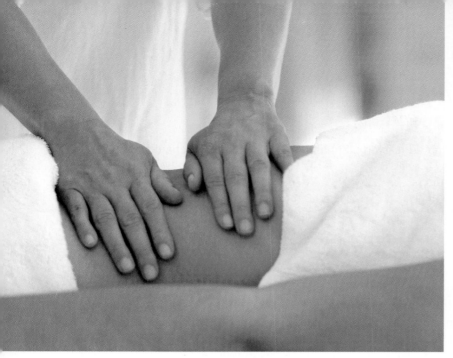

Goal-Oriented Planning

LEARNING OUTCOMES

After studying this chapter, you will have information to:

1. Appreciate the importance of planning.
2. Use the six-step process for planning goal-oriented massage sessions.
3. Develop long-term, individual session, and treatment plans for meeting clients' goals.
4. Perform intake interviews to gather client information for planning.
5. Use basic evaluation tools to collect objective information for planning.

KEY TERMS

Biomechanical analysis	Goal-oriented planning	Observation	Range of motion evaluation
Clinical reasoning	Individual session planning	Palpation	Treatment planning
Gait analysis	Long-term planning	Posture analysis	

Ideas in Action

On your CD-ROM, explore:

▶ Goal-oriented, 6-step planning
  process
▶ Observations
▶ Posture analysis

▶ Biomechanical analysis
▶ Gait analysis
▶ Interactive video exercises

⤳ THE IMPORTANCE OF PLANNING

Every massage needs a plan. This is true whether you are giving a set massage routine to a healthy client, or designing a session to meet specific client goals. Session planning is the logical process of thinking through the massage. It includes collecting relevant information, assessing the situation and setting goals, choosing massage applications, performing the massage, and evaluating results.

Session planning is like planning a vacation. You decide on your destination, research the area for things to do, line up your transportation, pack the clothes and other items you'll need, and then set out on your trip. If things go wrong or other options surface on the way, you adjust your plans. Leaving room for spontaneity keeps things interesting. Keeping a journal and taking photos as you go lets you review and evaluate your trip afterward. It makes sense that reaching your destination and getting the most out of your journey takes some planning.

For massage, the thoroughness of the session planning process varies with the situation. At a minimum, a short verbal or written intake to screen for contraindications may be sufficient before giving a standard massage routine. This is a common situation when offering sample massage at a health fair, post-event massage at a sports event, or signature massage to one-time clients at a destination spa. Planning in those cases is done quickly. Modifications to the routine are made during the session from client feedback. The *plan* in that case involves performing the standard massage and making changes necessary for the safety, comfort, and satisfaction of the client.

Goal-Oriented Planning

Goal-oriented planning focuses on meeting specific client needs, rather than giving a standardized massage routine. Planning to achieve client goals provides a focal point for organizing massage sessions and choosing appropriate techniques. It increases both practitioner and client awareness of positive results and improves satisfaction of regular clients. Goal-oriented planning is an intellectual process that provides a foundation for the artful and intuitive side of massage.

Clients come for massage for a reason. It is either to improve feelings of wellbeing, rejuvenate the mind/body, relax, reduce pain, improve mobility, alleviate symptoms of a disease, or some other specific desire. Goal-oriented planning can be applied to the entire Wellness Massage Pyramid (WMP). Figure 6–1 ◀ lists some of the many goals clients have related to massage therapy. The more aware you are of your clients' goals, the better you can serve them.

Clinical reasoning, the cognitive process used in goal-oriented planning, is essentially a problem-solving exercise. The client presents you with a problem to be solved (e.g., stress, muscle tension, pain), and you devise a plan using massage therapy to solve the problem. According to Holey and Cook, the major steps in problem solving are problem recognition, problem definition, problem analysis, goal formation, data management, development of a solution, solution implementation, and outcome evaluation (2003, pp. 103–108). This is a cyclical process. Outcomes evalua-

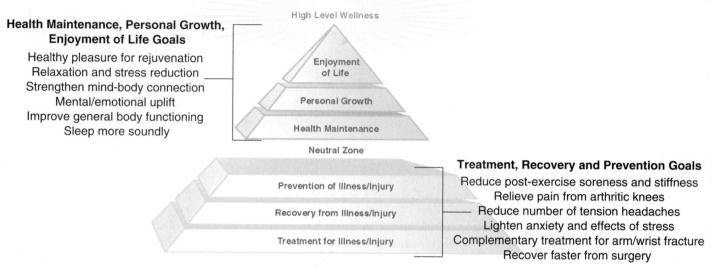

Health Maintenance, Personal Growth, Enjoyment of Life Goals

Healthy pleasure for rejuvenation
Relaxation and stress reduction
Strengthen mind-body connection
Mental/emotional uplift
Improve general body functioning
Sleep more soundly

Treatment, Recovery and Prevention Goals

Reduce post-exercise soreness and stiffness
Relieve pain from arthritic knees
Reduce number of tension headaches
Lighten anxiety and effects of stress
Complementary treatment for arm/wrist fracture
Recover faster from surgery

▲ **Figure 6–1** Sample client goals from the Wellness Massage Pyramid.

tion can lead to revisiting previous steps, such as redefining the problem or devising new solutions. This algorithm for problem solving is reflected in the steps for goal-oriented planning outlined below.

Three basic variations of goal-oriented planning are long-range planning, individual session planning, and treatment planning. The steps in the process are the same, but are applied differently for the different circumstances.

STEPS IN GOAL-ORIENTED PLANNING

Goal-oriented planning involves six steps with a feedback loop for making adjustments. The general process is outlined in Figure 6–2 ◄.

◄ **Figure 6–2** Six-step process for goal-oriented planning.

↳ **Step 1: Gather information from the client.** Obtain subjective information from the client via written forms and verbal interviews.

↳ **Step 2: Collect information through observation and measurement.** Compile objective information through practitioner observations, tests, and measurements.

↳ **Step 3: Assess the situation and set goals.** Analyze the subjective and objective information, obtained, make your conclusions, and determine client goals.

↳ **Step 4: Develop a plan to reach goals.** Design a long-term program to achieve client goals. If it is an individual session, choose massage applications to achieve the day's goals.

↳ **Step 5: Implement your plan.**

↳ **Step 6: Evaluate the results.** Analyze the outcomes of a series of sessions, or of one specific session.

↻ **Adjust goals and/or plans based on new information and results.**

✎ Document the process in session notes (SOAP notes).

Planning is presented here as *steps*, which implies a linear process. In practice, however, the thinking involved is not entirely linear. For example, subjective and objective information is gathered continuously as you listen to and observe your client before, during, and after a massage session. Information acquired during a massage from palpation or client feedback may signal a need to modify your session goals or massage application. Goal-oriented massage sessions are works in progress with adjustments as part of the process. Talking about the process as *steps* simply provides an orderly way to grasp the basic concepts, and stay focused on the goals.

Taking time for goal-oriented planning is important. However, in most cases it does not need to be lengthy. For most wellness applications, a 5- to 10-minute interview in the initial massage session will suffice, followed by brief check-ins before subsequent sessions to review goals for the day. Treatment of injuries and the use of massage as complementary to medical treatment require more planning and discussion with the client. More time is taken for tests, measurements, and assessment in the initial and progress evaluation sessions for those clients. Some massage therapists schedule an extra 30 minutes for new client intake and interview.

⟶ LONG-TERM PLANNING

Long-term planning is typically part of an initial massage session. It is focused on gathering subjective and objective information to get a big picture of the situation, determining overall client goals, and planning out a series of massage sessions to reach those goals. The term *long term* is used here to mean more than one session, or the interval between an initial session and a progress session to check the extent to which goals have been reached. The interval might be anywhere from 1 to 8 weeks. The steps in long-term planning are detailed on page 323 in Appendix E: Goal-Oriented Planning.

Steps 1 and 2

Subjective information for Step 1 is gathered from the client intake form, health history form, and initial client interview. Objective information for Step 2 is collected from observing things like the client's posture, movement, expression, and stress level. Tests are conducted and measurements are taken related to the client's stated goals, complaints, or written referral or prescription for massage. Tools for information gathering are described in more detail later in this chapter. Their purpose is to collect enough information to assess the situation and identify reachable goals.

Step 3

In Step 3 you assess the situation and establish long-term goals. Wellness goals that can be addressed with massage are identified, as well as problems for which massage is indicated. Also part of assessing the situation is identifying contraindications for massage and cautions to take into consideration later in planning. It may be determined at this point that the client should be referred for medical diagnosis before proceeding with massage.

For clients who receive regular massage as part of their general wellness plan, setting goals depends on what is happening in their lives at the time. They may go through a particularly stressful time, or participate in a seasonal activity like gardening or skiing. They may sustain injuries or get a new job with different physical requirements. Check in with regular clients on an ongoing basis for a continuous updating of long-term goals, or goals for a particular session.

An important aspect of Step 3 is prioritizing goals with the client. This helps you determine what to focus on the most without losing sight of the bigger picture. It also

CASE FOR STUDY

Kate and Long-Term Planning

Kate has decided to add regular massage to her overall wellness lifestyle. She contacts a massage therapist recommended by a friend and schedules her first massage. She is not sure what to expect but believes that massage will be beneficial for her.

The massage therapist has Kate fill out intake and health history forms. Kate reports that she is taking medication for allergies, but otherwise has no major medical conditions. She broke her left arm a few years ago, but it has healed. She is also adjusting her diet for healthier eating and plans to exercise more.

The massage therapist observes that Kate has some limitation in motion in the upper extremities around the past fracture. She checks with Kate about her sensitivity to certain massage oils and lotions. They briefly discuss the potential health benefits of massage and Kate's expectations. They agree to focus on stress reduction and relief of tension in the left arm and shoulder for the next few sessions.

Kate plans to come for massage every other week. Before each session, the massage therapist checks on the effects the massage sessions are having. Additional goals are expected to be set as the client learns more about massage and expands her ideas about how it can help her achieve optional wellness.

The massage therapist will apply Swedish massage techniques, adding trigger point therapy and stretching to the shoulders and arms, for the first few sessions. She writes intake information, observations, assessment, and the long-range plan in the session notes for the day. After 2 months, the massage therapist will evaluate progress toward the original goals, and modify them as needed as the therapeutic relationship develops over time.

Questions for Planning:

▶ What subjective information did Kate provide?

_____

▶ What objective information was gathered by the massage therapist?

_____

▶ What were the agreed upon goals for massage therapy?

_____

▶ What was the resulting long-range plan?

_____

brings the client into the process as he or she participates consciously in planning with you. Remember that it is the client's massage, and it is his or her goals that direct the sessions.

Step 4

With the results of Steps 1 through 3 in mind, an action plan is developed to achieve the client's goals. For a long-term plan, this means suggesting the frequency and length of massage sessions. For example, to reduce chronic stress, the plan may be for the client to receive a 1-hour massage weekly at the end of the work week. Or during a competitive season, the plan may be for an athlete to get a weekly maintenance massage with an additional recovery massage the day after an event. Or to facilitate rehabilitation of soft tissue injury such as a sprain, a half-hour massage twice a week for 3 weeks may be the plan.

The action plan includes selecting a general approach such as relaxation massage sessions, trigger point therapy, myofascial massage, passive joint movements, or some combination. Perhaps polarity therapy, shiatsu/acupressure, lymphatic massage, or some other form of bodywork is called for. Massage therapists survey their repertory of techniques and methods to see which ones are most likely to effectively address client goals. Obviously, the larger your repertoire, the more choices you have. Also, the more knowledgeable you are about the effects of different techniques and approaches, the better able you will be to choose an approach to help clients reach their goals.

Home care is another important aspect of Step 4. Note that massage therapists do not *prescribe* activities for their clients, which is outside of their scope of practice. But they can suggest different activities to be done on the clients' own time at home that may help them achieve their goals more quickly or effectively. Common home care activities include self-massage techniques, hot and cold applications, stretching, active exercises, and relaxation techniques.

Step 5

Implementing a long-term plan entails reviewing the plan with the client and making appointments. Being an educator is part of being a massage therapist as you teach your clients how to do their home-care activities.

Step 6

Long-term planning involves taking time to evaluate the results of a series of massage sessions and answering the question, "How well are the client's goals being met?" This is done in special progress sessions for well-defined goals, or on a less formal basis in pre-session interviews with the client, or with observations made during sessions.

The important point is to keep goals in mind, and be aware of positive results toward those goals as time passes. You will thus gain from your experiences and become a better massage therapist than if you just give massage sessions without paying attention to the results. Your clients benefit from achieving their goals, and you benefit as you learn from your experiences.

Loop

After the evaluation of results, the process loops to one or more steps above as more information is gathered, and goals and plans are updated. Goal-oriented planning is less a linear process and more of a looping spiral.

Long-term plans are documented in notes that go into client files. These notes are essentially a recap of the steps in the planning process. Chapter 7: Documentation and SOAP Notes on page 166 explains in detail what goes into the notes and how to write them.

A client who comes for massage to achieve a specific goal (e.g., to reduce tension headaches) may stop appointments once that goal is met. Many clients, however, benefit from regular massage to achieve high-level wellness, or to address a chronic health problem. Working with a client over time is a continuous process of assessing the situation and modifying your approach accordingly.

CRITICAL THINKING

Explore the truth of the statement: "Every massage needs a plan." Consider these questions:

1 What purpose does planning serve?

2 Can you give a massage without a plan?

3 How detailed does a plan for massage need to be?

4 When is a more detailed plan appropriate? When is an abbreviated plan a better choice?

⟶ INDIVIDUAL SESSION PLANNING

Each individual massage session is a step toward achieving long-term client goals. Some basic questions to ask for individual session planning are, "Where are we today, and what can we do in this session to move closer to the long-term goals?" The goal-oriented planning process for massage sessions is summarized on page 323 in Appendix E: Goal-Oriented Planning.

Step 1

Before a client arrives, it is useful to do a quick review of previous session notes, and in some cases, his or her intake and health history forms. Reacquaint yourself with the long-term goals and the results of the last session. From that point of orientation, you greet your client and perform a brief pre-session interview. In that interview, you ask the client about any changes in health status or medications and any progress or regression related to his or her goals since the last massage session.

Step 2

As you greet and interview your client, observe general posture, facial expression, voice quality, and other outward indicators of his or her state of being. Either before or during the session when the client is on the massage table, use brief tests and

CASE FOR STUDY

Steve and Individual Session Planning

Steve signs up for a massage at the health club about once a month. He believes that regular massage helps him relax and relieves the aches and pains from his sports activities. Steve has been getting massage at the club for about 2 years. He sees whichever massage therapist is available at the time he wants to schedule the session.

While the massage therapist is waiting for Steve to arrive, he quickly reviews Steve's health history. He also looks at past session notes, especially from the last four massage sessions. He is looking for contraindications, past injuries, recent goals for sessions, and notes about results.

When Steve arrives, the massage therapist screens for changes in health status and current medications, and asks about Steve's specific goals for the session. Steve reports that his legs and feet are a little stiff, and that he has some bruises on his legs from a hiking trip the past weekend. Steve is looking for general relaxation, reduced stiffness, and overall rejuvenation.

The massage therapist plans a full-body basic maintenance sports massage session. He will spend a little extra time on the legs and feet, but will avoid deep pressure over bruised areas. The session will include effleurage and

kneading techniques, trigger point therapy, and myofascial massage as needed. Joint mobilizing and stretching, especially in the lower extremities, will be done. Problems found through palpation and range-of-motion evaluation will be noted and addressed if there is time. The massage therapist writes observations, techniques applied, and results in the individual session notes.

Questions for Planning

▶ What subjective information did Steve provide?

_____

▶ What objective information was gathered by the massage therapist?

_____

▶ What were the agreed upon goals for massage therapy?

_____

▶ What was the resulting session plan?

_____

measurements to collect objective information (e.g., evaluating flexibility during a stretch, tissue quality while performing massage techniques, or ability to relax and let go of tension).

Step 3

Prior to beginning the massage, assess the current situation and prioritize the day's goals with the client. Determine any contraindications and cautions to be taken into consideration in this session. This may include long-standing conditions or temporary conditions, such as a recently acquired bruise or aspirin taken an hour before for a minor headache. Agree on goals for the session, and briefly review your general plan for the day with the client.

Step 4

While assessing the situation in Step 3, begin formulating your plan for the day. This is a good example of the steps in the planning process as overlapping and blending, rather than being discrete, sequential steps. The goals for the session will lead logically to an appropriate session organization and choice of techniques. While the client is undressing and getting onto the table, you can go over the plan in your mind, start your notes for the day, or prepare adjunct modalities such as hot packs.

Step 5

Begin the massage with the action plan in mind. For example, you begin at a certain place on the body using techniques chosen to achieve specific client goals. During the session, you might see reactions or results that either support the approach planned or signal a need to modify the plan. As you become aware of additional subjective and objective information, you will modify the original action plan for best results.

Step 6

Evaluating progress during a massage session is an essential part of the implementation phase (Step 5) as explained above. A post-session evaluation is also important. When you are saying good-bye to the client, you can make general observations, and conduct a brief post-session interview. Questions should be open-ended and designed to elicit information useful to evaluating the outcomes of the massage, for example, "How is your arm feeling now?" or "Are you feeling more relaxed?"

Each session is documented in notes that go into client files. The SOAP note format described in Chapter 7: Documentation and SOAP Notes on page 161 is well suited for capturing the goal-oriented planning process. The notes from the last session become a point of departure for planning the next time the client comes for massage.

⟶ TREATMENT PLANNING

Treatment planning is a form of goal-oriented planning in which the goal is alleviation of symptoms, or facilitation of healing of a pathological condition. It is used for medical, clinical, and orthopedic massage applications, and the treatment and recovery levels of the Wellness Massage Pyramid. A treatment plan is sometimes called a *plan of care*. See Appendix E: Goal-Oriented Planning on page 324.

CASE FOR STUDY

Angela and Treatment Planning

Angela comes for massage complaining of frequent tension headaches. In the client intake interview, she reports having headaches at least 3 times a week. She mentions that her neck is stiff. The massage therapist notices that she has trouble turning her head from side to side. Angela takes aspirin, but that is becoming less effective. The headaches are more likely to occur in the afternoon after she works at her desk for a long period of time.

She has not been in an accident lately and has no other signs of contraindications for massage. Her doctor has ruled out any underlying medical conditions that might cause frequent headaches and prescribed moist heat and a pain reducer to alleviate the headache pain.

It appears to be a typical case of chronic tension headache with no contraindications for massage. After discussion, the massage therapist and Angela both agree that the goal for massage will be to reduce the intensity and frequency of the headaches. The plan is for Angela to come for massage twice a week for 2 weeks and perform home care of self-massage and stretching, as well as hot applications. She will also begin using a headset for the telephone, and reposition her computer screen to achieve better neck alignment when working.

The general approach for massage sessions will be to focus on the shoulder, neck, and head muscles most often associated with tension headaches. General relaxation will be included for the beneficial effects of the relaxation response. Techniques will be drawn from Swedish massage, trigger point therapy, and myofascial massage.

The plan is to reassess the situation after 2 weeks to see if there are fewer or less severe headaches. Before and after each session, the massage therapist asks Angela to rate her headache pain on a scale from 1 to 10 (1 = no pain; 10 = severe pain). She also notes days when headaches occurred and how severe they were.

As her headaches subside, Angela reduces her sessions to once a week, and then to twice a month. Regular massage and home care activities help keep shoulders and neck muscles relaxed, and reduce the number of headaches and their intensity.

Questions for planning:

▶ What subjective information did Angela provide?

_____

▶ What objective information was gathered by the massage therapist?

_____

▶ What were the agreed upon goals for massage therapy?

_____

▶ What was the resulting treatment plan?

_____

Treatment planning requires a greater knowledge of pathology and massage research, as well as more advanced assessment and manual skills than other massage applications. Massage therapists who treat structural problems learn advanced musculoskeletal anatomy, biomechanics, and kinesiology, the study of human movement.

The terms *clinical massage*, *medical massage*, and *orthopedic massage* are sometimes used to describe advanced specialties within the broader field of massage therapy that focus on treatment. These terms do not refer to a unique set of techniques, but rather to the application of massage in a treatment planning process (Lowe, 2004; Rattray & Ludwig, 2000).

One major difference between treatment planning and other types of goal-oriented planning is in Step 3, that is, assessment of the situation. In medical settings, assessment typically means identifying or diagnosing a pathological condition. Since massage therapists may not diagnose according to state laws, assessment is more about measuring function or loss of function (e.g., range of motion), or evaluating the condition of tissues (e.g., fibrosis and adhesions). It may be determining how massage can alleviate symptoms like pain or facilitate healing. Clients often come to massage therapists seeking complementary care for a condition already medically diagnosed and under treatment by other health care professionals.

Yates sums up the critical competencies for developing treatment plans for medical conditions. First is the "ability to accurately *assess* the cause of the patient's presenting complaint in order to select and plan appropriate treatment." Second is the "capacity to *recognize* conditions for which some therapeutic approaches are contraindicated and to modify treatment accordingly." And third is "mastery of a sufficient variety of soft tissue techniques and other modalities to be able to safely and effectively *perform* the most appropriate form of treatment" (2004, p. 13).

Another difference in treatment planning is the end point of treatment. Medical settings that take their lead from health insurance companies often define the point of discharge or end of treatment as reaching the neutral point. The neutral point is the point at which symptoms are relieved (e.g., pain), normal function is restored, or sign of illness undetectable. However, in the wellness model, that is the jumping-off point toward high-level wellness.

Collecting subjective and objective information from the client is the foundation of the goal-oriented planning process. These essential steps are explained in greater detail in the remainder of this chapter.

↪ COLLECTING SUBJECTIVE INFORMATION

Intake is the process of gathering relevant information from a new client. This is considered to be subjective information. Intake forms are usually filled out by the client without direct help from the massage therapist. They contain general information about the client (e.g., name, address, phone, occupation); identification of the primary health care provider and insurance company, if relevant; and the reason for the initial visit.

Intake forms also explain the nature and scope of the massage practice and fees and policies (e.g., fees, payment, and cancellation policy). Intake forms usually include a privacy statement explaining confidentiality policies and consent for care. Sample intake forms can be found in business practices books.

Give a copy of this form to the client to take home for reference, and keep a signed copy for his or her client file. A basic intake form for massage therapy can be found in Appendix F: Intake and Health History Forms on page 327.

Health/Medical History

A general health history is also filled out by the client as part of the intake process. The purpose of the health history is to learn more about the client's health and medical history, as well as to identify potential contraindications and cautions for massage. In treatment planning, information about medical conditions, diagnoses from health care providers, and treatment goals help massage therapists plan sessions specifically to address the condition for which massage is indicated.

A sample health history form for general wellness applications and a different form for more medically oriented situations may be found in Appendix F: Intake and Health History Forms on page 330. The medically oriented form has more detail about past and current injuries, surgeries, diseases, and medications.

There are situations when intake forms and health histories are impractical or unnecessary, for example, for a short massage at a health fair, trade show, or sports event. In these cases, a minimum amount of information is necessary to provide a safe massage session. Some basic screening questions to ask are:

▶ Have you ever had massage before? (If no, provide more explanation)
▶ Have you had any recent illnesses?

- ▶ Do you have any skin conditions, injuries, or bruises I should avoid?
- ▶ Have you taken any medication today that affects your blood pressure or circulation?
- ▶ Have you taken any pain relievers today?
- ▶ If a woman: Are you pregnant?
- ▶ Is there any area that is especially tense that you'd like me to spend more time on?

The main purpose of these screening questions is to identify specific areas to focus on, and contraindications or places to avoid massaging. A short consent statement and liability release form should also be signed before giving even a short massage. A sample intake form for massage events can be found in Appendix F: Intake and Health History Forms on page 334.

Intake Interview

After the client fills out the intake and health history forms, the massage therapist conducts a short intake interview. The purpose of the interview is to clarify items on the forms, and fill in any gaps of information. For example, if a client says that he or she was in a car accident last week, you would want to ask further questions about medical treatment received, injuries sustained, or lingering aftereffects. This is also the opportunity to confirm the client's top priorities for massage, and collect more specific information about problems the person may be having.

Interview skills include a variety of methods for eliciting useful information from clients. Communication skills discussed in Chapter 5: Social and Communication Skills on page 119 include techniques like asking open-ended questions, multiple-choice questions, rating scales, and using body charts.

⟶ COLLECTING OBJECTIVE INFORMATION

Objective methods of collecting information include the massage therapist's own observations, evaluations, and measurements. These methods do not rely on a client's subjective view, but come from the practitioner's objective and outside perspective.

The type of information collected will vary according to the client's reason for seeking massage or to his or her initial complaint. Initial sessions and progress evaluation sessions will contain more measurement than ongoing sessions. Methods for collecting objective information include making general observations about the client, palpation of the client's tissues, range-of-motion evaluation, posture analysis, biomechanics analysis, and gait analysis.

Be mindful that there is a difference between what you observe and your interpretation of those observations. For example, you might observe that a client is moving slowly and stiffly. It will take further investigation to assess why this might be the case. The cause might be any number of things such as osteoarthritis, low mood, habitual movement pattern, a recent accident, or the marathon the individual ran the day before.

Be careful that you do not jump to conclusions or diagnose, that is, put the name of a pathology or medical condition to what you observe. Massage therapists are limited in their interpretations by their level of training. Beginning massage therapists have less knowledge to make interpretations than those with more training and experience. This means that you should sharpen your skills at observation, while understanding your limitations at interpretation of what you see.

General Observations

Observation is a basic tool for evaluation of the client's condition. Massage therapists use their senses to "observe" clients, that is, with their eyes, ears, noses, and hands. Some general observations and examples of descriptors are listed below.

- ▶ Skin: dry patches, blotches or red spots, acne, unusual marks or moles, rashes, bruises, wounds, scars
- ▶ Movement quality: slow, stiff, fluid, controlled, unstable, guarded
- ▶ Facial expression: smile, frown, nervous tick, furrowed brow, blank, serene
- ▶ Level of communication: nonstop talking, talkative, quiet, nonresponsive, silent
- ▶ Voice quality: loud, soft, weak, raspy, high pitched, low pitched
- ▶ Breathing: relaxed, diaphragmatic, chest breathing, labored, rapid, sighing, congested, wheezing, coughing
- ▶ Mental clarity: sharp, alert, fuzzy, vacant, distracted, forgetful, sleepy
- ▶ Emotional state: relaxed, agitated, nervous, angry, worried, anxious

For session notes, general descriptors are more useful if accompanied by specific or detailed descriptions of behaviors. For example, "The client seemed nervous and was tapping her pencil through the whole interview" is more informative than "The client seemed nervous." Another example, "The client's breathing was relaxed, from the diaphragm, and even" tells more than "The client seemed relaxed." Note that the simpler descriptions (e.g., nervous and relaxed) are actually interpretations of more specific behaviors that you observed.

Be as specific as you can in your notes. You may find out later that your interpretation of what you observed was incorrect. It is useful to be able to refer back to the original observation when reinterpreting or reviewing a situation. Although you observe many things about the client during the course of a massage, notes written about the session are limited to information used in planning and evaluating the current or future massage sessions. Session notes are discussed in more detail on page 160 in Chapter 7: Documentation and SOAP Notes.

Palpation

Palpation is the act of sensing information about the client through touch. Palpation is about the *feel* of tissues and of movement at joints. Biel explains palpation as "an art and skill which involves 1) locating a structure, 2) becoming aware of its characteristics, and 3) assessing its quality or condition so you can determine how to treat it" (2001, p. 14). A fourth aspect of palpation is to detect changes in quality or condition of tissues as a result of massage.

Palpatory sensitivity can only be developed through hands-on practice, aided by describing in words what is felt. Chaitow states, "we need to unleash a torrent of descriptive words for what we feel when we palpate" and "to obtain a thesaurus and to look up as many words as possible to describe accurately the subtle variations in what is being palpated" (1997, p. 9). The physical skill of sensing qualities and the verbal skill of describing them accurately make up palpatory literacy.

The first step in palpatory literacy for massage therapists is to be able to locate specific structures, that is, to feel where anatomical structures are located on the body. This is usually learned in anatomy class with a hands-on lab. Focus is on muscles, bones, joints, and related tissues and structures. This is useful knowledge for any type of massage therapy.

As palpation skills develop, you become more aware of differences in tissue temperature, texture, and firmness. You sense the ease of movement in healthy tissue and joints.

You are then able to detect abnormal tissue conditions. Descriptors for abnormal tissues include *spongy*, *hard*, *grainy*, *stringy*, *taut*, *taut bands*, *nodules*, *thick*, *congested*, *dehydrated*, and *adhering*. When assessing fascia, you feel for restrictions to movement or sticking. Abnormal joint movements may be described as *stiff*, *clicking*, *shortened*, *grinding*, or *bound*.

Some forms of massage therapy key into the body's rhythms that can be felt in the tissues. Body rhythms include circulatory rhythm or pulse, respiratory rhythm or breathing, and craniosacral rhythm in the circulation of cerebral-spinal fluid. Practitioners of Chinese medicine read the subtle radial pulse and detect the health of each organ and flow of energy, or *chi*, in the body.

Some forms of energy bodywork rely on detection of the body's energy field and the flow of energy in and around the body. These include polarity therapy, reiki, and therapeutic touch.

Developing palpation skill takes time and attention. Biel offers three principles of palpation (2001, p. 18):

1. Move slowly. Haste only interferes with sensation.
2. Avoid using excessive pressure. Less is truly more.
3. Focus your awareness on what it is you are feeling. In other words, be present.

The more conscious hands-on time you log, the better your palpation skills will be. Palpation skills develop throughout your entire career as a massage therapist. Examples of useful terms to describe palpation findings are listed in Figure 6–3◀.

Range-of-Motion Evaluation

Objective information about the general condition and degree of flexibility at a specific joint can be obtained by a **range of motion evaluation**. This is done by active or passive

◀ **Figure 6–3** Descriptors for documenting palpation findings.

Words used to describe palpation findings are presented below in relative terms. Although most of these terms have inexact definitions, but are useful in describing the general palpation findings.

Skin
hot / warm / cold
dry / damp / oily
hairless / hairy
smooth / rough
loose / taut
thin / thick
elastic / mobile
scarred

Soft Tissues (General)
spongy / firm
hard / tough / pliable / soft
dehydrated / puffy / swollen
congested
grainy / smooth

Muscles and Tendons
hypertonic / hypotonic
hard / firm / pliable
taut / taut bands / lax
knotty / smooth
ropey or ropelike
stringy
spasm / relaxed

Fascia
adhering / sticking / moving freely
restricted / unrestricted

Joint Movement
stiff / easy / free
clicking / hitches / glitches
crepetations
grinding / grating
stuck / bound / freely moving

Pulses
strong / weak
fast / slow
even / uneven
regular / irregular

Energy
stagnant / blocked / free flowing
pooled
fluid
excess/deficient

movement of the joint through its range, while observing any restrictions or shortening and any discomfort experienced by the client.

For evaluating active range of motion (AROM) at a joint, first demonstrate the movement you want the client to perform. Ask him or her to move slowly and steadily. Observe the client's ease of movement and any limitations or weakness. The client may report pain or discomfort verbally or by facial expression. Compare movement on both sides of the body. Document any deviation from normal, pain-free movement in your session notes.

Three simple AROM tests for the shoulder are described by Hoppenfeld in *Physical Examination of the Spine and Extremities* (1976, p. 21). These are the Apley Scratch Test and two tests for internal rotation and adduction shown in Figure 6–4◀. Tests like these are simple for clients to perform and offer quick, objective evaluations.

For evaluating passive range of motion (PROM) at a joint, have the client relax the muscles surrounding the joint while you move the joint through its range or apply a mild stretch. A passive stretch offers a good estimate of the degree of motion at a joint. For upper and lower extremities, compare the degree of flexibility on both the right and left sides. Note any restrictions in movement, differences in left and right sides, or discomfort experienced by the client. Document any positive findings, that is, any deviations from normal, pain-free movement at the joint.

You can also measure the range of motion quantitatively using an instrument called a goniometer, which is similar to a protractor used in geometry to measure angles. There are specific protocols for measuring range of motion with this instrument that take some practice to master. The goniometer is used primarily for medical applications and research.

Range-of-motion evaluation offers clues to potential muscle and tendon problems (AROM), or problems with ligaments and joint structures (PROM). Swelling, discoloration, or severe pain with passive joint movement signals that massage is contraindicated in the area. For any suspected joint injury, the client should see a health care provider for a diagnosis of his or her condition.

On the other hand, restricted range of motion may simply be a sign of tense, shortened muscles that can benefit from increased circulation in the area, muscle relaxation, and lengthening of muscle fibers. Mobilizing techniques and stretches for the spine and upper and lower extremities are described in *Tappan's Handbook of Healing Massage Techniques* by Patricia J. Benjamin.

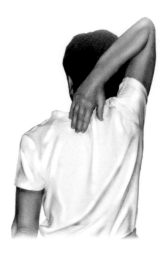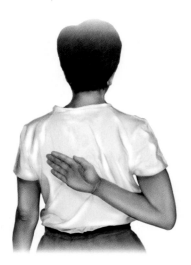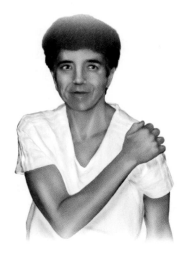

▶ **Figure 6–4** ▶ Active range-of-motion (AROM) tests for the shoulder.

Posture Analysis

Posture, or body alignment, tells a lot about a client's physical and emotional state and reveals habitual patterns that can cause problems in the musculature. Standing, sitting, and sleeping posture are three basic points of reference for evaluating a client who complains about back, neck, and shoulder tension or pain. The evaluation of the body's structural alignment is called **posture analysis**.

Important guidelines for good posture include standing straight and tall while avoiding locking the knees. The weight of the body should be mostly over the balls of the feet, not back on the heels. The head should be in alignment on top of the neck and spine and the chin not pushed forward. To keep the head level, the chin can be tucked slightly. The arms hang naturally down at the sides of the body. The shoulders are relaxed.

Standing posture analysis can be as simple as asking a client to stand for a moment and observing his or her alignment. This can be done with the client clothed, shoes off, standing comfortably with feet slightly apart, and arms hanging at the sides. View the client from the front, back, and sides. Look for uneven height in shoulders or hips, leaning, head and chin forward, stooping, head tilted to one side, twisting, one arm hanging lower than the other, and any other deviation from good body alignment. A vertical point of reference such as a door frame can be used to identify leaning or other asymmetry.

Wall grid charts are essential for formal postural analysis and are useful for structurally focused massage therapists. Grid charts have both vertical and horizontal lines to measure more accurately any deviations from balanced posture. Photos taken of clients standing in front of grid charts are useful for the initial analysis, client education about posture, and evaluation of progress toward goals of improving posture. Body charts that show bony landmarks are useful for visual charting of posture deviations (see Figure 6–5 ◀).

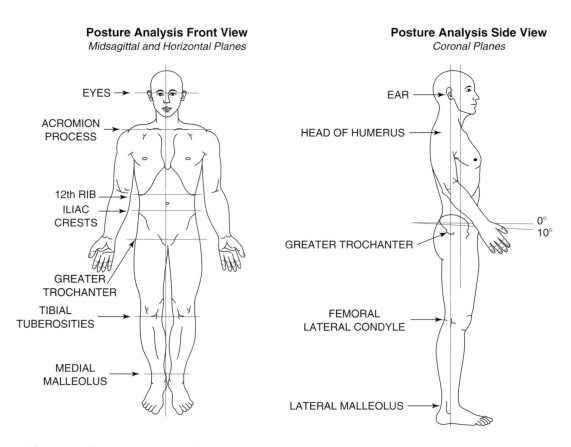

▲ **Figure 6–5** Body chart for standing posture assessment.

▶ **Figure 6–6** Good alignment for sitting posture.

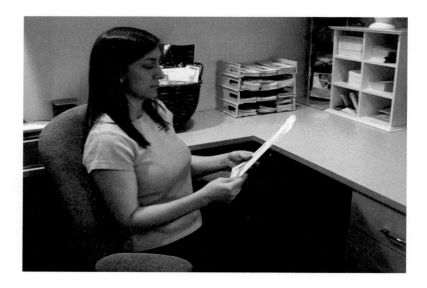

Sitting posture analysis is especially important for clients who work at desks or tables and complain of neck and shoulder tightness or pain. Some guidelines for good sitting posture are that the back is supported by the back of the chair, and the knees are aligned evenly with the hips, or slightly higher. Both feet are flat on the floor, or on a foot support. Slouching or sitting forward should be avoided, and the head should be aligned over the shoulders with the chin tucked slightly, as in good standing posture. If working at a desk, the arms should be flexed at a 75- to 90-degree angle, with shoulders squared and relaxed. Stretching breaks should be taken to avoid sitting in one position too long. Aligned sitting posture is shown in Figure 6–6 ◀.

A client's sleeping posture may also cause problems. Subjective information about sleeping habits may reveal a source of muscular aggravation. Firm mattresses are generally better than soft ones for proper back support. Sleeping on the side or back offers better alignment than sleeping on the stomach, which can strain the neck and lower back. Pillows should help keep the natural curvature of the neck and not cause hyperextension or flexion. While the client is supine on the massage table, you can demonstrate using a neck roll for added support and the use of a pillow under the knees to relieve pressure on the lower back. You can also show proper use of pillows for good alignment while in the side-lying position.

Biomechanical Analysis

Biomechanics is the study of movement in living organisms. It takes into account principles of motion and the structure and function of the human body, especially the muscle and skeletal systems. Whereas posture analysis looks at the body at rest, biomechanics looks at the body in motion. It is a branch of kinesiology and an important aspect of sports medicine.

Biomechanical analysis of your own movements while performing massage is an important aspect of your training. It can help you avoid injuries from poor body mechanics and serve as a starting point for understanding your clients' body mechanics. Good body mechanics and self-care for massage therapists are discussed in Chapter 4: Personal Development and Professionalism on page 89.

Knowledge of biomechanics is essential for massage therapists who work with athletes, dancers, musicians, artists, craftsmen, and others who use their bodies in their daily activities. Massage therapists who specialize in musculoskeletal complaints or structural bodywork should also be well versed in analyzing how the body moves, and how it applies and absorbs force.

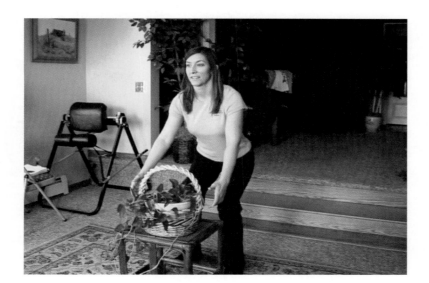

◀ **Figure 6–7** Good body mechanics for lifting heavy objects.

Biomechanical analysis is the examination of common movements, such as lifting, and job-related movements, such as using a computer keyboard, and can help massage therapists identify points of stress and strain on their clients' bodies. This is especially helpful in providing objective information about clients with overuse injuries.

Biomechanical analysis can not only point to specific structures affected by a movement (e.g., muscles, tendons, joints, ligaments), but also can suggest ways of correcting movement patterns that may be causing a client musculoskeletal problems.

Biomechanical analysis of lifting a heavy object with good alignment is shown in Figure 6–7◀. Notice that the knees bend to reach the object, with the back bending as little as possible. In proper alignment, the leg muscles do the lifting, and not the lower back or arm muscles. Keep the weight of the object as close as possible to your center of gravity. Poor alignment when lifting puts strain on the lower back.

Advise your clients to carry heavy objects close to the body, and switch arms frequently if carrying something in one hand, such as a suitcase. Balance equal weight on both sides if possible when carrying more than one object. When carrying a backpack, avoid leaning forward and rounding the shoulders. If unable to keep good alignment, consider using a pack or case with wheels.

Gait Analysis

Gait analysis looks at biomechanics while walking or running. Gait analysis starts when your client walks into the room, and you begin to observe his or her movement pattern. For further analysis, watch the client walk away from you and toward you. Figure 6–8◀ shows the phases of walking.

The phases of walking for each foot include a stance phase (heel strike, flat foot, push-off, and acceleration), and a swing phase (toe-off, midswing, and deceleration). While one foot is in the stance phase, the other foot is in the swing phase. Points to look for in walking are base width (2–4 inches from heel to heel), vertical movement of the center of gravity, knee flexion, lateral shifting, length of step, and pelvis rotation.

Deviations from normal include slow gait, limping, shuffling, twisting at the waist, dragging the feet, waddling (lateral movement), wide base, lurching. Compensations may also be made for arthritic or fused joints in the feet or legs. Some of the common causes of walking gait deviations are listed in Table 6–1. More detailed analysis of gait is found in biomechanics, clinical massage, and orthopedic massage texts.

▶ **Figure 6–8** Phases of the normal walking gait.

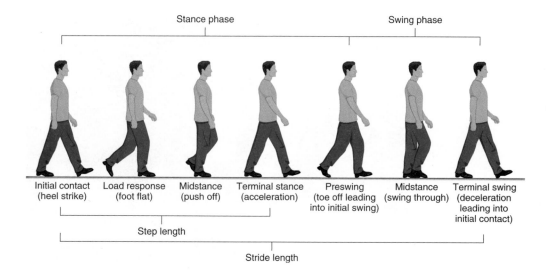

ORTHOPEDIC TESTS

A number of orthopedic tests are available to assess pathology in musculoskeletal structures, movement and locomotor disorders, and sources of soft tissue pain and dysfunction. Use of these tests is shared with other professionals, such as physical therapists, athletic trainers, and orthopedic doctors. Massage therapists use orthopedic tests to evaluate current function for goal-oriented planning.

Orthopedic or clinical massage is an advanced specialty for massage therapists that focuses on the use of massage to treat orthopedic conditions. Details about orthopedic massage and assessment skills are outside the scope of this foundations book, but can be found in other texts (see Appendix I: References and Resources on page 352).

Massage therapists who apply these tests do so in the context of their scope of practice. They do not diagnose pathologies. The purpose of massage therapists using orthopedic tests is for observation of function, ruling out conditions and injuries that may be contraindications for massage, and for decisions about referrals to doctors for medical diagnosis.

	TABLE 6-1
Common Causes of Walking Gait Deviations	
Gait Deviation	**Common Causes**
Slow walk	Old age, neurological disorder, joint disease, or injury
Limping	Injury to foot or leg, short leg
Shuffling	Weak quadriceps, Parkinson's disease, neurological disorder
Twisting	Arms crossing midline during walk
Dragging	Tibialis anterior weakness (also called drop foot, toe scraping)
Waddling	Pain in lower back, hips, lower extremities
Wide base	Unsteadiness, dizziness, general weakness, vision problems
Lurching	Weakness in gluteal muscles

PRACTICAL APPLICATION

Use the goal-oriented planning process to plan a one-hour individual massage session with a practice client. Implement the plan. Afterwards, write down your experience with each step. Ask yourself the following questions:

1 How long did it take to gather enough subjective and objective information to determine client goals for the session?

2 During the session, did you learn any information that caused you to modify the original plan?

3 Do you think that the approach and techniques you used helped achieve the goals for the session?

4 Did the practice client report results consistent with the goals you agreed on before the session?

Chapter Highlights

▶ Session planning is the logical process of thinking through the massage from beginning to end.

▶ Goal-oriented planning focuses on achieving specific client goals, as reflected in the Wellness Massage Pyramid.

▶ Clinical reasoning is the cognitive process used in goal-oriented planning and is essentially a problem-solving exercise.

▶ The six steps in goal-oriented planning are (1) collecting subjective information from the client; (2) collecting objective information through observation, tests, and measurements; (3) assessing the situation and setting client goals; (4) devising a plan to achieve client goals; (5) implementing the plan; (6) evaluating the results. The plan is revised as needed based on the results obtained.

▶ Three basic variations of goal-oriented planning are long-range planning, individual session planning, and treatment planning.

- Long-range planning is done in the initial session and in progress evaluation sessions.
- Individual session planning is done before each massage session.
- Treatment planning is done when the goal is the alleviation of symptoms, or facilitating healing of a pathological condition.
- Each of the variations uses the six-step session planning process, modified for their specific application.

▶ Intake is the process of gathering relevant information from a new client.

▶ Intake involves the client filling out an intake form and a health history form, and the therapist conducting a new client interview.

- A health history provides information to identify contraindications and as background for planning sessions.
- When providing routine massage at an outreach event, the intake process can be shortened to a few relevant questions and signing a consent form.

▶ Objective methods of collecting information include the massage therapist's own general observations, palpation, range of motion evaluation, posture analysis, biomechanical analysis, gait analysis, and orthopedic tests.

▶ Subjective and objective information gathered in Steps 1 and 2 of the session planning process is used in Step 3 to asses the situation and prioritize client goals.

Exam Review

Learning Outcomes

Use the learning outcomes at the beginning of the chapter and shown here as a guide to the major topics covered. Perform the task given in each outcome, and share your results with a study partner. Check off the tasks as you complete them.

❏ Appreciate the importance of planning.

❏ Use the six-step process for planning goal-oriented massage sessions.

❏ Develop long-term, individual session, and treatment plans for meeting clients' goals.

❏ Perform intake interviews to gather client information for planning.

❏ Use basic evaluation tools to collect objective information for planning.

Key Terms

To study the key terms listed at the beginning of the chapter, choose one or more of the following exercises. Writing or talking about ideas helps you better remember them, and explaining them to someone else helps deepen your understanding.

1. Write a one-sentence definition of each key term. Put the term in a general category, and then distinguish it from other terms in that category. For example, "*Clinical reasoning* is a problem-solving process used in goal-oriented session planning." Or "*Palpation* is the act of sensing information about the client through touch, and through the feel of tissues and movement at joints." Try to capture the essence of each term in a concise statement.

2. Make study cards by writing the key term on one side of a 3 × 5 card and a concise definition on the other side. Shuffle the cards and read one side, trying to recite either the explanation or word on the other side.

3. Pick out two or three terms and explain how they are related. For example, how is gait analysis related to treatment planning?

4. With a study partner, take turns explaining key terms verbally.

5. Make up sentences using one or more key terms. Variation: Read your sentences to a study partner who will ask you to explain unclear statements.

Memory Workout

The following fill-in-the-blank statements test your memory of the main concepts in this chapter.

1. Session planning is the _____ process of thinking through a massage session.

2. Step 2 in the goal-oriented planning process is collecting _____ information through observations, tests, and _____.

3. The phrase *long term* is used to mean _____ than one session, or the _____ between the initial session and a progress session.

4. Step 4 of a long-term plan is determining the _____ and _____ of massage sessions needed to achieve client goals.

5. In the interview before a regular massage session, ask about any _____ in the clients' health status or medications, and any progress or _____ related to their goals.

6. The goal of treatment planning is the alleviation of _____, or the facilitation of _____ of a pathological condition.

7. The main purpose of a short intake interview before giving massage at outreach events is to identify possible _____.

8. Palpation is the act of sensing information about a client through _____, and through the _____ of tissues and movement at joints.

9. Signs that massage and movement might be contraindicated at a joint include _____, _____, or severe pain with _____ joint movement.

10. In good standing posture, the head is in alignment over the shoulders, and the chin is _____ slightly.

11. In proper lifting mechanics, power comes from the *leg* muscles, not the _____ muscles.

12. Walking includes a _____ phase, and a _____ phase for each foot.

Test Prep

The following multiple choice questions will help to prepare you for future school and professional exams.

1. Which of the following is a method of collecting subjective information from clients?

   a. Range-of-motion evaluation
   b. Gait analysis
   c. Health history forms
   d. Palpation of tissues

2. Suggesting activities to be done outside of the massage session on the client's own time is correctly referred to as:

   a. A prescription
   b. Home care
   c. Contraindication
   d. An assignment

3. The goal-oriented planning process is best described as:

a. Rigid and linear

c. Linear and disorderly

b. Logical but disorderly

d. Looping spiral

4. Which of the following is *not* typically within the massage therapist's scope of practice?

a. Measuring function or loss of function

c. Diagnosing a medical condition

b. Assessing the condition of tissues

d. All of the above

5. At what point in a massage session does the massage therapist clarify the client's top goals for the massage?

a. Pre-session interview

c. Mid-point in the session

b. Post-session interview

d. When writing post-session notes

6. Which of the following tends to reduce the ability to feel or palpate the condition of tissues?

a. Moving slowly

c. Using heavy pressure

b. Being focused and present

d. Putting descriptive words to what you feel

7. In good sitting posture, the knees should be aligned with the hips or slightly:

a. Lower

c. Turned in

b. Higher

d. Turned out

8. Which of the following occurs in the *swing* phase of walking?

a. Heel strike

c. Push off

b. Flat foot

d. Deceleration

Video Challenge

Watch the appropriate segment of the video on your CD-ROM and then answer the following questions.

Segment 6a: Goal-Oriented Planning

1. What does the massage therapist interviewed in the video say about collecting subjective information from the client? What is she looking for in the client interview?

2. What does the massage therapist say about the massage she offers? Is it the same for each client?

Segment 6b: Observation: Posture, Biomechanics, and Gait

1. What do the massage therapists interviewed in the video describe as important observations for planning massage sessions? When do they start observing their clients?

2. Review scenes from the video explaining good posture. What are important instructions for assessing a client's standing and sitting alignment?

3. List the different occupations illustrated in the video in the section on biomechanics. Identify potential musculoskeletal problems clients in these occupations might develop.

Comprehension Exercises

The following exercises provide questions for you to answer and tasks you can do to enhance your understanding of the material presented in this chapter.

1. List the six steps in the goal-oriented planning process. Give an example of using the process for planning an individual massage session.

2. Describe at least four general observations about a practice client that offer clues to his or her state of well-being. Include possible observations within each category (e.g., skin: dry patches, scars, moles, bruises, etc.).

3. Describe good standing posture. List some anatomical markers for evaluating proper alignment when viewed from the front and from the side.

For Greater Understanding

The following exercises are designed to give you a deeper understanding of the subjects covered in this chapter. Action words are underlined to emphasize the active nature of this approach to learning.

1. <u>Have a massage</u> as a new client at a spa, clinic, or private practice. <u>Notice</u> the intake process, the forms you are asked to fill out, and the pre-session interview. <u>Describe</u> your experience of the session using the 6-step session planning process. <u>Report</u> your findings to the class or a study partner. Did it seem like a goal-oriented process?

2. <u>Interview</u> a family member or friend after he or she has filled out a health history form. <u>Lead</u> the person in a discussion of the potential benefits of massage in helping to improve his or her overall wellness using the Wellness Massage Pyramid. <u>Help</u> the individual determine his or her top three goals for getting massage in the future.

3. <u>Go</u> to a pubic place where you can observe people without being intrusive. Public parks, shopping malls, and downtowns or city centers are good "people watching" places. <u>Observe</u> individuals standing, sitting, walking, and moving in different ways, their facial expressions, and other objective factors. <u>Make</u> brief notes about what you observe, using concise descriptive terms. Be careful not to stare or be too intrusive.

4. <u>Perform</u> a posture, biomechanical, or gait analysis of a classmate's movements. <u>Describe</u> what you observe, and <u>offer instructions</u> for more balanced alignment or biomechanically sound movement.

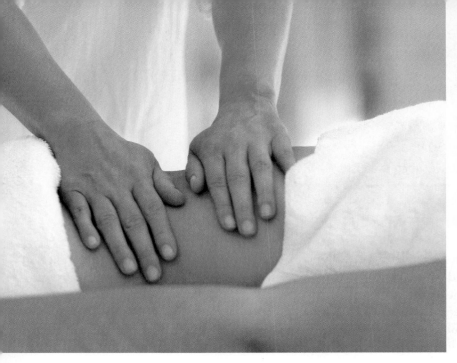

Documentation and SOAP Notes

LEARNING OUTCOMES

After studying this chapter, you will have information to:

1. Appreciate the importance of documenting massage sessions.
2. Describe four types of SOAP notes.
3. Write SOAP notes clearly, concisely, and correctly.
4. Write simplified notes when appropriate.
5. Design a documentation system for a massage practice.
6. Identify legal and ethical issues related to documentation.

KEY TERMS

Assessment	Documentation	Objective	Simplified note
Continuing notes	HIPAA Privacy Rules	Plan	SOAP notes
Discharge notes	Initial note	Progress notes	Subjective

Ideas in Action

On your CD-ROM, explore:

▶ Writing SOAP notes

▶ Interactive video exercises

IMPORTANCE OF DOCUMENTATION

Documentation is the process of writing massage session records for future reference. It is also called note-taking or charting. Session notes are kept on paper or in electronic form in client files.

Notes can be considered legal documents when used for insurance reporting, or may be subpoenaed as evidence in court cases. Notes are official client health records. In clinical settings they are protected by **HIPAA Privacy Rules**. HIPAA stands for the Health Insurance Portability and Accountability Act, which was passed by the U.S. Congress in 1996 to protect the privacy of medical records. (Find more information about HIPAA on page 218 in Chapter 9: Therapeutic Relationships and Ethics.)

Notes are also very practical. Notes assist the massage therapist in remembering what happened the last time a client came for massage and may show meaningful patterns over time. If two or more massage therapists share clients, they can review each other's notes while planning an upcoming session. Notes demonstrate the care taken to ensure a client's safety and well-being. Well-written SOAP notes also reflect a logical or clinical reasoning process by presenting information in an organized way and keeping the focus on goals for the massage sessions.

Documentation is not an extra chore or optional task. It is an important part of every massage session. Time can be set aside either between sessions or at the end of every day for completing client records.

Each massage practice or business creates its own system of keeping client notes. It is common for all regular clients to have personal files with an official record of their massage sessions. The systems of note-taking explained in this chapter contain the essential elements of documentation that can be adapted for your own or a specific employer's requirements. The goal-oriented SOAP note format, as well as simplified formats for note-taking, are presented in the remainder of the chapter.

SOAP NOTE OVERVIEW

SOAP notes have become a standard for charting massage sessions. *SOAP* refers to the format used to write the notes, and is an acronym for *subjective*, *objective*, *assessment*, and *plan*. The SOAP format helps sort information into meaningful categories and provides a standard outline for reports. SOAP notes are written in a kind of shorthand using standard abbreviations.

SOAP notes capture the relevant information in a goal-oriented session plan. The SOAP format also serves as a guideline for planning sessions from the beginning. If you understand the planning process well, SOAP notes will be easier to write.

The SOAP format records the elements of logical and clinical reasoning. You start with **subjective** (S) and **objective** (O) information about the client, come to an **assessment** (A) of the situation (either the nature of a condition and/or goals for sessions), and create a general **plan** (P) for achieving the goals and a plan for each massage session. The initial session plan is followed in continuing sessions, and progress is evaluated regularly.

Even if you see a client for only one session, or have limited time for interviews, the session organizing and logical reasoning reflected in SOAP notes help you to aim the session at meeting client needs instead of giving exactly the same 1-hour routine to everyone. And even if the record forms or charts you use have only blank lines for recording session notes, you can use the SOAP format to better organize your thoughts about the client and the session.

Four types of notes are commonly reported on SOAP charts. These are intake notes, continuing session notes, progress notes, and discharge notes. The four types of notes reflect different stages in planning massage sessions. The **intake note** is a comprehensive note that includes the client's stated reason for massage or specific complaint, related subjective and objective information, agreed-upon long-term goals, and a general plan. **Continuing session notes** are briefer and record the session-by-session history of a client's visits. **Progress notes** are for special sessions that reevaluate a client's progress related to his or her long-term goals. Progress notes contain more assessment information than regular session notes and may identify new goals and plans. **Discharge notes** are a final summary of the client's progress and any comments about a course of treatment. A summary of the different types of notes is found in Table 7–1 ◀.

SOAP Note Format

Although originally designed for medical record keeping, the general format for SOAP notes can be adopted for nonmedical settings. The SOAP format is useful in settings such as health clubs, spas, and private offices. However, the detail required and abbreviations used in different settings may vary. Insurance companies may require that certain terms be used in SOAP notes to qualify for reimbursement.

Massage therapists working in the same office or with the same clients should use standard abbreviations so they can read each other's notes. The elements in notes are generally the same; however, a specific type of information may appear in different sections in different systems. Follow the format established and used in your current location.

Some massage therapists have adopted a variation called a *SOTAP note*. The *T* stands for *treatment*, and provides a separate section in the note for recording the massage and related techniques used in the session. In the SOAP format, the *T* description is often included in the *P* or *plan* section of the note.

SOAP Note Content

S stands for *subjective* and refers to subjective information reported by clients. It includes things like what clients say about their reasons for getting massage, how they feel overall, where they feel pain or tension, stresses in their lives, and recent accidents, illnesses, or other changes in health status. For continuing session notes, the *S* section summarizes complaints on the day of the session and any changes clients perceive from their last sessions to their current ones.

O stands for *objective* and refers to what the practitioner observes about the client. Objective information provides clues about the client's state of well-being. It includes observations (for example, facial expression, general posture, or skin conditions); qualitative measurement from palpation of soft tissues or movement at joints; or results of standardized tests (quantitative measurement) for range of motion, muscle strength, posture, or specific muscle injuries.

TABLE 7-1

Four Types of SOAP Notes

Type of Note	Elements of the Note
Intake note	Timing: Client's first visit for massage
	Purpose: To record essential intake information, general client goals, and general plan for achieving those goals
	Sections: (S) Initial reason or complaint, health history, initial interview, referral, diagnosis, symptoms, contraindications and cautions, (O) observations, tests and measurements, (A) long-term client goals, (P) general plan for subsequent massage sessions, and self-care homework
Continuing session note	Timing: Each massage session after determination of long-term client goals
	Purpose: To record individual massage sessions and results
	Sections: (S) Pre-session interview, subjective feedback, (O) current observations, (A) goals for the day, (P) session plan (organization and techniques), results of the session, self-care homework
Progress note	Timing: After initial and several continuing sessions
	Purpose: To record progress toward achieving general client goals, and to revise general goals and plans as needed
	Sections: (S, O) Evaluation of progress toward goals using subjective and objective information, (A) revised general goals, (P) revised general plan
Discharge note	Timing: At end of series of massage sessions or at end of prescribed treatment
	Purpose: To summarize the client's progress toward achieving general goals, and make comments about the course of massage overall
	Sections: (S, O) Final subjective and objective assessment of progress, (A) general comments about the course of massage

A stands for *assessment*, and in medical charting, is the practitioner's conclusions from the subjective and objective record. It is the assessment of the situation. For example, in an initial visit, a doctor may conclude that a patient has an arthritis flare-up that is causing a swollen, painful knee. That is the diagnosis that goes into the *A* section of the note. Since diagnosis is *not* in the scope of practice of massage therapists, the *A* section can be used for other information.

A good use of the *A* section, from a wellness perspective, is to identify long-term goals for the client. Goals follow from an assessment of the client's needs (based on subjective and objective information), and ideally are agreed upon by the practitioner and client. This provides a basis from which to plan sessions that meet defined goals.

Examples of goals include reducing chronic muscle tension in the forearm, improving flexibility in the hip joint, or alleviating chronic stress or anxiety. Goals could be higher up the Wellness Massage Pyramid (see Figure 6–1 on page 137), e.g., maintaining overall health, or body–mind–spirit rejuvenation. Another use suggested for the *A* section is to "summarize the patient's functional ability: limitations, previous ability, and current situation; and to set goals that, when accomplished, demonstrate functional progress" (Thompson, 2005, p. 139).

For health care professionals whose scope of practice includes diagnosis of pathologies, the *A* section is fairly straightforward. *A* is used to record the diagnosis and prognosis of a medical condition as a prelude to writing a treatment plan. For wellness practitioners, the goals identified in the *A* section might fall anywhere within the full scope of the Wellness Massage Pyramid from treatment to health maintenance to life enjoyment.

P stands for *plan* and refers to the strategy for meeting the goals in the *A* section. It includes the plan as carried out for the current session, as well as long-term, general plans.

Additionally, *P* includes a description of the immediate massage application, including the length of the session, techniques used, and parts of the body massaged. Record specific work in more detail, such as when addressing neck and shoulder tension within the context of a general wellness massage.

In medical settings, *P* is the treatment plan for the diagnosed pathology. In massage therapy, the long-term plan might include the number and frequency of massage sessions to meet the goals; details about the massage and related therapies to be used; home care such as self-massage, relaxation exercises, or stretching; and a reevaluation date.

For regular massage clients in nonmedical settings, the *A* and *P* sections can be revisited regularly to provide continuous focus on client needs and goal-oriented massage sessions. Although the goals of the regular sessions may change over time and may be special in any one session, meeting long-term client needs is the foundation of a successful practice. The more conscious you are of your clients' needs, the better you will be able to serve them. A summary of the SOAP note content appears in Table 7–2 ◀.

→ WRITING SOAP NOTES

Correctly placing information into the different sections of a SOAP note requires an understanding of the logical and clinical reasoning behind the system. And writing concise, accurate, and useful notes takes practice. The following sections provide further instructions about writing SOAP notes by discussing each part of the note in detail and reviewing the important elements of style for good note-taking.

Writing the *S* or Subjective Section

Subjective information is obtained by listening to what clients have to say when they call or come in for sessions. Subjective information appears on health history forms, is collected in initial client interviews or intake sessions, and is updated when clients

TABLE 7-2

Summary of SOAP Note Content

SOAP Note Section		Content Possibilities
S	Subjective	Client's stated reason for massage
		Initial and subsequent complaints
		Health history information
		Report of medications taken
		Report of recent illness or injury
		Description of symptoms (e.g., pain, trouble sleeping)
		Report of functional limitations (e.g., walking, sitting)
		Qualitative description (e.g., tension, pain, numbness, stress)
		Quantitative rating (e.g., tension, pain, numbness, stress)
		Diagnosis from health care provider
O	Objective	Visual observations (e.g., posture, skin color, facial expression)
		Palpation (e.g., tissue quality, joint movement quality)
		Range-of-motion measurement
		Posture analysis
		Gait analysis
		Orthopedic tests of function
A	Assessment	Summary of conditions or limitations
		Identification of contraindications and cautions
		General goals for a series of massage sessions
		Goals for a specific massage session
P	Plan	General plan to achieve general goals
		▶ Number of sessions and frequency of massage
		▶ Use of adjunct modalities (e.g., hot/cold packs)
		▶ Home care (e.g., stretching, relaxation exercises)
		Plan for specific massage session
		▶ Time spent on each body area
		▶ Techniques used
		▶ Adjunct modalities used
		▶ Results

Logical/clinical reasoning behind SOAP notes: *Subjective* information from the client and *objective* information gathered by the massage therapist are used in an *assessment* of the situation to set goals for the massage sessions, followed by the development of *plans* to achieve those goals.

arrive for each of their sessions. The *S* section of a SOAP note is not a transcription of clients' words, but a summary of the pertinent information they offer related to their goals for the massage session.

The *S* section might also include a subsection with diagnoses, prescriptions, and test results from other health care providers. This is the *problem section* of a medical documentation system known as Problem-Oriented Medical Record, or POMR. If you routinely accept referrals from health care providers, you may want to adopt a PSOAP note system that documents the *P* or problem as a separate category. Otherwise it can appear clearly marked in the *S* section of a SOAP note.

An important aspect of the *S* section is the client's response to the theoretical question, Why are you here? Because people seek massage for a variety of reasons, don't assume you know what an individual's goals for massage are. For example, a client may indeed be recovering from a fractured arm, but wants a massage for relaxation. On the other hand, that person might have been referred for massage by his or her doctor, who expects massage to be focused on the arm and related musculature. Once you know why the client has come for massage, you can proceed to ask questions pertinent to establishing goals for the session.

A client's description of symptoms is recorded in the *S* section. In the interview, ask the client to be as specific as possible, including a general description (e.g., pain, tension, weakness, swelling, cramping, or insomnia), location, intensity, duration, frequency, onset, and activities that aggravate or relieve the symptoms. Also ask the client what has been done thus far to address the problem and how successful it has been.

Qualify or quantify subjective information when possible. For example, ask if the pain reported is mild, moderate, or severe; or dull, sharp, shooting, or throbbing. Or use quantitative methods such as asking the client to rate the pain on a scale from 1 to 10, with 1 being very mild and 10 being most severe. This allows you to track changes for ongoing evaluation, and helps the client become aware of any progress that is being made toward established goals.

SOAP charts that include diagrams of the body are effective for obtaining subjective information. Clients are asked to indicate on the charts where they are feeling pain, numbness, tension, and other subjective information. Body charts are good visual aids, helping clients to pinpoint problem areas more specifically and massage therapists to focus their efforts and establish useful goals.

Also note potential contraindications for massage mentioned by the client and medications being taken that may affect this particular session or sessions in the future. This information should be continuously updated for regular clients. Over time, people develop and recover from diseases, have accidents and recover from injuries, and go on and off medications.

Record anything that has potential safety implications. Some note-keeping systems have a separate page to track important information like contraindications and medications so that a massage therapist does not have to weed through other notes to find critical safety information.

Writing the *O* or Objective Section

Objective information comes from you, the practitioner. It includes what you observe about the client, results of measurements you take and tests you give, and qualitative judgments you make. Measurements taken should be related to the client's stated reason for coming for massage, or what you think is pertinent to the person's goals for the session.

Although diagnosis of pathologies is not in the scope of massage therapy, certain general evaluations or measurements may be appropriate. These include analysis of posture, observations of movement or gait, and active and passive ranges of motion. Simple orthopedic tests may reveal a potential contraindication for massage, or lead to a referral to a health care provider for medical diagnosis. Take care not to imply either verbally to a client or in a written record that you have diagnosed a medical condition. Measurements simply give you more information for your eventual assessment of the situation and for planning the session.

Visual information related to the skin may include noting red spots, moles, rashes, bruises, scratches or cuts, or other significant conditions. Dry skin or conditions like eczema might be important in planning a session.

Some of the most valuable objective information is obtained through palpation of tissues during the massage. For example, the texture of the soft tissues may feel soft and pliable, or grainy, hard, spongy, ropey, or restricted. Trigger points feel like small knots or nodules that elicit pain when pressed. Tissues may be cold, warm, or hot. Quality of movement at a joint might indicate something significant. When noting palpation information, be sure to include the location as well as qualitative descriptions.

Writing the *A* or Assessment Section

The *A* or assessment section flows from the subjective and objective information. The reasoning is, "given the subjective and objective information gathered, this is the client's situation, and therefore, these are our goals for the massage sessions."

For primary health care providers, the *A* section records the diagnosis and prognosis for the pathology. For them, the goals are implicit, that is, to reduce symptoms or heal the pathology.

Since massage therapists do not diagnose medical conditions, and work within the entire wellness scope, this is the section in which goals for the massage sessions are laid out. The goals might be as simple as "general relaxation," or "relieve neck and shoulder tension," or "improve flexibility in legs and hips." Goals might be stated in more functional terms such as "faster recovery and fewer injuries during marathon training," or "reduce tension headaches," or "reduce effects of asthma through general relaxation and release of muscular tension in upper body."

The idea of setting a goal implies that it will be reached at some point; for example, that an injury will heal, tension will go away, or circulation will improve now and forever. Of course, life is not always like that. In many cases, the goal for massage is to help manage a chronic situation, or massage is part of a general wellness strategy. Even in the case of regular massage in the latter situation, specific goals for an individual session can be identified and a session tailored to meet immediate client needs.

The *A* section may include long-term goals, short-term goals for the next few weeks, and the immediate goals of this particular session. Goals should be revisited before every session, and if related to healing an injury or illness, progress should be reevaluated at specified times. Contraindications and cautions may be identified in the *A* section of an intake note or continuing notes, as well as "red-flagged" elsewhere in the client's file.

Writing the *P* or Plan Section

The *P* section reflects how massage is applied to meet client goals as recorded in the *A* section. The reasoning here is, "given the agreed-upon goals for the massage session, massage was applied in the following way, and with these results."

In an intake or progress session note, a short-term (1- to 6-week) or long-term (7- to 12-week) plan is laid out. For example, a short-term plan for relieving tension headaches might be for a 30-minute massage session 2 times a week focusing on trigger points in the neck and shoulders followed by a cold pack application, with reevaluation in 3 weeks; immediate adjustment of workstation to allow for better sitting posture; self-massage, stretching, and cold packs as home care activities.

In continuing session notes, the *P* section describes the massage application on that day. The client's comments made before the session are recorded as Subjective information, while how the client felt after the massage is recorded in the Plan section.

Results are important to record so that effective applications can be continued and ineffective approaches eliminated or adjusted in subsequent sessions. Adaptations made for local contraindications are recorded here.

ELEMENTS OF STYLE

SOAP notes are written in shorthand using brief descriptions, abbreviations, and symbols. They tell a lot with few words, like text messaging on cell phones. With some practice, they can be written quickly using little space. However, they must be readable and able to be transcribed by others. Notes that cannot be read are not very useful. Common abbreviations and symbols used in SOAP notes are listed in Figure 7–1◀.

For greater ease of use, highlight terms used most often in your practice and keep the list handy when you are writing or reading notes.

▶ **Figure 7–1** Common abbreviations and symbols used in SOAP notes.

Term	Abbreviation/Symbol	Term	Abbreviation/Symbol
General			
As soon as possible	ASAP	Equals, is	=
At	@	Excessive	xs
Client	Cl, CL	Fibrous tissue	FT
Contraindication	CI, contra	Headache	HA
Date of birth	DOB	Hearing impaired (hard of hearing)	HOH
Diagnosis	Dx	High blood pressure, hypertension	HBP
Did not keep appointment	DKA	Hypertonic, tense muscle	tens, ≡, HT
History	Hx	Leading to, resulting in	→
Homework	HW	Lengthened, longer than normal	↔
Long term goal	LTG	Light, low, mild	L
Massage therapist	MT	Low back pain	LBP
Massage therapy session	MTx	Mobility	mob
Medications	meds	Moderate	mod
Not applicable	N/A	Normal	N
NO, none	∅	Numbness, tingling	≋
Number	#	Pain	●
Prescription	Rx	Pain and burning	P & B
Recommendation	rec	Pain on motion	POM
Reported	rpt	Primary	1°
Short term goal	STG	Secondary, due to	2°
Symptoms	Sx	Severe	sev
Times, repetitions	X	Shortened, shorter than normal	>-<
Treatment, therapy	Tx	Sleep disturbance	SD
Unknown	unk	Soft tissue injury	STI
With	w/	Spasm, cramping	SP, ≈
Without	w/o	Stiffness	st
		Inflammation	INFLAM, ✳
Descriptions, Symptoms		Tender point	TeP, ●
Abnormal	Abn	Trigger point	TP, TrP, ⊗
Activities of daily living	ADL	Up, increase	↑
Adhesion	adh, X	Very good health	VGH
After	post		
And	&, +	*Massage & Related Techniques*	
Approximate	~	Active assisted stretching	AAS
Backache	BA	Active range of motion	AROM

◀ **Figure 7–1** (continued)

Term	Abbreviation/Symbol	Term	Abbreviation/Symbol
Before	pre	Acupuncture, acupressure	ACU
Change	Δ	Aromatherapy	aroma
Complains of	c/o	Cold packs	CP
Continue same treatment	CSTx	Connective tissue massage	CTM
Crepitus	crep	Craniosacral therapy	CST
Date of injury	DOI	Cross fiber friction	XFF
Decrease, down	↓	Deep tissue	DT
Degenerative disk disease	DDD	Direct pressure	DP
Degenerative joint disease	DJD	Effleurage	eff
Edema	ed	Energy work	EW
Elevation	/	Exercise (active movement)	Ex
Friction	Fx	Posterior superior iliac spine	PSIS
Full body massage	FBM	Quadratus lumborum	QL
Full body relaxation massage	FBRM	Quadriceps femoris	quads
Hot packs	HP	Rhomboid muscles	rhomb
Hydrotherapy	hydro	Scalene muscles	scal
Ice, compression, elevation,	ICES	Soft tissue	ST
support		Sternocleidomastoid muscles	SCM
Manual lymph drainage	MLD	Sacroiliac	SI
Massage	Ⓜ	Thoracic, thoracic vertebrae	T, T1-12
Muscle energy technique	MET	Tensor fascia latae	TFL
Myofascial release	MFR	Temporomandibular joint	TMJ
Neuromuscular therapy	NMT	Trapezius muscles	traps
Palpation	palp	**Locations, Directions, Movement**	
Paraffin bath	PB	Abduction	abd
Passive range of motion	PROM	Adduction	add
Petrissage	pet	Anterior	ant
Positional release	PR	Bilateral, both	BL, Ⓑ
Proprioceptive neuromuscular	PNF	Circumduction	circ
facilitation		Depression (e.g. scapula)	dep
Reciprocal inhibition	RI	Dorsiflexion	DF
Reflexology	reflex	Elevation	ele
Soft tissue mobilization	SFT	Eversion	ever
Strain, counterstrain	SCS	Extension	ext
Stretching	str	External	ext
Swedish massage	SwM	Flexion	flex
Tense and relax	T&R	Internal	int
Anatomical Terms		Inversion	inv
Abdominals	abs	Lateral	lat
Anterior crutiate ligament	ACL	Lateral flexion	lat flex
Anterior superior iliac spine	ASIS	Left	Ⓛ
Cervical, cervical vertebrae	C, C1-7	Medial	med
Connective tissue	CT	Plantarflexion	PF
Deltoid	delt	Posterior	post
Erector spinae	ES	Pronation	pro
Gastrocnemius	gastroc	Proximal	prox
Gulteal muscles	gluts	Range of motion	ROM
Hamstrings	hams	Active range of motion	AROM
Iliotibial band	ITB, IT band	Passive range of motion	PROM
Latissimus dorsi	lats	Resisted range of motion	RROM
Levator scapulae	lev scap	Rotation	rot
Low back	LB	Right	Ⓡ
Lumber, lumber vertebrae	L, L1-5	Sidebending	SB
Muscles	mm	Supination	sup
Pectoralis muscles	pecs	Within normal limits	WNL

Notes do not contain complete sentences. They are typically strings of descriptions separated by commas and semicolons, or bulleted lists.

Notes contain anatomical terms for locations, adjectives, symptoms, measurements, and ratings. They might report quotes from the client such as "can't get to sleep at night," or "trouble turning my head when driving." Some examples of SOAP note entries are found in Figure 7–2◀.

Intake SOAP Note – Example 1

S: CL 1° reason for M = stress ↓; 2° c/o is mild LBP with st in legs; Hx of LB ≈ 2 weeks ago; ↓ with use of CP and rest; CL walks and gardens for Ex; does mod lifting in job; previous M = 0.

O: CL walks slowly w/ st and mildly bent over; mm in LB felt ≡; flexibility in hams = poor; Mild ed in ST around knees; mm in shoulders and neck ≡ and short.

A: 1° LTG = stress ↓; 2° LTG = ↓ st in LB, legs, shoulders, neck.

P: GP = FBRM 1 X per wk w/ M for ↓ ≡ in mm in extremities and LB; HW of str in legs and back & gen relax Ex; CP if spasm in LB returns.

Continuing Session SOAP Note – Example 2

S: CL c/o ↑ stress at job from ↑ in workload; ↑ in # HA from ↑ ≡ in shoulders and neck; sev bruise on R lower arm; rpt ↑ mob in lower legs after str last M.

O: CL face looked ↑ tired; rubbed his neck; bruise on R lower arm ~ inch in diameter + dark color.

A: 1° goal = gen relax & ↓ ≡ in shoulders and neck; 2° = flex in hips and legs; bruise on R arm = local contra.

P: 1 hr M + NMT; 40 min on upper body + 20 min on hips & legs; DP to TrP in traps and neck mm + str; deep eff, pet & str to legs; used neck roll; enjoyed relax music; rpt feeling ↑ relax overall after M; HW: HP on shoulders and neck 2X day & str at night.

Continuing Session SOAP Note – Example 3

S: CL rpt feeling ↑ depression this wk; not heard from son in days; SD; yesterday in house all day & 0 visit w/ friends; skin dry; c/o cramp forearm mm.

O: Looked tired & sad; CL rated energy very L; skin dry; forearm mm ≡ on palp; held fist.

A: 1° goal ↑ feeling well-being & ↑ energy; 2° lube skin & ↓ forearm mm ≡.

P: 1 hr FBRM w/ mod pace & eff + gentle pet; 15 min M forearms and hands; music upbeat; oil & lotion to FB w/ more in dry areas; HW: relax Ex and str for forearms; CL ↑ talk and alter post Tx.

▶ **Figure 7–2** Examples of SOAP note entries.

SOAP charts that include diagrams of the body are useful to manual therapists. They show front, back, and side views. Symbols can be used to locate problem areas visually, and indicate the general symptoms felt there, such as pain, numbness, inflammation, adhesions, or shortening. Elsewhere on the form there is space for the narrative SOAP notes. Figure 7–3 ◀ is an example of a SOAP chart with body diagrams.

Entries are descriptions, *not* diagnoses, unless reporting a diagnosis made by a health care provider. In that case, the note would read something like, "client reported a diagnosis by his physician of arthritis in the R knee." A client's self-diagnosis should be reported as just that; for example, "client complained of arthritis in knees—not diagnosed by physician." The massage therapist's note might read, "R knee infl and P," meaning, "right knee inflamed and painful." This is a subtle but important point and must be observed to stay within the scope of practice of massage therapy.

◀ **Figure 7–3** Example of SOAP chart with body diagram.

SOAP NOTE CHART
CONTINUING MASSAGE SESSION

Practitioner's Name _____ Date _____

Client's Name _____

S: Reason for massage, complaints, reports

O: Observations, qualitative/quantitative measurements

A: Primary and secondary goals for the session; contraindications

P: Duration of massage; areas addressed; techniques used; results; suggested home care

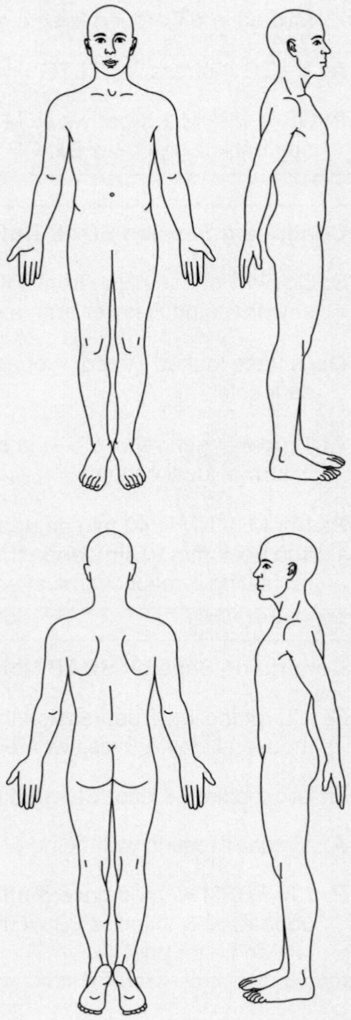

Practitioner Signature _____ Date _____

Symbols:

Primary 1°	Secondary 2°	Change Δ	Increase ↑	Decrease ↓	Tension ≡
Adhesion **X**	Pain **P**	Numbness ∿∿	Inflammation ✳	TrP ⊗	

If you or a client will be filling out health insurance claim forms for massage sessions, use terminology in your notes that will be recognized by the insurance company, and learn current medical codes that apply. This is important because medical codes are used to process claims, and your records might be subpoenaed to support a client's insurance claim. Massage therapy covered may include hot and cold packs, massage, and manual therapy.

The medical codes change periodically, so if you do insurance billing, check with your state licensing or other appropriate agency for which codes currently are legally acceptable for massage therapy. Be aware that code numbers for physical and occupational therapy may be different from code numbers for massage therapy.

Guidelines for Writing SOAP Notes

The following guidelines summarize standard procedures for writing SOAP notes. They approach SOAP notes as legal documents and reflect some of the same standards used for legal contracts and accounting. With a little practice, these procedures can become second nature.

- ▶ Write legibly and in ink.
- ▶ Write in concise, clear language using standard abbreviations and symbols; no need for complete sentences.
- ▶ Do not use so many symbols or abbreviations that the meaning of the note is lost; abbreviations make the most sense in context.
- ▶ Aim for spending only 5–10 minutes writing each SOAP note. Writing concise, useful, readable notes comes with practice.
- ▶ Start your note right after the last note entered so that it will always be in chronological order, and difficult for notes to be altered or added to.
- ▶ Date the note clearly at the beginning, or in the space provided on the form.
- ▶ Print your name and initial or sign your note at the end.
- ▶ If you make a mistake, draw a single line through the mistake, write "error" next to or above the area, and initial it. This makes it clear what was originally written and who altered the record. Never scribble over a note or use correction fluid over a mistake.
- ▶ Be objective, impersonal, and respectful in your notes.
- ▶ Stick to descriptions of symptoms and conditions (e.g., swollen, red, warm, painful), and do not make statements that could be mistaken for a medical diagnosis (e.g., tendonitis).
- ▶ Do not write anything that is personal, slanderous, or that you would not want the client to read. Clients have a legal and ethical right to see what is in their official records.
- ▶ Keep client records for at least 7 years, even if the client has stopped coming to you for massage. The records may be needed for legal or insurance purposes.
- ▶ Follow HIPAA Privacy Rules for storage and access to client records when applicable.

⟶ SIMPLIFIED DOCUMENTATION

There are circumstances in which documentation of a massage can be minimized, and post-session notes can be shortened or dispensed with altogether. However, at the very least, it is a good idea to keep a record of who received massage and to have clients sign a legal release form.

At venues like health fairs, trade shows, sports events, and outreach events where people are receiving short, standard massage routines and will not be seen by the practitioner again, no post-session notes are necessary. An example of a form used at outreach events where massage recipients sign their names after reading a statement at the top is found in Appendix F: Intake and Health History Forms on page 334.

A simplified form can also be used for walk-in clients at a street venue, at a stand within a store or mall, or in public places like airports. In those cases, adequate documentation might consist of a short intake form with a general statement about the massage to be given, a few questions asking for information about major contraindications, and the client's signature granting permission for the massage. This provides a record of who received massage and evidence that they knew what to expect. See Figure 7–4◀. This type of form works well with 1-time clients.

Thompson describes a **simplified note** system called a HxTxC note for situations where full SOAP documentation is unnecessary. *Hx* stands for *history*, *Tx* for *treatment*, and *C* for *comments*. *Hx* records relevant health history, medications, contraindications, and cautions. *Tx* describes the massage application and techniques used. *C* is for comments about things like personal preferences, variations from a routine, unusual reactions, results, and progress (2005).

▶ **Figure 7–4** Simplified note for one-time client.

SHORT INTAKE and NOTE FORM

Client _____ Date _____

Address _____ Phone _____

Massage Therapist _____

Please answer the following questions to ensure a comfortable and safe massage session:

1. What is your primary goal for this massage?
   ☐ Relaxation, stress reduction
   ☐ Relieve muscle tension, specify area: _____
   ☐ General health and wellbeing
   ☐ Other, please specify _____

2. Have you had any illness, accidents, or injury recently? ☐ No ☐ Yes

   If so, please explain briefly _____

   _____

3. Are you experiencing any of the following today? Check all that apply.

   ☐ pain or soreness   ☐ numbness or tingling   ☐ dizziness
   ☐ stiffness   ☐ swelling   ☐ nausea

4. Do you have any allergies, especially to oils or lotions? ☐ No ☐ Yes

   If so, please explain briefly _____

   _____

5. For women – Are you pregnant? ☐ No ☐ Yes ☐ Maybe

6. Have you taken any medications today? ☐ No ☐ Yes

   If so, please list _____

I have answered the above questions to the best of my ability. I acknowledge that massage therapy does not include medical diagnosis and that I should see an appropriate health care provider to diagnose and treat medical problems. I give my consent for the massage session.

_____ Date _____
Signature

Plan:

Comments:

SHORT NOTE CHART

Client's Name _____

Date _____ Practitioner's Name _____

S: Comments, complaints, reports, recent illness or injury, medications

O: Visual observations, palpation

P: Length of session, routine given, significant modifications

C: General comments

MT Initials _____

Date _____ Practitioner's Name _____

S: Comments, complaints, reports, recent illness or injury, medications

O: Visual observations, palpation

P: Length of session, routine given, significant modifications

C: General comments

MT Initials _____

Date _____ Practitioner's Name/Initials _____

S: Comments, complaints, reports, recent illness or injury, medications

O: Visual observations, palpation

P: Length of session, routine given, significant modifications

C: General comments

MT Initials _____

◀ **Figure 7–5** Example of simplified note form for routine massage.

This type of simplified system is adequate when a standard routine is given and then modified for a client's safety and/or preferences. It might be appropriate at a spa or health club where clients come for massage periodically, but have no long-term goals in mind. Figure 7–5◀ shows an example of a simplified note form with space for more than one date on a page for use with regular or periodic clients.

The short form contains some of the elements of a SOAP chart (e.g., subjective and objective information), but the *A* section is unnecessary, and a *C* section for general comments is added. The *P* section documents the length of the session, the routine performed (e.g., relaxation massage routine), and significant modifications made to address contraindications and cautions. If a client comes for a more goal-oriented massage, a regular SOAP chart can be used to document that session.

As with all documentation, it is recommended that even shortened and simplified records be kept for a period of 7 years. Entries must be legible and understandable.

PRACTICAL APPLICATION

Obtain a blank copy of the documentation form used in student clinic at your school. Examine the form to see how it is formatted and what information is requested for each massage session. Use the form to document practice sessions in preparation for your student clinic experience. Answering the following questions will help you with student clinic documentation.

1. What level of detail will be required at student clinic?

2. Is there a chart of standard abbreviations used in student clinic?

3. Does the clinic have specific guidelines related to completing documentation, e.g., what information goes in each section and how each entry should be signed?

DESIGNING A SYSTEM OF DOCUMENTATION

Consider several factors when designing a note-taking system for your own practice. You may develop a few different forms for different circumstances. For example, if you have an office, do house calls, and work trade shows you may want to use three different forms. Or if you have an office and offer routine massage as well as medical treatment, you may use two different forms.

As a general rule, use SOAP notes for goal-oriented or treatment sessions. A simplified form can be used for routine massage or for one-time, walk-in clients. For a trade show or health fair, a signature list following a short statement might be adequate. Sample note forms can be found in business practices books. See Appendix F: Intake & Health History Forms on page 327.

If you process claims for insurance reimbursement, be sure to document the services performed in claims. Design your note forms to include all the information required by the insurance companies you deal with.

Make a separate file for each regular client. File folders with fasteners are useful for keeping papers in order. In a file with two fasteners, general information (e.g., intake form, signed privacy and policy statement, health history, referral letter) can be kept on one side, and individual session notes on the other side.

Records for one-time clients can be kept in alphabetical order in a group file. If they become regular clients, you can make an individual file for them. Signature lists from events can have their own file in chronological order. The important thing is to have a system that allows you to locate records easily, and one that works for your type of practice.

LEGAL AND ETHICAL ISSUES

Legal and ethical issues related to documentation and note-taking revolve around scope of practice, accuracy, honesty, confidentiality, and respect for the client. Since diagnosis is not in the scope of practice of massage therapists, no diagnoses by them should appear in session notes. References to others' diagnoses need to be clearly identified, e.g., "condition as diagnosed by client's physician," or "client self-diagnosis." This is a legal as well as an ethical matter.

Write session notes to accurately reflect what happened in the session. Writing notes as soon as possible after a session increases the likelihood of complete and

CRITICAL THINKING

Obtain examples of three or four different note-taking forms used by massage therapists. Compare, contrast, and analyze the forms to determine which forms might be appropriate for different settings (e.g., spa, health club, clinic, private practice, outreach event). Redesign the forms to improve their appearance or usefulness. Consider the following:

1 Is the form complete? Is all important information included?

2 Is it easy to use? Is the format logical?

3 Is the form useful for the intended setting?

4 Does the spacing allow for writing entries?

accurate documentation. Only record procedures that were performed in the session. Defrauding an insurance company is unlawful and unethical.

Keep session notes in a secure place such as a locked cabinet, and do not leave them lying around for others to see. Follow all HIPAA rules related to privacy of health records where applicable. Share the contents of clients' files only with their permission. See Chapter 9: Therapeutic Relationship and Ethics on page 218 for more information about HIPAA confidentiality rules.

Write notes using respectful and professional language. Omit opinions and personal comments about clients that are unrelated to their massage session. Remember that clients have a right to look at their notes and others may someday have access to the notes as well. Your notes are a reflection of your level of professionalism.

CASE FOR STUDY

Jennifer and Simplified Documentation at the Salon

Jennifer, a massage therapist with a small practice within a community beauty salon, uses a simplified format for documentation of massage sessions given there. She has informed clients that the massage offered in the salon is primarily for relaxation and rejuvenation, and refers clients to other massage therapists for more clinical massage applications. The form she developed has three sections to document each massage session.

▶ The *H* section is for recording relevant health information including contraindications.

▶ The *MT* section is for a description of the massage therapy application for the day.

▶ The *C* section is for comments, including noteworthy events and results.

Jennifer can fit notes for four sessions with a client on one page and has learned to be concise in her documentation.

Session with Martha
Martha came in for her regular massage and in the brief pre-session interview reported that she had been to the doctor in the past week for a skin rash on her leg. The doctor thought it might be an allergic reaction and prescribed some oral medication and some anti-itch cream. Martha was stressed out from a family situation and was looking forward to relaxing. Jennifer gave her the relaxation massage as usual, but switched to a hypoallergenic lotion. She spent more time on the neck and shoulders, where Martha had reported tension, and avoided massage around the rash. Martha was a little more talkative than usual, and Jennifer tried to help her focus on her breathing and letting go of tension. She played special relaxation music for a calming atmosphere. Jennifer sensed that Martha was distracted, but did seem a little more relaxed at the end of the session. Martha thanked Jennifer and reported feeling less anxious.

Write notes for this session using Jennifer's system of documentation.

H_____.

MT _____

C _____

Date _____ Time _____

Chapter Highlights

▶ Documentation is the process of writing massage session records for future reference; also called note-taking or charting.

▶ Session notes are kept on paper or in electronic form in client files.

▶ Notes are legal documents, are used for insurance reporting, and may be subpoenaed as evidence in legal cases.

▶ Notes are official client health records.

 • Notes may be protected by HIPAA Privacy Rules.
 • Notes are practical as an aid to memory and in planning sessions. Writing notes is an important part of completing a massage session.

▶ SOAP notes have become a standard for charting goal-oriented massage sessions.

▶ The SOAP format reflects a logical or clinical reasoning process.

 • Four types of SOAP notes are intake, continuing session, progress, and discharge notes.
 • Massage therapists working in the same office should use standard abbreviations and symbols, and follow the format required by their employer.

▶ SOAP is an acronym for subjective, objective, assessment, and plan.

 • The *S* or subjective section contains information provided by the client.
 • The *O* or objective section contains observations, tests, and measurements made by the massage therapist.
 • The *A* or assessment section identifies the goals for the massage session(s).
 • The *P* or plan section lays out the steps planned to achieve identified goals and session results.

▶ SOAP notes are written using brief descriptions, abbreviations, and symbols.

 • Notes are not complete sentences, but are strings of descriptions separated by commas or semi-colons, or are bulleted lists.
 • Diagrams of the body are useful in writing notes.
 • Entries are descriptions and not diagnoses of conditions.

▶ SOAP notes are written legibly in clear, concise language. They conform to standards for legal documents related to making and initialing changes, and are dated and initialed at the end.

 • Personal comments about clients should not be written.
 • Clients have the right to see their files.
 • Files are kept for at least 7 years.

▶ Simplified note formats may be used when routine massages are given and with 1-time, walk-in clients.

 • Documentation can include at a minimum a short intake form asking about contraindications, a description of the massage to be given, a date, and a signature from the client giving permission for the session.

▶ Massage therapists design systems of documentation and note-taking appropriate for the type of practice they have.

 • Therapists can design their own charting forms or use premade forms.
 • A separate file is created for each regular client.

▸ Legal and ethical issues related to documentation revolve around scope of practice, accuracy, honesty, confidentiality, and respect for clients.

▸ Clients files should be kept secure and shared only with the client's permission.

- The way you keep your files is a reflection of your level of professionalism.

Exam Review

Learning Outcomes

Use the learning outcomes at the beginning of the chapter and shown here as a guide to the major topics covered. Perform the task given in each outcome, and share your results with a study partner. Check off the tasks as you complete them.

❏ Appreciate the importance of documenting massage sessions.
❏ Describe four types of SOAP notes.
❏ Write SOAP notes clearly, concisely, and correctly.
❏ Write simplified notes when appropriate.
❏ Design a documentation system for a massage practice.
❏ Identify legal and ethical issues related to documentation.

Key Terms

To study the key terms listed at the beginning of the chapter, choose one or more of the following exercises. Writing or talking about ideas helps you better remember them, and explaining them to someone else helps deepen your understanding.

1. Write a one-sentence definition of each key term. Put the term in a general category, and then distinguish it from other terms in that category. For example, "The *assessment* or *A* section in a SOAP note is a record of the massage therapist's assessment of the situation and agreed-upon goals for massage." Or, "A *progress note* is a type of SOAP note that records a special session to evaluate the degree of achievement of a client's general goals." Try to capture the essence of each term in a concise statement.

2. Make study cards by writing the key term on one side of a 3 × 5 card, and a concise definition on the other side. Shuffle the cards and read one side, trying to recite either the explanation or term on the other side.

3. Pick out two or three terms and explain how they are related.

4. With a study partner, take turns explaining key terms verbally.

5. Make up sentences using one or more key terms. Variation: Read your sentences to a study partner who will ask you to explain unclear statements.

Memory Workout

The following fill-in-the-blank statements test your memory of the main concepts in this chapter.

1. Documentation is the process of writing detailed _____ of massage sessions for future reference. It is also called _____ taking or _____.

2. The acronym SOAP stands for S_____, O_____, A_____, P_____.

3. The initial SOAP note is a comprehensive _____ note, which results in _____-term plans for a series of massage sessions.

4. SOTAP is a variation of the SOAP note, and the T stands for _____.

5. Body charts are good _____ aids for collecting subjective information.

6. Start your note right _____ the last note entered.

7. Print your name and _____ or _____ your note at the end.

8. In a simplified note system called HxTxC, the acronym stands for _____, _____, _____.

9. Records for one-time clients can be kept in _____ order in a group file.

10. Signature lists from events can have their own file in _____ order.

11. Only share contents of a client's file with his or her _____.

12. Do not write personal comments about the client _____ to the massage sessions.

Test Prep

The following multiple choice questions will help to prepare you for future school and professional exams.

1. The S section of a SOAP note contains:

   a. A transcription of the client's words from the intake interview
   b. A summary of subjective information from the client
   c. A summary of measurements taken during the intake interview
   d. A summary of the session plan

2. In the PSOAP variation of SOAP notes, the first P contains:

   a. Possible contraindications
   b. Plans developed in a prior session
   c. Permission to send records to the insurance company
   d. Prescription or diagnosis from a primary health care provider

3. In which section of SOAP notes for an individual massage session are the results of the day's massage typically recorded?

   a. S
   b. O
   c. A
   d. P

4. Once you have mastered writing SOAP notes, about how much time would you expect to spend after each massage session writing an entry?

   a. 1–2 minutes
   b. 5–10 minutes
   c. 25–30 minutes
   d. 45–50 minutes

5. Which of the following instructions for correcting a mistake made in SOAP notes is *not* acceptable?

   a. White-out or erase the mistake
   b. Put a single line through the mistake
   c. Write "error" above or next to the area
   d. Initial the correction

6. What is the recommended number of years that client records are kept?

   a. 1
   b. 3
   c. 5
   d. 7

7. Under which of the following circumstances, could post-session notes be omitted?

   a. After sessions with regular clients
   b. After brief sessions at outreach events and health fairs
   c. After sessions at spas
   d. After sessions for relaxation

8. The most acceptable place to store client records securely in a massage office is:

   a. In a locked file cabinet
   b. In a desk drawer
   c. In a box in the closet
   d. On a shelf behind the desk

Video Challenge

Watch the appropriate segment of the video on your CD-ROM and then answer the following questions.

Segment 7: Documentation and SOAP Notes

1. What do the massage therapists interviewed in the video say about the importance of writing SOAP notes?
2. List the many practical uses for session notes mentioned in the video.
3. Identify where the massage therapist gets the information contained in each section of the SOAP note as explained in the video.

Comprehension Exercises

The following exercises provide questions for you to answer and tasks you can do to enhance your understanding of the material presented in this chapter.

1. What does the acronym *SOAP* mean? Briefly describe what type of information goes into each section of SOAP notes.

2. What is the difference between a *diagnosis* and a *description* of a complaint by a client? Which is within the scope of practice of massage therapists? Give an example.

3. In what situations can documentation of massage sessions be omitted? Give an example of adequate documentation at a health fair where you are giving short massage sessions.

For Greater Understanding

The following exercises are designed to give you a deeper understanding of the subjects covered in this chapter. Action words are underlined to emphasize the active nature of this approach to learning.

1. Critique samples of notes from a student or professional clinic. Be sure that the names of clients and massage therapists have been removed. Rewrite the notes as needed so that they conform to the guidelines for good documentation.

2. Design a SOAP note chart, or choose one you like from a business practices resource manual. Document a practice massage session using the chart. Revise the chart as needed for ease of use for your purposes.

3. Write a sample SOAP description in complete sentences without abbreviations or symbols. Give that description to a study partner and ask him or her to translate the longer descriptions using the SOAP shorthand format. Now give the abbreviated SOAP notes to a third study partner, and see if he or she can translate the note correctly back into longhand.

4. Visit a massage clinic or spa and ask the manager to explain the facility's system of documentation. Obtain blank copies of its note forms if possible. Report your findings to the class or study group. Compare and contrast the documentation used in different settings. Discuss the appropriateness of each system to the setting in which it is used.

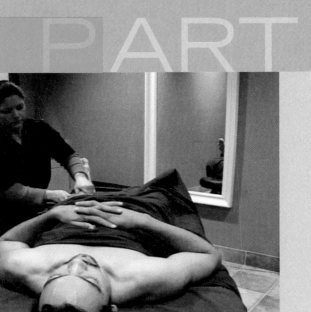

PART IV

| PROFESSIONAL ETHICS

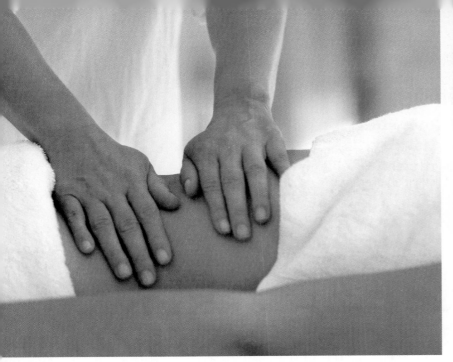

Foundations of Ethics

LEARNING OUTCOMES

After studying this chapter, you will have information to:

1. Explain the relationship between professional ethics and values, rights, and duties.

2. List ways to minimize vulnerability to unethical behavior.

3. Describe the role of professional organizations in developing ethical codes and standards.

4. Find examples of codes of ethics and standards of practice for massage and bodywork practitioners.

5. Describe the role of government in enforcing ethical standards through law.

6. Identify major ethical principles for massage therapists.

7. Use a decision-making model to address ethical questions.

8. Continue development of ethical judgment.

KEY TERMS

Codes of ethics	Ethical dilemmas	Ethics	Rights
Duties	Ethical judgment	Personal temptations	Standards of practice
Ethical decision-making model	Ethical questions	Professional ethics	Values

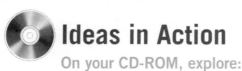

Ideas in Action

On your CD-ROM, explore:

▶ The ethical decision-making model
▶ Ethical judgment
▶ Interactive video exercises

NATURE OF ETHICS

Ethics is the study of moral behavior; that is, determining the *right* thing to do in a specific situation. Ethical behavior conforms to certain values like honesty and fairness, upholds human rights like privacy and safety, and reflects the duties inherent in being in a position of power. Ethical codes and standards translate moral values into guidelines for daily living.

Laws are sometimes enacted by governments to enforce ethical behavior. These laws are passed for the protection of the public. However, many behaviors considered unethical are perfectly legal. For example, gossiping about a client may not land you in jail, but is considered unethical.

Professional ethics is the study of moral behavior relative to a specific occupation such as massage therapist. Because massage therapy falls into the categories of service, helping, and therapeutic professions, standards of behavior are high. Although the first rule is "to do no harm," professional standards also take into consideration what is best therapeutically for the client, as noted by Taylor (emphasis added):

> Such standards specify those behaviors which have proven counter-therapeutic and are therefore considered unacceptable by the professional community. In other words, sets of ethical guidelines *encourage* behavior that is most effective therapeutically and *discourage* behavior that is ineffective or therapeutically harmful. (1995, p. 5)

Professional organizations develop codes of ethics and standards of practice to clarify the values of the group and serve as references for ethical decision making. These documents contain the collective wisdom of the profession regarding ethical behavior among its members. "Establishing an ethical code is an exercise in self-reflection and clarification of values for those who write, review, and approve such documents" (Taylor, 1995, p. 233). See Appendix G for NCBTMB Code of Ethics and Standards of Practice on page 335.

Business ethics concern the commercial aspects of being a massage therapist and the treatment of clients as consumers. Business ethics encompasses areas such as advertising, payment policies and procedures, keeping proper licenses, and other business matters. It can be thought of as that part of professional ethics that has to do with having a private practice. Chapter 10: Business Ethics will specifically focus on business ethics.

VALUES, RIGHTS, AND DUTIES

Ethical principles are founded on the values, rights, and duties deemed important in society. Professionals apply these factors in determining acceptable conduct in the practice of their work.

Values

Values are principles, traits, or qualities considered worthwhile or desirable. Ethical codes and standards are developed to protect the values that give meaning and direction to the profession. For example, the standard that massage therapists represent their qualifications truthfully stems from the value of *honesty*.

Values that have come to the forefront in the massage and bodywork profession include *compassion,* or the wish to relieve suffering, and *selfless service,* or giving clients' well-being top priority. For example, "refuse any gifts or benefits intended to influence a referral, decision, or treatment that are purely for personal gain and not for the good of the client" (National Certification Board for Therapeutic Massage and Bodywork [NCBTMB], 2005).

Honesty is speaking the truth and avoiding deception, while *integrity* is living up to our values consistently. Being *trustworthy* includes being reliable, honest, and principled.

Equality, *fairness*, and *nondiscrimination* entail treating others with equal respect and not playing favorites. *Unconditional regard for others* calls for being nonjudgmental and giving our best efforts to everyone regardless of who they are. An item in the NCBTMB Code of Ethics (2005) directs massage therapists "to respect the inherent worth of all persons."

For every positive value, there is an opposite or negative, which is often the thing that catches our attention. People have inner voices or consciences that tell them that something is wrong. For example, you might have an uncomfortable feeling when talking about one of your clients to a friend. Knowing about the principle of *confidentiality* helps you sort out which actions are ethical and which are not.

A better sense of important values can be cultivated by study and discussion. Some values, like honesty, are widely recognized and deeply ingrained. But how these values are applied in a specific profession may not be so obvious at first, like applying the concept of honesty to making health claims for the benefits of massage therapy. By being more aware of values and how they affect our behavior, they become more relevant to real-life situations.

Values provide a moral compass to point the way when we are lost or confused. Having an awareness of the values held by the profession is a prerequisite for making ethical decisions as massage therapists.

Rights

Rights also come into play when discussing ethical behavior. Rights are claims to certain treatment or protection from certain treatment. Rights are expected to be honored by others and enforced by standards or laws, if necessary. For example, clients have a right to privacy, which is the basis for draping practices and confidentiality policies. They also have a right to freedom from violations like sexual misconduct, which requires clear professional boundaries. Client rights that play an important part in ethical standards for massage therapists are the clients' rights to privacy, self-determination, and safety.

The client's *right to privacy* is the root of several ethical standards. Draping procedures and the practice of leaving the room while clients are undressing preserve their privacy. Prohibitions against revealing information about clients to others, or *confidentiality*, also protects their privacy. Confidentiality rights related to medical records are protected by law through HIPAA (Health Information Portability and Accountability Act). For more information about HIPAA, see page 218 in Chapter 9: Therapeutic Relationship and Ethics.

The client's *right to self-determination*, also called *autonomy*, affirms that clients should have the opportunity to make informed choices about what happens to them. Self-determination is protected by standards about massage therapists obtaining informed voluntary consent from clients to perform certain massage techniques or to work in certain body areas. Another is "the client's right to refuse, modify, or terminate treatment regardless of prior consent given" (NCBTMB, 2005).

The client's *right to safety* is the basis of hygiene standards and regulations. Clients have a right to expect cleanliness and a germ-free environment in a massage room, as well as that tables and other equipment be in good repair. Also related is the standard that massage therapists "provide only those services which they are qualified to perform" (NCBTMB, 2005).

In recent years, the consumer rights movement has led to a crackdown on deceptive business practices and the enactment of a number of consumer protection laws. How these relate to massage therapists will be discussed in Chapter 10: Business Ethics.

Massage therapists have rights, too; for example, the right to fair compensation for their work and the right to a safe environment. They have the right to create and enforce policies for their practices. The NCBTMB Code of Ethics recognizes the right "to refuse to treat any person or part of the body for just and reasonable cause."

Duties

Duties or responsibilities are obligations to act in a particular way. Duties arise out of being in a certain position in relationship to others, or as the result of some action. Massage therapists have duties related to their clients, colleagues, coworkers, employers, and others. Duties reflect *moral bonds* that are generally recognized in a society and deeply felt as obligations or "oughts" by individuals (Purtilo). They are intricately related to the values and rights discussed above.

A basic duty of massage therapists is to maintain professional boundaries that clarify and preserve the roles inherent in the therapeutic relationship. It is the massage therapist's responsibility to establish good boundaries regardless of what the client wants. This potential dilemma will be discussed further in Chapter 9: Therapeutic Relationship and Ethics.

Duties can arise out of the rights of others; that is, if individuals have a right to something, and a massage therapist is in a position to influence what happens to them, then that massage therapist has a duty to protect those rights. For example, given that clients have a right to a safe environment when receiving massage, massage therapists have a duty to keep their spaces clean and remove potential safety hazards.

Duties related to being a health professional include *nonmaleficence* (refraining from harming anyone), *beneficence* (doing good for those in our care), *fidelity* (keeping promises—explicit or implicit), and *veracity* (telling the truth). Causing harm or wrong to someone else calls for *reparations*, while *gratitude* is due when someone is good to us (Purtilo).

Just as with values and rights, there is no finite list of duties for massage therapists. However, the concept of duties is useful when discussing ethical behavior for two reasons. First, duties have the weight of moral obligations. Second, when values, rights, and duties are in conflict, creating an ethical dilemma, critical thinking about such a situation calls for consideration of all sides of the issue, including the duties involved. Figure 8–1 ◀ lists many of the foundation values, rights, and duties on which ethical principles are based.

➔ VULNERABILITY TO UNETHICAL BEHAVIOR

Almost everyone considers him- or herself a moral, ethical person. However, if people are honest with themselves, everyone can think of instances when they didn't live up to ethical standards, or in retrospect, would have acted differently (i.e., more eth-

VALUES	RIGHTS	DUTIES
Compassion	*Client*	Beneficence
Equality	Personal respect	Avoid harm
Fairness	Privacy	Professional boundaries
Honesty	Self-determination	Gratitude
Integrity	Safety	Veracity
Nondiscrimination	Fair treatment	Reparation
Selfless service	Honest advertising	Fidelity
Unconditional regard for others	Best effort of massage therapist	Trustworthy
	Massage Therapist	
	Fair compensation	
	Respect	
	Safe environment	
	Practice policies	

◀ **Figure 8–1** Values, rights, and duties on which ethical principles for massage therapists are based.

ically) in a given situation. Admitting our human vulnerability and making a conscious commitment to be ethical massage therapists is the first step on the path to building ethical practices.

The next step is to learn about ethical standards in the profession and take them seriously. Ignorance of ethical standards leaves one vulnerable to unethical behavior. Codes of ethics and standards of practice are documents that open the door to discussion of ethical issues in the profession. They should be familiar to all massage and bodywork practitioners. Codes of ethics and standards of practice are discussed further in the next section.

A key principle for behaving ethically is to hold your client's well-being above your personal gain. This principle is sometimes expressed as "selfless service." This does not mean that you work for free, since you have a right to make a living as a massage therapist. It means that when making decisions that might affect your clients' well-being, you do nothing that has the potential to cause them harm, even if for you it means a loss of money, power, or other desirable gain. For example, you do not expose your clients to illness by dragging yourself to work when you are contagious with the flu.

For personal ethical development, it is important to know your weaknesses as well as your strengths. Issues related to money, power, and sex are the usual culprits in unethical decisions. But less obvious roots of unethical behavior might be found in a need to feel loved and accepted, a need to be right, a lack of assertiveness, or even sloppy bookkeeping. Unexamined personal issues may also trip you up in the therapeutic relationship, for example, transference and countertransference, in which negative or positive feelings toward someone in their pasts are brought into the therapeutic relationship by either the client or therapist. Transference and countertransference are discussed in greater detail on page 201 in Chapter 9: Therapeutic Relationship and Ethics.

Self-care in all facets of life reduces vulnerability to unethical behavior. Wellness in the physical, mental, emotional, social, spiritual, and financial realms is a foundation for clear, ethical thinking. Even good time management plays a role, since caregiver burnout can lead to poor judgment when making decisions.

Lack of skill in ethical decision making also leaves one vulnerable. Knowing standards and possessing the ability to apply them in specific situations are very different. It is also harder to think clearly when in the midst of difficult or emotional circumstances. Practicing the steps in ethical decision making in simpler situations is good preparation for the more difficult and complex issues that come up. The process of ethical decision making is explained in more detail in a following section.

ETHICAL CODES AND STANDARDS

Most major professional organizations for massage therapists have published codes of ethics, and some have developed standards of practice. **Codes of ethics** are usually stated in broad terms as general principles that reflect commonly held values. **Standards of practice** are longer, more detailed documents that go into specifics in interpreting ethical principles. These documents can be found on organization websites. The Code of Ethics and Standards of Practice for the National Certification Board for Therapeutic Massage and Bodywork (NCBTMB) are in Appendix G on page 335.

Ethical codes and standards are the products of the collective thinking of a group of professionals. They take into consideration the traditional values and recognized clients' rights related to the profession. These ethics documents are updated from time to time to reflect current issues and new awareness. For example, the concept of "informed voluntary consent" was not on the collective radar screen for massage therapists until a few decades ago. As ethical understanding evolves, so do the documents that codify the latest thinking on the subject.

Professional organizations organize and display their codes of ethics differently. Some go into more detail than others in a combined codes/standards document. However, the values and clients' rights contained in the codes are very similar. The summary of ethical principles for massage therapists found in Figure 8–2 ◀ is based on the major common themes from current massage therapy organization codes of ethics.

The summary of ethical principles is a good overview for discussing ethics for entry-level massage therapists. Some items present general principles that can be expanded (e.g., "Give your best effort to each client"), and others describe specific behavior (e.g., "Refrain from alcohol and recreational drugs when performing massage") to give more pointed guidance to students. This list can be used along with other standards for ethical decision making.

ETHICS AND LAW

Ethics and law are related but are not the same. Both ethics and law are based on values, rights, and duties recognized by a community, but they are enacted and enforced in different ways by different entities.

Professional ethics are the province of associations, which adopt codes of behavior related to the practice of the profession. These are enforced within the group, usually by disciplinary action against members who violate the accepted code of behavior. Disciplinary actions for ethical code violations generally range from letters of reprimand, to probation, to suspension of membership for a period of time, to cancellation of membership in the organization. The decision usually follows a hearing in which the accused is given the opportunity to defend him- or herself. This enforcement of values within the group is referred to as *self-regulation* within a profession.

Laws, on the other hand, are passed by governmental bodies at the local, state, and federal levels to protect the public from harm or to ensure fair practices. Laws are usually only passed when there is a compelling public reason. Violations of law are determined by a judge or by trial and are punishable by fines, community service, or time in jail.

Some of the ethical principles recognized by professional associations have been given the force of law. An example is the federal HIPAA privacy law that ensures confidentiality of medical records. This law lifts the ethical principle of confidentiality to a legal status and specifies what that means under federal law.

Summary of Ethical Principles for Massage Therapists

Massage Therapist

1. Give your best effort to each client.
2. Hold your clients' well-being above your own personal gain.
3. Present a professional image.
4. Present your credentials honestly.
5. Perform only those services for which you are trained and qualified.
6. Stay within your legal scope of practice.
7. Refrain from alcohol and recreational drugs when performing massage.
8. Keep licenses to practice massage therapy current.
9. Stay up-to-date in your field by continued education.

Therapeutic Relationship

10. Set clear professional boundaries with clients.
11. Treat all clients equally with courtesy and respect.
12. Honor your clients' physical, intellectual, and emotional boundaries.
13. Practice good draping skills for client privacy and comfort.
14. Get clients' informed voluntary consent for all massage therapy performed and for touching sensitive body areas.
15. Do not perform massage when it is contraindicated for a client.
16. Acknowledge your limitations, and refer clients to other health care professionals as appropriate.
17. Keep your professional and social lives separate.
18. Do not engage in sexual activities with clients, or sexualize a massage session in any way.
19. Keep your clients' information confidential.

Business Practices

20. Do not make claims for massage therapy that are not true or that you cannot reasonably defend.
21. Do not sell or recommend health products or services outside of your area of expertise.
22. Develop written policies about time and money, and make sure clients understand them.
23. Keep the massage room, equipment, and yourself sanitary.
24. Do not solicit tips.
25. Keep accurate client and financial records.
26. Abide by all local and state laws related to your practice.

Based on the codes of ethics of major massage therapy organizations (American Massage Therapy Association – AMTA; American Organization for Bodywork Therapies of Asia – AOBTA; Associated Bodywork and Massage Professionals – ABMP, National Certification Board for Therapeutic Massage & Bodywork – NCBTMB).

◀ **Figure 8–2** Summary of ethical principles for massage therapists.

CRITICAL THINKING

Examine a code of ethics or standards of practice document for massage and bodywork therapists. Analyze the underlying values, rights, and duties for each item.

1 Do some values, rights, or duties appear more than others?

2 Are there any relationships among these values, rights, and duties?

3 What does your analysis say about the ethical principles most important to massage therapists?

In addition, laws licensing massage therapists usually have sections dealing with ethical issues. For example, the Illinois Massage Licensing Act, Section 45 Grounds for Discipline prohibits "advertising in a false, deceptive, or misleading manner" and "making any misrepresentation for the purpose of obtaining a license." If convicted of an offense, a massage therapist licensed in Illinois can be assessed a fine, be put on probation, or have his or her license suspended or revoked. Disciplinary actions are matters of public record. Currently 38 states in the United States have similar provisions for regulating massage therapists (see Appendix D: Massage Licensing Laws in North America on page 317.

Whereas violations of association codes of ethics can result in censure by the organization a person belongs to, violations of the law can lead to losing a license, paying fines, and/or spending time in jail.

Another connection between professional ethics and law is found in legal cases where the standard of behavior is based on the accepted practices in the profession. An example would be a massage therapist who is being sued for injury to a client during a massage session. If by professional standards the massage therapist should have known about a contraindication for the massage technique used, or if it was outside of the therapist's scope of practice, then the judgment may be in favor of the person making the complaint. In other words, the judge may use a recognized professional standard to decide a case when no specific law pertains to the situation.

ETHICAL DECISION MAKING

Massage therapists make ethical decisions every day. Most are small, uncomplicated issues like keeping client records secure, staying within the scope of practice, and giving their best effort to each client. Other situations can be complex and pose a dilemma about the best way to act. The ethical decision-making model explained below provides a step-by-step method of sorting out the answers to ethical questions and dilemmas.

Ethical Questions and Dilemmas

Ethical issues are most often framed like questions; for example, "Is it ethical to ....? **Ethical questions** are frequently followed by qualifiers; for example, "Is it ethical to (do something), if (this is the situation)?" Many ethical questions can be answered by reviewing a code of ethics or standards of practice to find the profession's view of the subject. However, as in all complex human interactions, the variables of the situation can influence a decision and make it a judgment call.

It is important to distinguish between ethical questions and legal questions. As mentioned before, something may be quite legal, but unethical by professional standards. However, if something is illegal, it is automatically unethical since an all-encompassing ethical principle is to abide by all local, state, and federal laws related to the practice of massage.

Ethical dilemmas occur "when two or more principles are in conflict, and regardless of your choice, something of value is compromised" (Benjamin & Sohnen-Moe, 2003, p. 9). Put another way, no matter what you do, some harm will result or some good will not happen. The ethical dilemma is in selecting the lesser harm or greater good.

Ethical dilemmas are in a different league than **personal temptations** to act unethically. For example, it may be a personal temptation to mix your social and professional lives, and that may be a personal dilemma ("What am I going to do?"), but it is not an ethical dilemma ("What is the most ethical action to take?"). Those are two different questions.

Temptations often involve time and/or money. Working when sick, skimping on hygiene, not completing session notes, constantly arriving late for appointments, and keeping a client who should be referred to another health professional are all personal temptations. These should take a backseat to doing what is best for the client.

The Ethical Decision-Making Model

The **ethical decision-making model** is a step-by-step process of thinking through an ethical question or ethical dilemma. It involves critical thinking, since you are analyzing the situation, and taking into consideration your own motivations and biases. Both external standards, like codes of ethics and laws, and internal standards, like your own sense of right and wrong, play a part. It is essentially a problem-solving process for an ethical situation.

A 10-step ethical decision-making model is summarized in Figure 8–3 ◀. Although the model is listed in steps, implying a linear sequential process, it is best thought of as a logical process that proceeds in an orderly manner. Information may be gathered, and steps revisited, at any time. For Step 9, selecting the course of action, it is useful to review the information gathered in Steps 1 through 8 in order to have a full picture of the situation.

The first step in ethical decision making is to define the ethical question or ethical dilemma. Remember that some choices are not ethical questions if no moral principle is involved. It might simply be a business decision or choice between two plans of action. Frame the situation by filling in the blanks: "Is it ethical to … (do something), if … (this is the situation)?" or "Is it more ethical to … (do something), or to … (do something else)?"

Next, determine if this is also a legal issue. Some situations are covered by consumer protection, privacy, licensing, zoning, or other laws. The overriding principle of abiding by local, state, and federal laws may apply.

Identify the values, rights, and professional standards relevant to the situation. For example, is it a matter of honesty, integrity, beneficence, fairness, or privacy? Look through the professional code of ethics and standards of practice for massage therapists to see if the ethical question is covered. If the situation is not specifically mentioned, is there a relevant principle, value, or right that can be applied in this case?

List the people who might be affected by the decision. They might include yourself, the client, the client's family or friends, your family and friends, coworkers, employers, or landlords. Remember that actions can have ripple effects.

PRACTICAL APPLICATION

An important way to learn ethical behavior and how to navigate ethical issues is by observing others who model ethical conduct. Interview a practicing massage therapist about his or her most memorable ethical issue or dilemma. Listen not only to the massage therapist's narrative, but also observe the body language while this person describes his or her ethical decision and its consequences.

Questions to consider:

1 What was the ethical question?

2 What were the most important factors in the situation?

3 What were the consequences of the therapist's actions?

4 Do you think this massage therapist handled the issue appropriately and made the best ethical decision? Why?

▶ **Figure 8–3** Ethical decision-making model. This is best thought of as a logical process that proceeds in an orderly manner. Information may be gathered, and steps revisited, at any time.

Ethical Decision Making Model

Ω **Step 1. Define the ethical question or ethical dilemma.**
"Is it ethical to… (do something), if… (if this is the situation)?"
"Is it more ethical to…(do something), or to…(do something else)?"

ΩↃ **Step 2. Determine if this is also a legal issue.**
Consumer protection laws
Privacy laws (e.g., HIPAA)
Licensing laws
Other laws (e.g., zoning)

ΩↃ **Step 3. Identify values, rights, and professional standards that apply.**
What values or rights are involved?
Is this situation mentioned in a code of ethics or standards of practice?
Does an employer policy apply to the situation?

ΩↃ **Step 4. List the people who might be affected by the outcome of the decision.**

ΩↃ **Step 5. List alternative courses of action.**

ΩↃ **Step 6. Identify the most important values, rights, standards, and other considerations.**
Is there an overriding principle that applies? (e.g., do no harm, selfless service, abide by laws)

ΩↃ **Step 7. Identify your own motivations or interest in the outcome, and any personal temptations.**

ΩↃ **Step 8. Consider advice from others.**
Consult colleagues, former teachers, or an association.
Consult coworkers or work supervisors.
Consult a professional supervisor.

Ω **Step 9. Select the course of action that maintains the highest values or that results in the greatest good with the least harm.**

Step 10. Evaluate the consequences of your decision, and learn from your experience.

List alternative courses of action. Include all possibilities even if you reject them later, since they may suggest new approaches you had not thought of at first. Consider creative solutions to the problem that preserve important values or rights.

Identify the most important values, rights, standards, and other considerations. This is especially important in ethical dilemmas where competing values or rights are at stake. An overriding principle, like "do no harm" or "abide by the law," may apply.

Before you choose an action, identify your own motivations or interest in the outcome. Look at your personal temptations related to time, money, power, or social advantage. Remember the overriding principle to "hold the client's well-being above your own personal gain."

Consult with others to get a more objective view of the situation, generate more options for actions, and check your own biases and temptations. Sometimes just talking it through with someone else can help you see things more clearly. People familiar with professional ethics and who have experience in the field are especially good to consult. They may have dealt with similar problems in the past and can help you sort out alternatives.

In the end, you have to decide what to do. Base your choice on the action you think will maintain the highest values, or that will result in the greatest good with the least harm. Then do the right thing. Knowing what to do and actually doing it are two different things. Get emotional support if you need it.

Finally, learn from the outcome. The end result will help you judge whether your decision was the best. Analyze the consequences of your decision. Did it uphold the values or rights as you thought it would? Was there something you didn't take into consideration that you should have? Were there any surprises? Would you do it differently next time? Talking with the same people you consulted previously about how the situation turned out can be helpful.

Learn from your successes and your mistakes. You will get better at making ethical decisions with experience. Chapters 9 and 10 contain examples of ethical decision making related to the therapeutic relationship and to business practices.

DEVELOPMENT OF ETHICAL JUDGMENT

The development of **ethical judgment**, that is, consistency in making good ethical decisions, is a lifelong process. Just being aware that decisions might have ethical consequences is important. Ethical behavior is strengthened by continued learning, including learning from successes and mistakes. Ethical judgment improves with critical thinking and evaluating results.

Codes of ethics can be framed and hung in offices to show a commitment to ethics in a practice. Keeping a code of ethics and standards of practice for massage therapists on file for reference makes it easier to consult when an issue arises.

Some licensing laws and certification programs require continuing education in ethics for renewal. Classes in ethics are offered through massage schools and by professional associations. Classes in ethics for health professionals and business ethics classes offer a wider perspective on the subject.

CASE FOR STUDY

Twila and the Flu

Twila works as a part-time massage therapist at a day spa. She woke up on Tuesday feeling weak and sick to her stomach. She was running a mild fever. Several people in her family had the flu over the past week, and she thought she might be coming down with it too. Twila is a responsible person and did not want to miss the four massage appointments scheduled for the day. She also did not want to lose the income if she stayed home from work.

Question:
Is it ethical for Twila to take some over-the-counter medicine to reduce her symptoms and help her get through her massage appointments?

Things to Consider:

▶ Is this situation covered in a code of ethics or standards of practice for massage therapists?
▶ What is Twila's responsibility to her clients in terms of their health and safety?

▶ Who might be affected by Twila's decision?
▶ What are the "worst-case" and "best-case" scenarios?
▶ What are her alternative courses of action?
▶ What might Twila's motivation be for going to work? For staying home?
▶ What would her supervisor advise her to do?
▶ What are the most important considerations in this situation?
▶ What decision would result in the greatest good with the least harm?

Your Reasoning and Conclusions

_____

_____

_____

_____

Networking with other massage therapists in professional associations increases awareness of ethical issues that come up in practices and consequences of certain actions. Reading professional journals helps massage therapists keep up-to-date on the latest thinking about ethical issues. Reports on individual cases dealing with ethics can be instructive.

Clinical supervision involves consultation about different issues that come up in the therapeutic relationship. It is done in a formal setting with a specially trained supervisor. Clinical supervision is an idea borrowed from mental health professionals that is catching on in the massage and bodywork community. Supervision sessions are an opportunity for massage therapists to process what is happening in their practices and their experiences with clients.

Group supervision of practitioners in similar circumstances can be especially useful. "In a group setting clinical supervision undertakes four functions: (1) addressing the relationship issues that arise between clients and practitioners; (2) functioning as a support group for the participants; (3) serving as a forum for didactic instruction on important psychological concepts (such as projection, transference, counter-transference); and (4) training the participants in supervisory skills so that they feel confident continuing this helpful type of coaching by themselves at a later date without a supervisor" (Benjamin & Sohnen-Moe, 2003, p. 243).

Good ethical judgment comes with learning and experience. Mistakes will most likely happen along the way. There might be errors in judgment or lapses of moral behavior. The important thing is to make a commitment to ethical behavior as a massage therapist, learn from successes and failures, and reenergize your ethical sense from time to time throughout your career.

Chapter Highlights

▶ Ethics is the study of moral behavior; that is, determining the "right" thing to do in a specific situation.

- Professional ethics is the study of moral behavior relative to a specific occupation such as massage therapist.
- Business ethics concern the commercial aspects of a massage practice.

▶ Values, rights, and duties provide the foundation for ethical principles.

▶ Values are principles, traits, or qualities considered worthwhile that serve as a moral compass.

▶ Rights are claims to certain treatment or protection from certain treatment.

▶ Duties are obligations to act in a particular way.

▶ Building ethical practices starts with acknowledging human vulnerability to unethical behavior. This vulnerability can be minimized by making a commitment to ethical practices and learning about ethical standards in the profession.

▶ A key ethical principle is selfless service or holding your client's well-being above your own personal gain.

▶ Two overriding ethical principles are *do no harm* and *obey the law*.

▶ Professional organizations develop codes of ethics and standards of practice that are updated periodically to reflect current thinking in the field related to ethics.

- Ethical standards are enforced within organizations through disciplinary action against members who violate the standards.

▶ Some ethical principles are given the force of local, state, or federal law.

   ● Violators of laws can be fined, lose their licenses, or end up in jail.

▶ Ethical questions can be framed in this way: "Is it ethical to … (do something), if … (this is the situation)?"

▶ An ethical dilemma occurs when two values or rights conflict.

▶ Personal temptations to act unethically should not be confused with true ethical questions or dilemmas.

▶ The ethical decision-making model is a step-by-step process of thinking through an ethical question or dilemma. It involves critical thinking, making ethical choices, and analyzing the consequences of the final decision.

▶ Development of ethical judgment is facilitated through having professional standards ready for reference, continuing education classes, professional networking, and clinical supervision.

Exam Review

Learning Outcomes

Use the learning outcomes at the beginning of the chapter and shown here as a guide to the major topics covered. Perform the task given in each outcome, and share your results with a study partner. Check off the tasks as you complete them.

❏ Explain the relationship between professional ethics and values, rights, and duties.
❏ List ways to minimize vulnerability to unethical behavior.
❏ Describe the role of professional organizations in developing ethical codes and standards.
❏ Find examples of codes of ethics and standards of practice for massage and bodywork practitioners.
❏ Describe the role of government in enforcing ethical standards through law.
❏ Identify major ethical principles for massage therapists.
❏ Use a decision-making model to address ethical questions.
❏ Continue development of ethical judgment.

Key Terms

To study key terms listed at the beginning of the chapter, choose one or more of the following exercises. Writing or talking about ideas helps you better remember them, and explaining them to someone else helps deepen your understanding.

1. Write a one-sentence definition of each key term. Put the term in a general category, and then distinguish it from other terms in that category. For example, "*Ethics* is the study of moral behavior" or "*Standards of practice* are documents describing the accepted and encouraged moral behavior of members of a profession." Try to capture the essence of each term in a concise statement.

2. Make study cards by writing the key term on one side of a 3 × 5 card and a concise definition on the other side. Shuffle the cards and read one side, trying to recite either the explanation or term on the other side.

3. Pick out two or three terms and explain how they are related. For example, explain the relationship of values to codes of ethics.

4. With a study partner, take turns explaining key terms verbally.

5. Make up sentences using one or more key terms. Variation: Read your sentences to a study partner who will ask you to explain unclear statements.

Memory Workout

The following fill-in-the-blank statements test your memory of the main concepts in this chapter.

1. Ethics is the study of _____ behavior.

2. Speaking the truth and avoiding deception is called _____.

3. The principle of *confidentiality* stems from a client's right to _____.

4. That clients get to make informed choices about what happens to them is based on their right to _____-_____.

5. Issues related to _____, _____, and _____ are the usual culprits in unethical decisions.

6. The ethical decision-making model is a _____-by-_____ process of thinking through an ethical question or dilemma.

7. Before making a final ethical decision, examine your own _____ or interest in the outcome.

8. Ethical judgment improves with _____ thinking and _____ from results.

9. Networking in professional associations increases awareness of ethical issues, and _____ of certain actions.

10. Clinical supervision involves consultation with _____ or a specially trained _____ about different issues that come up in the therapeutic relationship.

Test Prep

The following multiple-choice questions will help to prepare you for future school and professional exams.

1. Values are:
   a. Principles, traits, or qualities considered worthwhile
   b. Claims to certain treatment or to protection from certain treatment
   c. Obligations to act in a certain way
   d. Moral bonds with society

2. Integrity means:

   a. Telling the truth
   b. Keeping your promises

   c. Living up to your values consistently
   d. Learning from your mistakes

3. Unconditional regard for others calls for giving our best efforts to everyone and being

   a. Honest
   b. Critical

   c. Judgmental
   d. Nonjudgmental

4. In contrast to codes of ethics, standards of practice are

   a. Shorter
   b. More general

   c. More detailed
   d. Stated in broad terms

5. How do professional organizations typically enforce ethical standards?

   a. Criminal prosecution
   b. Disciplinary action like probation or revoking membership

   c. Jail time
   d. Filing lawsuits

6. An ethical dilemma occurs when

   a. Values, rights, or ethical principles are in conflict
   b. An overriding ethical principle is violated

   c. There is personal temptation to act unethically
   d. An ethical question is unclear

7. Which of the following is the *least* important consideration in making an ethical decision?

   a. Determining what will maintain the highest values
   b. Judging what will result in the greatest good overall

   c. Judging what will result in the least harm overall
   d. Determining what will produce the best monetary outcome for myself

8. Which of the following is an important reason to discuss an ethical situation with a colleague?

   a. To get a more objective view of the situation
   b. To generate more options for action

   c. To check my own biases and temptations
   d. All of the above

Video Challenge

Watch the appropriate segment of the video on your CD-ROM and then answer the following questions.

Segment 8: Foundations of Ethics

1. What do the massage therapists interviewed in the video say about the importance of ethics in their practices?

2. How did the massage therapist in the video handle the situation of a client who asked her out on a date? What are other possible endings to that situation? Which would be ethical and which would not be ethical?

3. What does the video say about developing good ethical judgment?

Comprehension Exercises

The following exercises provide questions for you to answer and tasks you can do to enhance your understanding of the material presented in this chapter.

1. Explain steps you can take to avoid unethical behavior.

2. Contrast ethical principles and the law. What are they based on? Who develops them? How are they enforced?

3. After collecting all of the information related to an ethical situation, how do you make your final choice for action? What two questions should you ask yourself?

For Greater Understanding

The following exercises are designed to give you a deeper understanding of the subjects covered in this chapter. Action words are underlined to emphasize the active nature of this approach to learning.

1. Locate an article about ethics in a professional journal for massage therapists. What ethical question or ethical dilemma is addressed? What values, rights, or duties are involved? What factors were considered in decision making? What did you learn from the situation presented?

2. Compare and contrast two or more codes of ethics and/or standards of practice from massage and bodywork organizations. How are they similar? How are they different?

3. Examine the massage licensing law in your state or a neighboring state for the section on ethics and discipline. What ethical principles are reinforced in the law? What are the consequences for violations of the law?

4. Examine the public record in your state or a neighboring state for specific violations of the massage therapy licensing law. How many violations were recorded in the past year? What were the most common offenses? What disciplinary actions resulted?

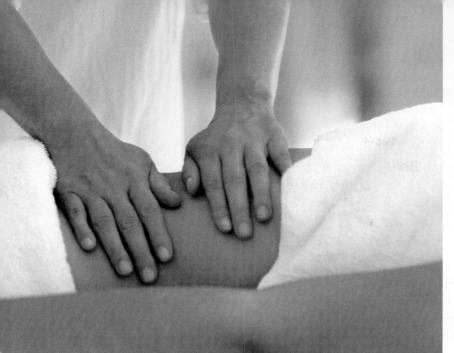

Learning Outcomes
Key Terms
The Therapeutic Relationship
Roles and Boundaries
Dual Relationships
Sexual Relationships
Sexual Misconduct
Relationships in School
Scope of Practice
Confidentiality and HIPAA
Chapter Highlights
Exam Review

LEARNING OUTCOMES

After studying this chapter, you will have information to:

1. Establish appropriate roles in the therapeutic relationship.
2. Recognize the potential impact of psychological factors on the therapeutic relationship.
3. Avoid boundary crossings and violations.
4. Evaluate the potential effects of dual relationships.
5. Avoid all levels of sexual misconduct.
6. Obtain informed voluntary consent when appropriate.
7. Use an intervention model to address inappropriate client behavior.
8. Stay within the scope of practice of massage therapy.
9. Keep client information confidential.
10. Comply with HIPAA rules regarding client records when appropriate.

KEY TERMS

Boundary crossing	Dual relationship	Personal boundary	Sexual misconduct
Confidentiality	Informed voluntary consent	Power differential	Therapeutic relationship
Defense mechanisms	Intervention model	Scope of practice	Transference

Ideas in Action

On your CD-ROM, explore:

▶ Roles and responsibilities   ▶ Intervention model
▶ Informed voluntary consent   ▶ Interactive video exercises

→ THE THERAPEUTIC RELATIONSHIP

The **therapeutic relationship** begins when a client seeks greater well-being through massage from a particular massage therapist, and the massage therapist agrees to provide that service. It is a special relationship based on specific roles and responsibilities.

In nonmedical settings like spas and health clubs, the relationship is *therapeutic* in a more general sense in that the goals are improved health and well-being of the client. In clinical settings, the therapeutic relationship may be part of the treatment itself and a key to the healing process. "The most healing aspect of a series or course of massage therapy sessions, especially in the longer term, can be the relationship between client and therapist. The massage therapist can facilitate this through building a trusting relationship by being non-judgmental, reliable, and supportive" (Greene & Goodrich-Dunn, 2004, p. 17).

Therapeutic relationships are very different from social relationships (e.g., between friends) and have a deeper dimension than simple business transactions. The therapeutic relationship in massage therapy is more intimate and personal than relationships in most commercial settings because clients are seeking help for their personal well-being from a service based on touch.

The intimacy in massage therapy is *physical* because it involves caring touch; *emotional,* as feelings of support and closeness develop; and *verbal* because there is disclosure of personal information. However, the appropriate intimacy in the therapeutic relationship is one-way.

> Practitioners physically touch their clients, allow them to disclose thoughts and feelings, and offer both verbal and physical support. The therapeutic relationship's function is not for the clients to do the same for the practitioner. (Benjamin & Sohnen-Moe, 2003, p. 112)

There is an inherent **power differential** between massage therapists and their clients in therapeutic relationships. That is, massage therapists have more power in the relationships by virtue of their training and experience, and by their being in a position of authority (Figure 9–1 ◀). It is similar to other familiar relationships such as teacher–student, boss–employee, and nurse–patient. "Even if the massage therapist does not want or seek out power, clients still ascribe power to the therapist because power *is an intrinsic element in the therapist–client relationship*" (Greene & Goodrich-Dunn, 2004, p. 13).

> Our clients come to us in pain or in need of help. Just by showing up at our offices, they make themselves vulnerable. They are hurting, and we are the authority. Even though they may not be conscious of it, we can become a doctor/parent figure in their eyes. Our responsibility is to meet that vulnerability with respect and kindness. (McIntosh, 1999, p. 17)

The massage therapist, therefore, has a fiduciary responsibility in the therapeutic relationship. Fiduciary is a legal term used to describe a relationship in which person A has placed a special trust in person B, who is then obligated to watch out

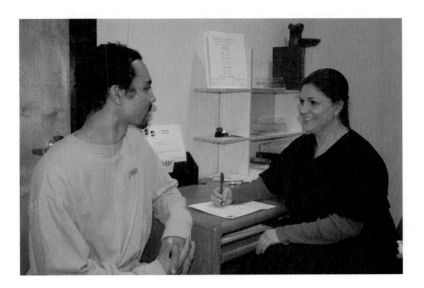

◀**Figure 9–1** There is an inherent power differential between massage therapists and their clients.

for person A's best interests. In other words, the client puts a special trust in the massage therapist, who is then obligated to look out for the client's best interests.

There are both explicit and implicit agreements in the therapeutic relationship. Explicit agreements are spoken or written, and include things like pricing information, payment policies, cancellation policies, and the type of massage and bodywork provided. Implicit agreements are those commonly understood for this type of relationship, which may be unspoken and unwritten. These include being on time, doing no harm, acting in the best interest of the client, keeping client information confidential, providing a safe environment, and staying within the scope of practice.

When a client comes for a massage, there is an implicit understanding that the massage therapist is upholding the standards of the profession. These standards are found in codes of ethics and standards of practice documents that outline what is expected of competent and ethical massage therapists.

As in any relationship, human interactions in the therapeutic relationship can be influenced by psychological factors. Massage therapists can learn to recognize those factors at work in their relationships with clients. In addition to improving the quality of their therapeutic relationships, awareness of the potential influence of psychological factors can help massage therapists make better ethical choices. Two factors with great potential to influence therapeutic relationships are transference and countertransference.

Transference and Countertransference

Transference occurs when a client transfers negative or positive feelings toward someone from his or her past into the therapeutic relationship. The feelings transferred would typically be about an authority figure like a parent, teacher, or other person important to the client when he or she was growing up. Transference has been called "a kind of spell generated by one's own psyche," with the result that the client "cannot see the therapist and/or the therapy as they actually are" (Greene & Goodrich-Dunn, 2004, p. 55).

A client who is experiencing *positive transference* projects good feelings toward the massage therapist. Positive transference can contribute to the therapeutic relationship by opening the door to acceptance, cooperation, and trust.

However, positive transference can also blind the client. For example, the client might place the massage therapist on a pedestal, thinking the therapist to be more knowledgeable than he or she actually is, or try too hard to please the therapist, or be overly submissive. A client in positive transference might give inappropriate gifts, or want to step over the line into a social or romantic relationship. The danger in positive transference is the temptation for massage therapists to relax professional boundaries, or to lose sight of who they (the massage therapists) really are.

Negative transference, or the projection of negative or bad feelings into the therapeutic relationship, can cause more obvious problems. A client thinking that the massage therapist doesn't like her, feeling like she just can't please the massage therapist, trying to argue with the massage therapist, or thinking that the massage therapist doesn't know what he or she is doing, all work against the massage therapy itself. If it is a case of transference, these negative thoughts and feelings have nothing to do with the reality of the situation with the massage therapist, but have been transferred from another relationship in the past.

Because massage therapists are not trained as psychotherapists, cases of positive and negative transference may be hard for them to identify. Suspect transference if you are uncomfortable with a client's behavior and you can say to yourself, "Her reaction doesn't make sense," or "This is not about me," or "This is not about this therapeutic relationship." When going through an ethical decision-making process as described in Chapter 8: Foundations of Ethics, on page 191, take the possibility of transference into consideration.

The best strategy when faced with a client's transference is to maintain your objectivity through critical thinking and getting someone else's viewpoint. Do not try to psychoanalyze your client, which is outside of your scope of practice. Keep good professional boundaries.

Countertransference occurs when massage therapists transfer positive or negative feelings toward others from their past into the therapeutic relationship. In this case, the massage therapists are under a "spell," and do not see the clients or the therapeutic situations as they really are. Trying too hard to please clients, relaxing professional boundaries against better judgment, and feeling more knowledgeable or powerful than they really are exemplify countertransference by massage therapists.

Being grounded in your role as a massage therapist, and in your own thoughts and feelings, helps minimize the effects of countertransference. Because it is an unconscious response, however, countertransference is difficult to detect in ourselves. Personal awareness, peer advice, and professional supervision can help sort out issues of transference and countertransference.

Defense Mechanisms

Defense mechanisms are behaviors or thoughts that help us cope with unwanted feelings like fear, anxiety, guilt, and anger. Both massage therapists and clients bring their defense mechanisms into the therapeutic relationship. These defenses can be amplified when receiving bodywork. Common defense mechanisms are projection, denial, repression, displacement, and resistance. Although there are subtle differences in these mechanisms, their common purpose is to protect the psyche from unwanted feelings.

Projection occurs when someone imputes to someone else a behavior that they themselves are doing, or a feeling that they are having. For example, a massage therapist who is attracted to a client might suppress that feeling within him- or herself, and instead perceive the client as seductive. Or a client may think of a massage therapist as a "know it all" instead of acknowledging his or her own feelings of superiority.

Denial is blocking out the existence of an unwanted feeling, or refusing to recognize the reality of a situation. For example, a massage therapist may not recognize that a valued client is taking advantage of him or her by frequently canceling at the last minute. Fear of losing the client may create a situation of denial. Or because of fear, a client may be unwilling to admit to him- or herself the pain he or she is feeling, and therefore not give useful feedback about pressure during a massage session.

Repression involves burying unwanted feelings, for example, by erasing them from conscious memory, or not allowing them to be felt. Repressed feelings can cause anxiety and depression unless and until they surface and are resolved. Either the massage therapist or client may have repressed feelings from past events or trauma.

Displacement is reacting to a feeling generated by one person or situation by acting out toward someone else or in a different situation. For example, bringing anger from something that happened at home or in your private life into the workplace is displacement. You're angry with your best friend, and you take it out on a coworker—that is displacement.

Resistance is "a failure of or refusal by the client to cooperate with the therapeutic process" (Greene & Goodrich-Dunn, 2004, p. 50). Resistance is usually unconscious and can take many forms, such as being unable to relax during a massage, missing appointments, or forgetting suggestions for self-massage at home. Resistance would be something that comes up with regular clients, or those coming for a series of massage sessions as treatment for a condition.

The resistance might have nothing to do with the massage therapist, but could be due to some other factor, such as transference. It is not massage therapists' place to psychoanalyze their clients' behavior, but just noticing resistance and bringing up observations with clients can be enough to bring it to a conscious level for resolution.

Defense mechanisms can cause problems in therapeutic relationships because they tend to deflect attention from the reality of a situation. The key is not to eliminate them (a near impossible task because they are habitual behaviors), but to recognize them when they surface and minimize their negative impact. Seeing through defense mechanisms can help massage therapists build healthier therapeutic relationships and avoid unethical behavior.

ROLES AND BOUNDARIES

Both massage therapists and clients have specific roles to play in the therapeutic relationship. The massage therapists' general role is to apply their training and experience within their scope and standards of practice to help clients meet their health goals. The clients' general role is to provide relevant information, participate cooperatively in massage therapy sessions, abide by policies and procedures, and pay the fees.

Professional boundaries maintain these roles within therapeutic relationships. As explained in detail in Chapter 5: Social and Communication Skills, on page 117, these include physical, emotional, intellectual, sexual, and energetic limits on what will and will not happen between the massage therapist and the client. It is the massage therapist's responsibility to create the framework that defines these boundaries, for example, with policies, rules, procedures, and the whole massage environment into which clients walk. Practical aspects of maintaining professional boundaries are discussed further in sections on dual relationships, sexual misconduct, and scope of practice found later in this chapter.

In addition to professional boundaries, massage therapists and clients have personal boundaries that must be respected. A **personal boundary** is a limit established by a person to maintain his or her own integrity, comfort, or well-being. For example, a client may ask a massage therapist not to touch his feet, or not to use oil with a fragrance. Or a massage therapist may prefer handshakes to hugs, or refuse to use petroleum-based oil. These are legitimate personal boundaries.

The NCBTMB Code of Ethics (see Appendix G: Code of Ethics and Standards of Practice for Massage Therapists on page 335) directs massage therapists to "respect the client's boundaries with regard to privacy, disclosure, exposure, emotional expression, beliefs, and the client's reasonable expectations of professional behavior. Practitioners will respect the client's autonomy." That includes the client's right to set personal boundaries.

"Stepping over the line," or boundary crossings and violations, can be ethical matters if they harm the therapeutic relationship or the individuals involved. According to Benjamin and Sohnen-Moe, a **boundary crossing** "is a transgression that may or may not be experienced as harmful," while a boundary violation "is a harmful transgression of a boundary" (2003, p. 39). So whether a boundary transgression is a crossing or a violation is a matter of degree and a matter of consequences. If a boundary crossing is not experienced as harmful, then it does not rise to the level of a violation, although it can be problematic. Boundary crossings can be annoying, intrusive, hurtful, or just uncomfortable. For example, a client answering a cell phone during a massage session might be annoying. A massage therapist may ask a client a question that seems intrusive or too personal. Or a client may be uncomfortable with a massage therapist massaging her neck but says nothing about it. These are examples of boundary crossings but probably not violations.

Violations leave one with a sense of being *violated*, a much stronger feeling than just feeling annoyed or uncomfortable. Integrity is compromised in some way, and the agreement within the therapeutic relationship is broken. Examples of boundary violations include a client who learns that his or her massage therapist talked to someone else about his or her medical condition without permission; a massage therapist whose client calls him or her at home to ask for a date; or a massage therapist touching a part of the body he or she was asked not to touch or for which there is an implicit agreement to avoid, such as a woman's breasts.

All professional and personal boundary violations are unethical, since some harm has been done. Even unintentional harm is still harm and may have adverse consequences. At a minimum, there will be negative consequences to the therapeutic relationship, and there may also be personal, professional, employment, or legal repercussions.

According to McIntosh, the majority of client complaints about massage therapists fall into two general categories of boundary violations: (1) blurring professional and social roles and (2) going beyond their expertise and training.

↪ DUAL RELATIONSHIPS

A **dual relationship** means that in addition to the therapeutic relationship, there are other social or professional connections between a client and a massage therapist. This applies to clients who are also family members, friends, coworkers, neighbors, fellow organization members, service providers like accountants and plumbers, or any other additional relationship.

In some cases a dual relationship can enhance a therapeutic relationship. This works if the two people involved are emotionally mature and "able to handle the multiple roles without confusion" (Benjamin & Sohnen-Moe, 2003, p. 86). For example, the familiarity between friends can give the massage therapist greater insight into what the client-friend is experiencing. However, a friend who becomes a client would have to agree to the role of a client during massage sessions and be comfortable with the appropriate professional boundaries set for that time. The same would apply to the massage therapist, who would have to set aside his or her own needs and wants, and keep to a professional role during the massage time.

In reality, most dual relationships have problematic dimensions. Issues are magnified if the power differential between the client and massage therapist varies in different situations. For example, in a client–neighbor dual relationship, the massage therapist holds a power role during massage sessions, but is an equal outside of the sessions. Or in a client–family member situation, family dynamics may come into play and affect the therapeutic relationship.

Financial or economic arrangements outside of the massage therapy relationship have their own potential problems. Two common scenarios involve bartering and employment. Bartering for services, such as accounting or website design, can be a mutually beneficial arrangement as long as both parties feel they are getting a fair deal and follow through on their agreement. The exchange might be hour for hour or session for session, regardless of time involved. Or for an accountant, it might be six massage sessions for doing the massage therapist's taxes for the year. A verbal contract for bartering needs to be crystal clear to avoid someone feeling taken advantage of. Exchanging invoices for services can reduce the potential for misunderstandings.

Being a massage therapist to a boss or an employee also calls for very clear boundaries because the power differential changes with the different roles. In the boss–client scenario, the boss is in a position of authority in the workplace, while during massage therapy, the practitioner is in charge. As long as both people can accept their roles in the different situations, the arrangement can work. However, it can become awkward if something happens that crosses boundaries, such as your boss asking you for information about your coworker while he or she is getting a massage.

Perhaps the most difficult lines to draw are those about socializing with clients. Degrees of socializing range from a cup of tea before a massage session, to meeting for coffee outside of the massage setting, to belonging to the same club or organization, to attending events together. Ethical issues that might come up during socializing are failing to protect other clients' confidentiality and offering too much self-disclosure about the massage therapist's personal life.

As mentioned previously, when people known in social settings become clients, strong professional boundaries can minimize problems. However, when a current client initiates a social invitation, a massage therapist must take into consideration the possibility of transference and consequences for the therapeutic relationship. The risk may outweigh any benefits, and romantic or sexual socializing would be unethical, as will be explained in more detail later in this chapter. A massage therapist whose personal social circle is heavily populated by clients is taking advantage of his or her practice for the wrong reasons. It is obvious that the variety of dual relationships is endless, and each one needs to be thought through carefully.

Evaluating Dual Relationships

For a massage therapist, deciding whether or not to enter into a dual relationship with a client, or to continue one already established, requires evaluating the potential benefits and risks. As the person in authority in the therapeutic relationship, it is the massage therapist's responsibility to make decisions in the best interest of the client. It is unethical to enter into or continue a dual relationship if there is high potential of harm to either party, or if the therapeutic relationship will be compromised.

One factor for consideration is the nature of the relationships involved. Are there conflicting power differentials? Do they involve money, friendship, love? Are they of short or long duration? Another factor is the maturity of the people involved. Are they good at keeping boundaries and cooperative in respecting limits? Do both parties understand the complexities involved? Experience says that:

> …both parties must allocate equal responsibility for the establishment, continuation, and if necessary, termination of any part of the dual relationship. Mutual and equal consent to all aspects of the dual relationship is shared by both parties. (Benjamin & Sohnen-Moe, 2003, p. 94)

Motivations for entering into the dual relationship need to be scrutinized. Does one party benefit at the possible expense of the other? Is there a possibility of transference or countertransference clouding the reality of the situation? Professional standards can help in certain situations. For example, the special case of sexual relationships, which is discussed in the next section.

The potential effects of the dual relationship on the therapeutic relationship are important to consider. Can both parties maintain their respective roles as massage therapist and client in relation to massage sessions?

"Worst-case" and "best-case" exercises are useful for making decisions about dual relationships. For example, a best-case scenario for a dual relationship in which the massage therapist hires a mechanic/client to repair his or her car is that the car gets fixed satisfactorily, and the therapeutic relationship continues unaffected. A worst-case scenario might be that the mechanic damages the engine and refuses to make fair compensation. Negative feelings from that scenario are likely to affect the therapeutic relationship, and possibly damage it beyond repair. The question to ask is this: Is hiring the client worth the risk, or can someone else do the job just as well without the complicating factor?

A good question for a massage therapist to ask him- or herself is, "If this dual relationship does not work out . . . am I willing to lose this person as a client? Or, am I willing to lose this person as a beautician (or accountant, friend, etc.)? Am I willing to jeopardize my other job (or membership in an organization, etc.)?" It is important not to underestimate the possible consequences of the dual relationship, but to enter into such relationships with thoughtfulness and clear vision. This is another case where discussing the situation with someone familiar with the complexities of dual relationships would be useful, for example, with a colleague, supervisor, or other professional.

→ SEXUAL RELATIONSHIPS

There are two general scenarios for professional relationships involving sexual partners. One is when a current client wants to become romantically or sexually involved with the massage therapist (and vice versa), and the other is when a current spouse or romantic friend becomes a client. These are two very different situations with different ethical considerations.

First of all, it should be noted that sexual activity with a client is strictly prohibited by professional standards and by massage therapist licensing laws. The NCBTMB Code of Ethics states that massage and bodywork practitioners should "refrain, under all circumstances, from initiating or engaging in any sexual conduct, sexual activities, or sexualizing behavior involving a client, even if the client attempts to sexualize the relationship."

That means no dating, or even socializing with clients who have romantic intentions. The power differential in the therapeutic relationship and the possibility of transference or other psychological factors having an influence make it unethical to enter into such a relationship. It can be dangerous emotionally for one or both parties and distorts the therapeutic relationship.

However, the NCBTMB Standards of Practice offers a solution for special cases that would minimize the dangers involved (see Appendix G: Code of Ethics and Standards of Practice for Message Therapists on page 335). It states that the massage practitioner should "refrain from participating in a sexual relationship or sexual conduct with a client, whether consensual or otherwise, from the beginning of the client/therapist relationship and for a minimum of 6 months after the termination of the client–therapist relationship"

CASE FOR STUDY

Rebecca and the Movie Invitation

Rebecca graduated from massage school and got a job at a local health club working part time. She likes to exercise and stay fit, so the setting was perfect for her. Dan comes to the health club to work out several times a week and gets massage regularly. He enjoys Rebecca's massage, so lately he has been going to her exclusively. They are both single and like each other. Dan asked her to go with him to a movie they both wanted to see.

Question:
Is it ethical for Rebecca to go with Dan to the movie?

Things to Consider:

> ▶ Does the health club have a policy about staff dating members?
> ▶ Is this situation covered in a code of ethics or standards of practice for massage therapists?
> ▶ Who might be affected by this decision?
> ▶ What are the "worst-case" and "best-case" scenarios?

> ▶ What are alternative courses of action?
> ▶ What are the most important considerations in this situation?
> ▶ What might Rebecca's motivation be for accepting the invitation? Declining it?
> ▶ What would a former teacher advise Rebecca to do?
> ▶ What decision would maintain the highest standards?

Your Reasoning and Conclusions:

_____

_____

_____

_____

(adopted September 1, 2000). The general ethical principle is to end the therapeutic relationship and wait for a period of time before beginning the romantic/sexual relationship. Waiting clearly separates the roles in time and provides perspective on the situation.

Developing a romantic relationship with someone special, who just happens to be a former client, can be perfectly ethical. However, dating a current client or regularly dating former clients is clearly considered unethical by professional standards.

If someone who is *already* a spouse, significant other, boyfriend or girlfriend, or a romantic or sexual partner later becomes a client, clear boundaries are a must. In addition to power issues coming into the therapeutic relationship, there is the potential for the association of massage therapy with sexual activity. During time set aside for massage therapy, there is no place whatsoever for sexual activity.

Engaging in sexual behavior during a time set aside for massage therapy, and especially on a massage table or in a space set aside for massage practice, is confusing on many levels even if the person is a spouse. Why? For the massage therapist, his or her professional role strictly prohibits sexual activity with a client, and so the situation is a blurring of roles. For the client-spouse, the association is made between massage therapy and sex, so they may feel uneasy, often unconsciously, about what their partner-therapist is doing with other clients. A clear separation of massage therapy and sexual activity in time and space is the only workable approach.

SEXUAL MISCONDUCT

Sexual misconduct involves any sexualizing of the relationship between a massage therapist and a current client. Sexual misconduct can occur before, after, or during a massage session and can be perpetrated by the massage therapist or by the client.

Forms of sexual misconduct range from those involving speech and body language to inappropriate touch to sexual contact to sexual assault. Figure 9–2 ◀ lists categories and examples of sexual misconduct encountered in massage practices.

The degree of severity of sexual misconduct ranges from relatively minor to very severe. How serious the offense is depends on the intentions of the initiator, the experience of the victim, whether physical contact is involved, and the resulting physical or psychological harm.

▶ **Figure 9–2** Forms of sexual misconduct.

Forms of Sexual Misconduct

Categories of sexual misconduct that grow progressively more serious:

↳ No touch involved: speech and body language
↳ Inappropriate touch involved
↳ Direct sexual contact
↳ Sexual assault

Examples of sexual misconduct of clients and massage therapists that grow progressively more serious:

Client
Flirting
Use of slang or crude words referring to the genitalia
Jokes with sexual content or innuendo
Talk about personal sexual experiences or problems
Seductive speech
Exposes his or her genitalia; woman exposes her breasts
Asks for sexual favors
⇩
Touches the massage therapist on thigh or buttocks seductively
Stimulates him- or herself sexually during massage
⇩
Assaults the massage therapist sexually; rape

Massage Therapist
Flirting
Use of slang or crude words referring to the genitalia
Jokes with sexual content or innuendo
Talk about personal sexual experiences or problems
Seductive speech
Exposes client through improper draping
Watches client dress or undress
Sexual fantasies about a client
⇩
Touches sensitive areas (e.g., upper thigh) without informed consent
Positions or braces the client using face or front of pelvis
Uses chest, head, face, lips, hair, pelvis, or breasts to massage a client

Outside of massage session
Dating or romantic socializing with a client
Sexual activity outside of massage setting

During massage session
Touches client's genitals or nipples
Fails to intervene when client sexually stimulates him- or herself
Stimulates him- or herself sexually during massage
Sexually stimulates client during massage
⇩
Assaults the client sexually; rape

The most common forms of sexual misconduct involve flirting, suggestive comments about a person's body or appearance, and off-color jokes or innuendo. Discussion of the sexual performance, preferences, or problems of either party sexualizes the situation. Seductive behavior is an open invitation to misconduct.

Sexual misconduct by a massage therapist also includes exposing clients' genitals or women's breasts. Good draping technique can prevent accidental exposure. Watching a client undress or dress, except in cases of advanced age or disability when assistance is needed, is also inappropriate. Respecting a client's privacy is essential.

Because of the physical contact involved, misconduct related to touch is especially harmful. Inappropriate touch by a massage therapist is a gross violation of the therapeutic relationship. Guidelines for appropriate touch include:

▶ Use only hands, forearms, elbows, and feet to massage a client.
▶ Never use the chest, head, face, lips, hair, pelvis, or breasts to massage a client.
▶ Use only knees, shoulders, lateral hip, and lower leg for bracing or stabilizing.
▶ Never use the face or front of the pelvis for bracing or stabilizing when applying techniques.
▶ Never massage in the nipple or genital areas.
▶ Never touch any part of your body to the client's genital area.
▶ Get informed consent to massage high on the thigh, around breast tissue, the buttocks, anywhere near the genitals, and on the abdomen. (Adapted from the *Report of the Sexual Abuse Task Force of the AMTA Council of Schools*, January 1991)

Informed Voluntary Consent

Informed voluntary consent is a process used by massage therapists to get the client's permission to touch areas that may have sexual associations (e.g., high on the thigh, buttocks, abdomen), or areas out of the scope of general care (e.g., ear canal, nasal passages, mouth, anal canal, and breast tissue). For some areas, the NCBTMB Standards of Practice further require *written* consent, and that the treatment be part of a plan of care (Standard VI: Prevention of Sexual Misconduct).

The words used to describe this process tell the story of its key elements. It is *informed* in that the client receives information about the proposed action and the reasons for it. It is *voluntary* in that the client freely agrees to the proposal. Finally, there is *consent* or permission by the client who exercises his or her right to self-determination.

The process of informed voluntary consent has five parts. First, the massage therapist informs the client about the nature and duration of the proposed action, that is, the body part to be touched, the technique to be used, or other relevant factors. Second, the massage therapist gives reasons for the proposed action. Third, the massage therapist describes what the client should expect. Fourth, the massage therapist gives the client the option to say no, either before beginning or at any time during the application. Fifth, the massage therapist explicitly asks permission to touch the area. This process is summarized in Figure 9–3 ◀.

For areas that are generally within the scope of a regular massage, but that may have sexual associations, verbal consent is usually adequate. Informed voluntary consent in these cases may be simple. For example, to an athlete complaining of tight thigh muscles, you might say, "I'd like to work the tendons to the muscles in your thighs closer to their points of insertion. That's a little higher than you're used to me working. But it should help those muscles loosen up better. I'll adjust the drape to make sure you're covered. The inner thigh can be sensitive so it may feel a little strange to you. If it gets uncomfortable at any time, just let me know. Is that all right with you? Shall I go ahead and start?" If the client says yes, remain aware of nonverbal commu-

▶ **Figure 9–3** Informed voluntary consent—permission to touch.

Informed Voluntary Consent

Obtain permission to touch areas with sexual association (e.g., buttocks, inner thigh) and areas outside of the norm for massage (e.g., nasal passages, mouth). Touching the genitals is never allowed even with consent.

Step 1 Inform the client about the nature and duration of the proposed action; for example, the body part to be massaged, the massage techniques to be used, the amount of time involved.

Step 2 Explain the reasons for the proposed action; for example, the goals and therapeutic benefits expected.

Step 3 Describe what the client should expect to feel.

Step 4 Invite the client to agree to the goals and methods for the proposed action; the client has complete freedom to accept or reject the proposed action or any part of it, before the massage is applied or anytime during the application.

Step 5 Ask permission to touch the area, and to begin the massage application; client signs written consent if applicable.*

* Written consent is advised for all massage treatments involving nasal passages, mouth, ear canal, anal canal, and women's breasts.

---

nication such as facial expression and muscle tightening that may signal discomfort. That could also signal "no" or "I changed my mind."

For body areas out of the general scope of massage, the ethical requirements are stricter. Special training is necessary to enter body orifices like the nose, mouth, and anus, and to massage the breasts. In addition, written consent must be obtained. Massage techniques for these areas are not usually taught in entry-level programs in the United States, or may be advanced treatments taught in longer, medically oriented programs. Working in these areas may also be outside of a massage therapist's legal scope of practice under his or her license.

The NCBTMB Standards of Practice require that massage treatments in these sensitive areas be performed within a *plan of care*. That means that there should be a medical reason for the special massage techniques, and the massage is part of an overall treatment plan. This also implies that other medical professionals may be aware of the massage treatment. The standards stop short of requiring a prescription from a doctor. However, such a prescription would validate the therapeutic necessity of the procedure and provide justification if needed. There are legal as well as ethical issues to consider.

Sexual Misconduct by a Client

Although the vast majority of clients respect the professional nature of massage therapy, massage therapists should be prepared to handle sexual misconduct by a client. This is a matter of safety as well as ethics for the massage therapist.

The importance of establishing a professional setting and boundaries cannot be emphasized enough. If the massage therapist is fuzzy about his or her boundaries, the client will also be unclear about where to draw the line on behaviors like flirting, jokes, and more overt sexual behavior.

Depending on where you work (e.g., spa, health club, clinic, office at home), and the amount of confusion in your city, town, or local area about the difference between legitimate massage and sexual massage, you may want to be more explicit about your standing. For example, when making appointments, you may want to state upfront "You understand that this is therapeutic and not sexual massage." Or you may wish to highlight a similar statement in the policy document that clients sign at their first appointment.

Client misconduct on any of the levels shown in Figure 9–2 should be addressed with directness and assertiveness. A client intent on sexualizing the massage will often begin testing the waters with minor misconduct like flirting and then escalate the sexual behavior with time. Stopping the misconduct early will clearly draw the boundary of acceptable behavior.

Minor misconduct can be addressed by clarifying boundaries. For example, "Seth, this is a professional setting. Please don't tell a joke like that again." Or "Barbara, I appreciate the invitation, but I am declining because socializing like that with clients can lead to problems in our relationship here." Or "Ricardo, you understand that as your massage therapist, I cannot go on a date with you. It is against our professional standards." If the client is mature and respects your professionalism, then that should be enough.

Clients looking for sexual gratification might come right out and ask for it. They might use euphemisms like "Do you give a *full* massage?" (with a vocal emphasis on *full*). Or "Do you give the 'happy ending'?" If that comes up before the massage, an assertive statement about your professional standards will usually send the client looking somewhere else. If it happens during the session, use the intervention model explained in the next section.

A client, either male or female, may become sexually aroused during a massage session with no prior intention of that happening. This might occur either in a cross-gender or same-gender session. While there is no exact formula for dealing with the situation, there are some guidelines to consider.

One possibility is that a technique that the massage therapist is performing, the body area he or she are massaging, or a combination of the two is causing an arousal response. If this is the case, changing the technique, tempo, or area being massaged can interrupt the process and the arousal may subside. Whether to talk to the client about the incident is a judgment call. It may be an opportunity to explain that sexual arousal can be a short-lived physiological response, and it need not be interpreted as deliberate or improper. However, it should be avoided if possible, interrupted if it occurs, and never acted on during massage therapy.

If a man has a partial or full erection during a massage session, it may or may not be necessary to intervene. If he shows no signs of embarrassment or sexual intent, it may be an innocent physiological response as described previously, and no formal intervention is necessary at that time. If he acts uncomfortable or embarrassed, even though he has not behaved inappropriately in any way, it is best to talk to him about it and assure him that you understand the physiological response involved. However, if he has made suggestive comments or other sexual overtures, touches himself, or asks you to touch him inappropriately, then you are ethically obligated to intervene and stop the session (Benjamin & Sohnen-Moe).

More extreme forms of sexual misconduct may also be illegal. Cases of assault, battery, gross indecency, and threatening behavior by clients should be reported to the local police. Massage therapists who have been victims of illegal client misconduct have been known to take their clients to court. This helps protect massage therapists and others in the community from becoming future victims of the perpetrator.

Intervention Model

The **intervention model** is a useful tool to address misconduct or suspected misconduct by clients. A seven-step approach is presented in Figure 9–4◀. For minor misconduct, an abbreviated version of the model may be all that is necessary. For more severe misconduct, all seven steps are recommended.

▶ **Figure 9–4** Intervention model—response to client miscondut.

Intervention Model
Step 1. Stop the session using assertive behavior.
Step 2. Describe the behavior you are concerned about.
Step 3. Ask the client to clarify the behavior.
Step 4. Restate your intent and professional boundaries.
Step 5. Evaluate the client's response.
Step 6. Continue or discontinue the session as appropriate.
Step 7. Document the situation and discuss it with a trusted colleague.*
*Assault, battery, gross indecency, and threatening behavior should also be reported to the local police.

First, stop the massage session or interrupt the behavior, using assertive verbal and body language. Assertive behavior signals that you are competent and in charge. If misconduct occurs during a massage session, remove your hands from the body and step away from the table. You want the client's full attention. Address the client calmly but firmly by name, and make a statement about why you are intervening. For example, say something like, "Peter, we need to talk about what just happened." Or "Vanessa, I'd like to talk about what you just said."

Second, describe the behavior you are concerned about. Be as specific as possible. For example: "That was the second time your hand brushed my leg. It seems to be intentional." Or "You keep removing the drape and exposing yourself." Or "You continue talking about your sexual relationship with your husband."

Ask the client to clarify his or her behavior, if appropriate. For example: "Are you trying to sexualize this massage?" Or "Are you looking for professional help with your sexual problems with your spouse?"

Restating your intent and professional boundaries may be all that is needed to get things back on track. For example, you can state, "This is a nonsexual massage, and you must stay draped at all times." Or "Sexual problems are outside of the scope of massage therapy, and I am not a psychotherapist. Please keep the conversation related to massage." Or "Touching me that way is not all right with me. Please stop."

Then evaluate the client's response. If you believe that the client will keep the reinforced boundaries, and you are comfortable and feel safe, you may continue the massage. If the client repeats the misconduct, or, in spite of what he or she says, you still feel uncomfortable or unsafe, you should terminate the session. Trust your intuition. This is a judgment call. You have a right to a professional, safe, and comfortable environment.

If you are in a public facility like a spa or clinic, you are less vulnerable to misconduct. If you have a private practice in an office or in your home, or are at a client's home or in a hotel, you are more vulnerable. Have an emergency plan in place including contacts, phone numbers, and an escape route. If you fear for your safety, leave the office or house and go somewhere people can help you.

Finally, document your experience either in the client's file or in a separate incident report file. Remember that clients have a right to see their personal files, and anything written in them should be descriptive (not interpretive) and professional. Other massage therapists who are scheduled with the client will appreciate knowing about what happened.

In terms of self-care, massage therapists who have experienced an incident of sexual misconduct by a client, especially one involving the intervention model, should talk about it with a trusted friend, colleague, or supervisor. Talking helps a person

PRACTICAL APPLICATION

The following client situations involve setting professional boundaries. With a friend or study partner, practice what you would say in these situations to maintain professional boundaries.

Responding to a client who:

▶ invites you out for social time
▶ you want to hire to do your taxes
▶ is habitually late
▶ talks through the whole massage session
▶ asks about another client's health
▶ tells off-color or ethnic jokes or uses profanity

1 How did you feel during each role-playing exercise?

2 Was your verbal and non-verbal communication about your professional boundaries clear?

3 How could you modify what you said to make it clearer?

4 What are some other boundary-setting situations in which it would be useful to rehearse your responses?

analyze and process the situation, which may have been upsetting. Getting it out in the open also helps to objectify the incident and use it as a learning experience.

RELATIONSHIPS IN SCHOOL

Massage therapy students have the potential for dual relationships with classmates, teachers and administrators, practice clients, and clients in student clinics and at outreach sites. Each of these situations deserves some careful thought. While some of these ideas were introduced in Chapter 4: Personal Development and Professionalism, they are discussed more fully here.

Classmates often get to know one another well during the course of a massage program. Relationships among classmates have some similarities to relationships with clients. Although these are not therapeutic relationships by a strict definition, they are special relationships based on giving and receiving massage and involve knowledge of personal information about the people in class. Classmates become somewhat vulnerable to one another, and a level of trust is established. Friendships also develop among classmates, and these are dual relationships with their own dimensions. Being a student of massage therapy is very different from other vocational and academic programs because of the intimate contact inherent in the learning situation.

There are implicit agreements among classmates involving confidentiality, trust, and respect just like in the therapeutic relationship. Figure 9–5 ◀ lists some of the important ethical aspects of relationships among classmates. It is a matter of integrity that ethical principles related to the therapeutic relationship carry over into massage school classmate relationships.

As in any school setting, friendships and socializing between students and teachers or school staff is a double-edged sword. On the one hand, learning may be enhanced through informal interactions; on the other hand, the inherent power differential can cause problems similar to problems in dual relationships between clients and massage therapists. In this case, students are in a position of lesser power. It is the teacher or staff member's responsibility to maintain appropriate social boundaries with students. Students can also recognize and avoid problems by limiting such socializing to official school events and group activities.

▶ **Figure 9–5** Ethical principles related to relationships with massage therapy classmates.

Ethical Principles Regarding Relationships with Classmates

To promote trust, respect, and harmony, and to avoid unethical behavior, classmates agree to:

1. Treat all classmates with equal respect, and avoid cliques and exclusive social groups during class time.
2. Keep personal information, including medical information, about classmates confidential, and refrain from gossiping about classmates with other classmates and with family and friends.
3. Respect classmates' privacy and modesty in hands-on technique classes while dressing and undressing, and by using proper draping.
4. Practice massage therapy techniques with care and attention to classmates' well-being, and respond promptly to their feedback about pressure, pain, and other concerns.
5. Observe precautions and contraindications with classmates regardless of a technique assignment, and consult with the teacher for necessary modifications to practice with a specific classmate.
6. Use informed voluntary consent as with any client.
7. Seriously consider the possible impact of transference and other psychological factors in relationships with classmates, and refrain from having sexual relations with classmates while in the massage program.
8. Report to school personnel about personally experienced or suspected cases of unethical behavior, especially inappropriate touching, intentional nudity, and other sexual misconduct of classmates during class time and practice sessions outside of class.
9. Do not ask or expect a classmate to lie, cheat, or cover up unethical behavior for another classmate.

Another dual relationship situation occurs when students become massage therapy clients of teachers. These relationships can be problematic, especially for the teacher–massage therapist who may have conflicting roles in the two settings. The positive and negative aspects of such a relationship need to be weighed before entering into it.

It is helpful to remember that after graduation, the relationships between graduates and teachers or school staff become more equal. Waiting to develop other relationships with teachers and school staff is much safer after graduation. It is wise to know and obey school policies about dual relationships between teachers and students.

A third type of dual relationship encountered by students is with family and friends who agree to be practice clients. Thinking of these people as a special kind of client, rather than as "practice dummies" or "guinea pigs" will help students understand how they should be treated. Practice clients should receive all the respect and care due to paying clients in the future. Practice time offers the opportunity to learn how to maintain professional boundaries and to internalize professional standards. Your practice clients will appreciate and respect the level of professionalism that you show during practice sessions.

Finally, providing massage therapy to the general public at outreach sites and in student clinics is usually a student's first encounter with "real" clients. Even though students may not be paid for these services since the experience is part of their education, these are real clients in every sense of the term, and all professional standards apply.

SCOPE OF PRACTICE

Massage therapists are required by their ethical standards and by law to stay within their scope of practice. **Scope of practice** means the range of methods and techniques used in a profession or by a professional, which may also include their intention in performing them (e.g., general wellness or treatment of a medical condition). Scope of practice is defined by professional organizations and licensing laws, often in their official definitions of massage therapy.

The scope of practice for massage therapists generally includes various soft tissue manipulation techniques, joint movements, and hydrotherapy. Different systems or modalities fall under the general scope of massage therapy, for example, trigger point therapy, polarity therapy, and lymphatic massage. A more broadly defined scope of practice might also include massage with mechanical and electronic devices, energy bodywork, relaxation techniques, and physical exercises.

The scope of massage therapy as taught in the United States today does not include "chiropractic adjustments" of the spine and other joints. It also excludes psychotherapy, nutrition, and methods designated exclusively for other professions by law (e.g., skin care by estheticians). Scope of practice can change over time; for example, colon therapy (colonics) was once within the scope of Swedish massage, but is now a separate profession.

A massage therapist's personal scope of practice is limited ethically by the extent of his or her training, that is, massage therapists "will provide only those services which they are qualified to perform" (NCBTMB Code of Ethics, 2005). For example, it would be unethical to accept clients for physical rehabilitation if a massage therapist's training was primarily relaxation oriented.

Scope of practice in any particular state, province, or country is defined by licensing or other laws. Massage therapists are prohibited from diagnosing medical conditions. For example, according to the Illinois licensing law, the purpose of massage is "to enhance the general health and well-being of the mind and body of the recipient" and "does not include the diagnosis of a specific pathology" (Illinois Massage Licensing Act [225 ILCS 57/], 2003). Even if massage therapists are well trained in a certain method, it might be outside of their legal scope of practice under their particular licensing law.

In its grounds for discipline, the Illinois Massage Licensing Act includes "practicing or offering to practice beyond the scope permitted by law or accepting and performing professional responsibilities which the licensee knows or has reason to know that he or she is not competent to perform" (Section 45). Massage therapists could face probation or lose their massage licenses if it is determined that they are practicing beyond their scope.

It is noteworthy that massage is within the legal scope of practice of several other licensed professions. Nurses, physical therapists, and athletic trainers typically use a limited amount of massage as part of the scope of their work. Cosmetologists and barbers are allowed to use massage during facials, manicures, and pedicures. However, the title *massage therapist* is usually restricted to those with professional training and credentials in massage therapy.

Some massage therapists are trained and licensed in more than one profession, for example, nurse–massage therapists. Other common professional combinations are massage therapist and chiropractor, athletic trainer, physical therapist, physical therapy assistant, psychotherapist, colon therapist, esthetician, or cosmetologist. Individuals with more than one license need to keep good boundaries about which "hat" they are wearing (i.e., which role they are playing) in a specific setting or with a specific client. When working under a license, a professional must keep within that particular license's legal scope of practice.

Staying in Bounds

To stay within their scope of practice, massage therapists need to understand two things. First, the legal scope for massage therapy in the specific jurisdiction, and second, the personal scope dictated by their training and experience. Keep a copy of the licensing law under which you practice handy for reference. Read the definition of massage therapy or scope of practice section carefully to understand what is allowed and not allowed under the law in your area.

Do not give advice to clients in areas outside of that scope, and refer clients to the appropriate professionals when their goals or conditions are outside of your scope. Three areas that massage therapists need to be especially clear about are their limits related to treating clients with musculoskeletal injuries and other pathologies, giving nutritional advice, and psychotherapy.

When clients come for massage with physical complaints such as pain or limited movement, it is the massage therapist's responsibility to determine if massage is indicated or contraindicated. Remember that the first principle is to "do no harm." Always ask clients if they have seen medical providers for diagnoses of their complaints. A medical diagnosis can tell you whether massage might do some good, or whether it should be avoided.

For undiagnosed musculoskeletal injuries accompanied by severe pain, deformity, or acute inflammation (redness, swelling, pain), it is best to refer clients to their health care providers or to an emergency room for evaluation. Symptoms for other pathologies that might be detected by massage therapists include skin diseases like cancerous moles, tumors, and misaligned vertebrae or ribs.

Do not verbally speculate about what you think is going on, especially using medical terms. While it is acceptable to observe things like swelling, redness, limited movement, or a client's level of pain, it is inadvisable to use diagnostic terms like *second-degree sprain, plantar fasciitis,* or *cancer.* Putting a label on a set of symptoms is considered diagnosis, and medical diagnosis is not within the scope of practice of massage therapists.

When clients' needs are within the scope of massage therapy, but not within your personal scope, refer clients to another massage therapist who does have the appropriate training and experience. Remember that you can widen your personal scope by getting advanced training and certifications.

Giving nutritional advice, including suggestions about food supplements like vitamins, is outside of the scope of massage therapy. It may be tempting to share with clients your personal beliefs and practices in the area of nutrition. But remember that to clients, you are a person of authority, and they may take what you say as expert advice. Do not say things like, "You should try this …" or, "Take two of these each day, and your joints will feel better."

You could use a qualifier like, "You might want to ask your doctor about …," or "You might want to read the research about …," or "Other clients have reported good results with …," to point them in a direction that you think might be helpful. You can also share information like an article or pamphlet, but avoid seeming like you are telling a client to do something specific outside of your area of expertise.

Massage therapists sometimes increase their incomes by selling food supplements or other products. It is unethical to pressure massage clients to buy anything you are selling, especially if it has the appearance of a prescription.

Mental and emotional wellness is another area in which scope of practice is important to define. When does listening to clients' emotional problems, which may also relate to their physical stresses and illnesses, step over the line of scope of practice? Or as Deane Juhan puts it in the Foreword to *Beyond Technique: The Hidden Dimensions of Bodywork,* what is the difference between "practicing professional psychology and the responsible handling of a range of psychological issues that are likely to emerge in the course of any bodywork practice?" (Kisch).

The massage therapist's role is to provide massage, which is fundamentally a hands-on therapy. As clients relax during massage and let down their defenses, buried emotions may surface. In the course of a massage session, massage therapists may

CASE FOR STUDY

Samantha and the Nutritional Supplements

Samantha is a massage therapist who works in a spa and has built a regular clientele among the spa customers. She has a side business selling nutritional supplements, some of which are advertised as aids to losing weight. Sara, one of Samantha's regulars, is overweight and has expressed an interest in finding a good weight-loss plan.

Question:

Is it ethical for Samantha to mention the nutritional supplements and offer to sell them to Sara?

Things to Consider:

- ▶ Does selling nutritional supplements fall under Samantha's scope of practice as a massage therapist?
- ▶ Are there different roles for Samantha as massage therapist and Samantha as sales representative for the supplements?
- ▶ How does the power differential in the therapeutic relationship impact this situation?
- ▶ Does the spa have a policy about staff selling their own products?

- ▶ Is this situation covered in a code of ethics or standards of practice for massage therapists?
- ▶ Is there potential for causing harm? For doing good?
- ▶ What are alternative courses of action?
- ▶ What are the most important considerations in this situation?
- ▶ What might Samantha's motivation be for selling the product to Sara?
- ▶ What would a former teacher advise Samantha to do?
- ▶ What decision would maintain the highest standards?

Your Reasoning and Conclusions

_____

_____

_____

_____

provide emotional support, listen to a client's concerns, or just be there when a client becomes emotional during a session.

The proper approach is to be supportive while not becoming too involved or trying to help the client resolve his or her feelings by talking. When discussing the client's emotional or mental issues becomes the focus of massage sessions, or the client looks to the massage therapist to resolve psychological issues, the scope of practice has been exceeded. Boundaries must be drawn "between intelligent, compassionate support on the part of the bodyworker and the recognition of the need for further discussion, clarification, and possible referral to various other forms of therapy" (Juhan in Kisch, 1998, p. vii).

Similar to not diagnosing physical pathologies, massage therapists should not diagnose psychological pathologies such as posttraumatic stress disorder, depression, bipolar disorder, disassociation, and psychotic episodes. These are specific medical diagnoses. Massage therapists can, however, recognize symptoms and refer clients to mental health professionals when appropriate.

Some forms of bodywork (e.g., Hakomi and Rosen Method) are specifically designed to help clients resolve psychological issues. These certified practitioners are highly trained in their approaches, and mental and emotional problems are within their scope of practice.

Education and Home Care

It is outside of the scope of practice of massage therapists to give prescriptions, sometimes abbreviated Rx. The word _prescription_ is a medical concept that implies a command on the part of the person making the prescription. Rx implies "do this" or "take this medication" and is sometimes called an "order." Prescriptions are written instructions that patients take to the pharmacy or to another health care professional. Doctors typically prescribe medications and sometimes physical therapy or even massage therapy. Prescriptions are given by doctors for medical conditions and may be paid for by insurance companies.

Massage therapists, on the other hand, provide information and education. They make suggestions to clients about home care for conditions within their scope of practice. For example, a massage therapist might show a client a self-massage technique for recovery after running, or a stretch to help relax and elongate a certain muscle group. Therapists may suggest an ointment for stiff joints or taking advantage of the whirlpool at the health club. Massage therapists do not give prescriptions for topical applications or anything taken internally.

This careful use of words is very important for clarity about scope of practice. Massage therapists do not prescribe, but do offer information, education, and suggestions for home care.

CONFIDENTIALITY AND HIPAA

Confidentiality is an implicit agreement between massage therapist and client, that is, there is an understanding and trust that the massage therapist will not reveal personal or medical information about the client to others without the client's permission. This principle is based on the client's right to privacy.

Confidential information includes what is written on health history forms, what is discussed in massage sessions, and observations about the physical, mental, and emotional health of the client. Even mentioning to someone else that a certain person is a client can be considered a breach of confidentiality. It is unethical to use people's names in advertising without their permission, especially celebrities or people prominent in the community, who prize their privacy. Gossiping about a client's personal life is a serious breach of trust.

The NCBTMB Code of Ethics states that practitioners must "safeguard the confidentiality of all client information, unless disclosure is required by law, court order, or is absolutely necessary for the protection of the public." In some states, licensed massage therapists may have responsibility for reporting cases of abuse of minors and the elderly.

In 1996, the U.S. Congress passed the Health Insurance Portability and Accountability Act (HIPAA) to protect the privacy of medical records. HIPAA requires health care providers to inform patients/clients about their privacy rights and how their information will be used. Providers must get permission in writing to contact insurance companies, and other third parties interested in the health records. Providers must implement procedures to ensure the confidentiality of records, and train employees to comply. In an office or clinic with more than one employee, a person must be designated as responsible for seeing that privacy policies are followed.

Patients/clients have the right to see their records and obtain copies upon request. They may ask for corrections to records if they find mistakes.

Patient/client records must be secured, and only those who need to see them should have access. For example, hard copies of records should be kept in locked files, preferably in isolated records rooms, and electronic files should be protected by passwords on office computers. Patients/clients must give written consent for the use and disclosure of information for treatment, billing, and other health care operations.

CASE FOR STUDY

Jason and His Former Teammates

Jason has accepted some of his former teammates from high school as massage clients. They have kept in touch over the years and get together periodically to watch basketball games. One of these clients, Bill, is a very sociable person. During every appointment, Bill wants to talk to Jason about what's going on with the others. Bill knows some of them come for massage and that Jason has probably seen them more recently than he has.

Question:
Is it ethical for Jason to discuss his other clients with Bill?

Things to Consider:

▶ Is this situation covered in a code of ethics or standards of practice for massage therapists?
▶ What is Jason's responsibility to his other clients in regards to confidentiality?
▶ What aspects of this dual relationship are problematic?
▶ Who might be affected by Jason talking to Bill about other clients during massage sessions?

▶ What if he just listened to what Bill had to say?
▶ What are the "worst-case" and "best-case" scenarios?
▶ What are alternative courses of action?
▶ What are the most important considerations in this situation?
▶ What might Jason's motivation be for talking about their mutual friends to Bill?
▶ What would a former teacher advise Jason to do?
▶ What decision would maintain the highest standards?

Your Reasoning and Conclusions

_____

_____

_____

_____

Client records in a massage therapy office may or may not fall under HIPAA. More clinically or medically oriented practices, especially those that keep records electronically and that take insurance payments, are more clearly subject to HIPAA requirements. In any case, HIPAA offers practical guidelines for ensuring client confidentiality, and massage therapists are encouraged to follow them.

PRACTICAL APPLICATION

It is the responsibility of massage therapists to protect their clients' rights to confidentiality, privacy, and safety. The following three activities explore ways that you might protect clients' rights in your practice.

1 Develop a written statement of policies and procedures related to confidentiality of client information. Include elements required by HIPAA rules for clinical and office situations. Visit the HIPAA Website (www.hhs.gov/ocr/hipaa) for details on the applicable rules.

2 Research the legal responsibility of licensed massage therapists in your state to report suspected cases of

child, spousal, or elder abuse. Discuss your ethical responsibility in these cases. Identify the agencies to which these reports would be made. How does the principle of confidentiality relate to these situations?

3 Research how and to whom to report a massage therapist whom you suspect is doing something unethical. When is it appropriate to make such accusations? What steps do you take to ensure that you approach the situation ethically, and protect yourself legally? After you've developed your answers in writing, discuss them with a group of classmates or a study partner.

HIPAA is administered by the U.S. Department of Health and Human Services (DHHS), and enforcement and complaints are handled by the DHHS Office of Civil Rights (OCR). Information about HIPAA can be found on the HHS website (www.hhs.gov/ocr/hipaa).

Chapter Highlights

▶ The therapeutic relationship between a massage therapist and client is based on specific roles and responsibilities.

- There is an inherent power differential between massage therapists and their clients, with the massage therapist in the position of authority and trust.
- Massage therapists have a fiduciary responsibility to act in the client's best interests.
- The therapeutic relationship involves both explicit and implicit agreements, and the massage therapist is expected to uphold the standards of their profession.

▶ Psychological factors can influence the therapeutic relationship.

- Transference and countertransference.
- Defense mechanisms such as projection, denial, repression, displacement, and resistance.
- Being aware of these psychological factors and their impact helps build healthier therapeutic relationships and avoid unethical behavior.

▶ It is the massage therapist's responsibility to ensure that professional and personal boundaries are respected.

- Boundary crossings may be annoying or uncomfortable.
- Boundary violations are crossings that cause harm.

▶ Dual relationships between massage therapists and clients should be avoided or entered into only after evaluating the potential benefits and risks. They can work only if both parties are emotionally mature and able to maintain appropriate roles in the therapeutic relationship.

▶ When an already established sexual partner becomes a client, it is important to enforce professional boundaries during massage sessions.

▶ Sexualizing the relationship with a current client is highly unethical. Professional standards require ending the therapeutic relationship and waiting a period of time before beginning a sexual relationship with a former client.

▶ Sexual misconduct ranges in severity from relatively minor to severe, and includes flirting, suggestive comments, jokes, discussing sex, seductive behavior, inappropriate touching, and sexual contact.

▶ Use the intervention model to deal with suspected sexual misconduct by a client.

- The intervention model includes interrupting the behavior, describing it, asking for clarification, restating your nonsexual intent, evaluating the client's response, and deciding whether to continue the session or to end it.

▶ Informed voluntary consent is used to get a client's permission to touch him or her in certain areas.

- Five parts of informed voluntary consent are informing, explaining, describing, agreeing, and consenting.

- Afterward, the massage therapist documents the incident in writing, and for self-care, discusses it with a friend or colleague.
- Illegal misconduct by clients should be reported to the local police.

▶ Relationships in school include those with classmates, teachers and administrators, practice clients, and student clinic clients. Ethical principles related to the therapeutic relationship may carry over into these relationships as well.

▶ The scope of practice of massage therapists is defined by professional organizations and by law.

- Massage therapists' personal scope of practice is limited by their training and experience.
- Massage therapists should know their legal scope of practice, and stay within that scope.
- Three areas to be especially clear about are limits on treating clients with illness and injuries, giving nutritional advice, and psychotherapy.
- Massage therapists do not give prescriptions (Rx) to clients, but do provide information, education, and suggestions for home care.

▶ Massage therapists are bound to keep client information confidential. Confidentiality is expected unless disclosure is required by law or necessary to protect the public.

- HIPAA was enacted in 1996 to protect the privacy of medical records.

Exam Review

Learning Outcomes

Use the learning outcomes at the beginning of the chapter and shown here as a guide to the major topics covered. Perform the task given in each outcome, and share your results with a study partner. Check off the tasks as you complete them.

- ❏ Establish appropriate roles in the therapeutic relationship.
- ❏ Recognize the potential impact of psychological factors on the therapeutic relationship.
- ❏ Avoid boundary crossings and violations.
- ❏ Evaluate the potential effects of dual relationships.
- ❏ Avoid all levels of sexual misconduct.
- ❏ Obtain informed voluntary consent when appropriate.
- ❏ Use an intervention model to address inappropriate client behavior.
- ❏ Stay within the scope of practice of massage therapy.
- ❏ Keep client information confidential.
- ❏ Comply with HIPAA rules regarding client records when appropriate.

Key Terms

To study key terms listed at the beginning of the chapter, choose one or more of the following exercises. Writing or talking about ideas helps you better remember them, and explaining them to someone else helps deepen your understanding.

1. Write a one-sentence definition of each key term. Put the term in a general category, and then distinguish it from other terms in that category. For example, "*Confidentiality* is a principle based on the understanding and trust that one person will not divulge private information about others without their permission." Or, "*Informed voluntary consent* is a process used to get the client's permission to touch areas of the body that may have sexual associations or areas out of the scope of general care." Try to capture the essence of each term in a concise statement.

2. Make study cards by writing the key term on one side of a 3 × 5 card, and a concise definition on the other side. Shuffle the cards and read one side, trying to recite either the explanation or word on the other side.

3. Pick out two or three terms and explain how they are related. For example, explain how dual relationships, boundary crossings, and informed voluntary consent may be related.

4. With a study partner, take turns explaining key terms verbally.

5. Make up sentences using one or more key terms. Variation: Read your sentences to a study partner who will ask you to explain unclear statements.

Memory Workout

The following fill-in-the-blank statements test your memory of the main concepts in this chapter.

1. The therapeutic relationship is a special relationship based on specific _____ and _____.

2. Failure or refusal of a client to cooperate in the therapeutic process is called _____.

3. A limit established to maintain a person's own integrity, comfort, or well-being is called a _____ _____.

4. Two issues likely to come up in dual relationships when socializing outside of the massage setting are _____ and _____-_____.

5. Sexual activity with a client is strictly _____ by professional standards.

6. When massaging areas outside of the general scope of massage (e.g., inside the mouth), a plan of _____ and written _____ is required.

7. After an intervention with a client related to sexual misconduct, _____ the incident in writing.

8. Time with _____ clients offers the opportunity to learn how to maintain good professional boundaries.

9. To stay within their scope of practice, two things massage therapists need to understand are the _____ scope in their jurisdiction, and their _____ scope dictated by their training and experience.

10. When discussing a client's emotional or mental issues becomes the _____ of massage sessions, or the client looks to the massage therapist to _____ their psychological issues, scope of practice has been exceeded.

11. Client information may be ethically disclosed if required by _____, or is absolutely necessary for _____ of the public.

12. According to HIPAA rules, medical records must be kept _____, and only those who _____ to see them should have access.

Test Prep

The following multiple-choice questions will help to prepare you for future school and professional exams.

1. Which of the following statements about the power differential in the therapeutic relationship is correct?
   a. The power in the therapeutic relationship is equal between adults.
   b. Clients have greater power in the therapeutic relationship because they are paying for the massage.
   c. Massage therapists have greater power by virtue of their perceived authority.
   d. Power is not an important factor in the therapeutic relationship.

2. Behaviors or thoughts that help us cope with unwanted feelings like fear, guilt, and anger are called
   a. Offense mechanisms
   b. Defense mechanisms
   c. Boundary crossings
   d. Self-disclosure

3. When a massage therapist transfers positive or negative feelings about someone in his or her past into the therapeutic relationship, it is called
   a. Countertransference
   b. Repression
   c. Projection
   d. Denial

4. A boundary transgression experienced as harmful is called a
   a. Boundary collapse
   b. Boundary violation
   c. Boundary crossing
   d. Faulty boundary

5. Which of the following factors is *least* important in determining the potential success of a dual relationship with a client?
   a. The emotional maturity of each person
   b. The ability of each person to maintain his or her proper role in the therapeutic relationship
   c. The power differential within the relationship outside of the therapeutic relationship
   d. How often you socialize outside of the therapeutic relationship

6. Before massaging an area that may cause the client embarrassment or discomfort, the following procedure should always be followed:
   a. Informed voluntary consent
   b. Intervention
   c. Informed intervention
   d. Written consent

7. What is the most ethical response for a massage therapy student to give to a student clinic client who asks him or her out for a dinner date?

    a. "Call me later this week when I am not working in the student clinic."

    b. "Yes, but don't let anyone here know about it."

    c. "Yes, but only as friends."

    d. "No, thank you. I prefer to keep my social and professional lives separate."

8. Which of the following is an example of a massage therapist who has clearly exceeded her scope of practice?

    a. One who refers a client to another health professional for a condition beyond her training

    b. One who gives advice about taking certain vitamins to improve a client's health

    c. One who listens to a client's concern about her situation at work

    d. One who instructs a client on self-massage for home care between appointments

Video Challenge

Watch the appropriate segment of the video on your CD-ROM and then answer the following questions.

Segment 9: Therapeutic Relationship and Ethics

1. Describe the situation involving informed voluntary consent depicted in the video. Identify the essential aspects of informed voluntary consent that are illustrated.

2. What steps in the intervention model are outlined in the video? Give examples of sexual misconduct by clients that may call for using the intervention model.

3. What do the massage therapists interviewed in the video say about maintaining good therapeutic relationships with clients?

Comprehension Exercises

The following exercises provide questions for you to answer and tasks you can do to enhance your understanding of the material presented in this chapter.

1. Explain how a therapeutic relationship is different from a social relationship. Include the concept of power differential in your explanation.

2. What is the purpose of establishing professional boundaries with clients? Give some examples of ways professional boundaries are created.

3. Explain the process of informed voluntary consent. When is it used?

4. Describe the intervention model. When is it used?

5. Define scope of practice. What is the scope of practice for massage therapists in the state you will be working in after graduation? Are there any restrictions on what massage therapists can do under their licensing law?

For Greater Understanding

The following exercises are designed to give you a deeper understanding of the subjects covered in this chapter. Action words are underlined to emphasize the active nature of this approach to learning.

1. Analyze the inherent power differential in your professional relationship with a past or present doctor, dentist, teacher, student, boss, or employee. What was the power based on? Was it ever abused? Compare it to the relationship you foresee with future clients.

2. Identify a personal example of when you used a defense mechanism to cope with a problem situation. Was it useful or counterproductive?

3. Think of a dual relationship that you have had in the past. Evaluate how well it worked out. Identify factors that led to its success or failure.

4. Discuss in small groups or with a study partner any boundary issues that you are having with practice clients. Define the problem and discuss how you are currently handling the issue and how you might approach it better in the future.

5. Research the scope of practice of massage therapists in your state and/or local area. What is the definition of massage therapy? What is allowed or prohibited? What are the disciplinary possibilities for massage therapists practicing outside of their scope?

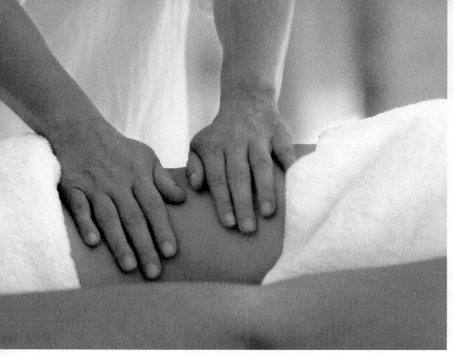

 LEARNING OUTCOMES

After studying this chapter, you will have information to:

1. Follow consumer protection laws.
2. Present your credentials honestly.
3. Make truthful claims for massage therapy.
4. Abide by copyright and trademark laws.
5. Set fair policies related to money.
6. Sell products with integrity.
7. Make and take referrals properly.
8. Increase client base ethically.
9. Report unethical behavior appropriately.

KEY TERMS

Business ethics	Deceptive advertising	Guarantee	Qualifying statements
Copyright	Defamation	Massage establishment ordinance	Trademarks
Consumer protection laws	Endorsements	Occupational license	

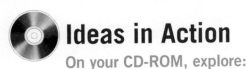

Ideas in Action

On your CD-ROM, explore:

- ▶ Claims for massage therapy
- ▶ Tips and gifts
- ▶ Selling products
- ▶ Interactive video exercises

BUSINESS ETHICS

Business ethics are moral and legal considerations related to commercial transactions (i.e., buying and selling of goods and services) and fair treatment of consumers. Because public safety and financial interests are involved, state and local governments enact business practices and consumer protection laws that give many ethical principles legal force.

Massage therapists, and the spas and clinics that employ them, are selling massage as a health service to customers. So in addition to treating people ethically as *clients* in the therapeutic relationship, they should also be treated fairly as *consumers* who pay money for advertised services.

Because massage therapy consumers are also clients, business ethics related to massage practices are stricter in some ways than in other commercial venues. The ethics of the therapeutic relationship give the massage therapist a fiduciary responsibility not necessarily present in other business transactions. For example, sales people in clothing stores, or servers in restaurants, do not have the same responsibilities to their customers as massage therapists do to their clients. It is a responsibility of all massage therapists to put their clients' well-being above their own personal gain. This is a departure from usual business thinking.

Health professionals usually speak of having a *practice* rather than a *business*. The concept of a practice blends the professional aspects related to relationships with clients and the business aspects of the operation. The professional and business sides together make up a massage therapy practice.

A massage therapist's practice is the totality of his or her work. A practice may range from 5 to 20 regular private clients a week. It may include work in several locations, for example, a few clients at a home office, a few days as an employee of a spa, and a shift at a chiropractor's office. Or a person may be a practicing massage therapist for 20 hours per week and a spa manager for 20 hours. A small, part-time practice may include 2 days' work at a spa. Depending on where they work and the hats they are wearing, massage therapists can have more or less involvement in the business side of massage.

LOCAL AND STATE REGULATIONS

It is a basic ethical principle that massage therapists comply with local and state laws. Therefore, knowledge of applicable laws is fundamental to developing ethical massage practices. There are four general types of laws to be aware of: those related to occupational licenses, zoning ordinances, business licenses, and special massage establishment licenses.

An **occupational license** is a credential issued by a government that gives a person permission to practice a profession in their jurisdiction. In the United States, state governments issue occupational licenses, although in the absence of a state license, some cities and counties issue their own occupational licenses. Thirty-eight states currently regulate massage therapy. Usually states have specific educational requirements and possibly others, such as passing a written examination and not having a criminal record. Licensing laws also specify scope of practice and advertising policies. Having a license for one location does not automatically mean that you can practice in a different place. Having a current occupational license, if one is required, in the location where you are working is a basic ethical principle. More on occupational licensing can be found on page 26 in Chapter 2: The Massage Therapy Profession.

A zoning ordinance is a law that specifies what type of housing or what kind of business can be in a particular location. For example, some areas are zoned for residential housing (e.g., single- or multifamily), and some for certain types of businesses like retail or manufacturing. Massage businesses are sometimes zoned in light industrial or adult entertainment areas, especially if a locality has had problems with massage parlors. Zoning for massage should be checked before signing a lease or other contract for practice space. Some places prohibit small businesses, like massage therapy practices, from operating out of private homes. Zoning variances that allow exceptions to the law may be available if applied for and approved. Zoning ordinances are passed by local governments like towns, cities, or counties.

A business license may be required by town or city government to operate a commercial enterprise in that jurisdiction. This way, government agencies know who is doing business in their area and can ensure that the businesses are complying with all related laws.

Some local governments have enacted special **massage establishment ordinances**, primarily to try to stop massage parlors from being used as a cover for prostitution. In localities where a massage establishment license is required, even health clubs and spas must have a license to offer massage therapy. Since an establishment is a place with an address, massage therapists who work for someone else or who have home visit practices are usually exempt from getting massage establishment licenses.

Establishment ordinances cover a variety of topics such as where the business can be located, hours of operation, shower and toilet facilities, sanitation, posted prices, and other factors related to the business operation. Some have requirements for STD (sexually transmitted disease) tests for persons performing massage, for clothes that may not be worn (e.g., see-through garments), unlocked massage room doors, unannounced inspections, prohibitions on serving liquor, and other regulations obviously aimed toward curbing prostitution, and not for legitimate massage therapists.

As offensive as some of these laws are, massage therapists must work for their revision rather than avoid getting a license to operate their practices. It has become easier to change restrictive establishment and zoning laws as more states adopt occupational licensing that limits the practice of massage to trained and ethical practitioners.

⌐▶ ADVERTISING

Advertising involves disseminating information about your massage therapy practice to potential clients. Advertising takes many forms and includes handing out business cards, putting flyers on community bulletin boards, displaying brochures, putting ads in newspapers and magazines, having a phone directory yellow pages listing, or posting a website on the Internet. Possibilities for advertising are discussed further on page 278 in Chapter 12: Private Practice and Finance.

The ethical principles of advertising are based on values of honesty and integrity. **Deceptive advertising** involves misleading the public about credentials, the nature of the service, its benefits, or how much it costs. The Federal Trade Commission (FTC) defines deceptive advertising as a "representation, omission or practice that is likely to mislead the [reasonable] consumer" (FTC Policy 1983) (www.ftc.gov/bcp/policystmt/addecept.htm). Consumer protection laws are designed to protect the public from unsafe products and services, and from deceptive advertising. Local regulations and licensing laws may also affect how massage therapy may be advertised.

Professional Image

The words and images used in advertising should convey a sense of professionalism (Figure 10–1 ◀). Some of the ethical principles of therapeutic relationships also apply to advertising, for example, those related to professional boundaries and confidentiality.

Using sexual suggestion in advertising text or images is highly unethical and may also be illegal. Unfortunately, many illusions to relaxation and pleasurable touch, which are perfectly ethical benefits of massage, also have sexual overtones. In the United States, the word "masseuse" has become associated with prostitution, so "massage therapist" is the preferred term for a professional massage practitioner.

Ads in big-city telephone books are instructive of what to avoid in advertising. For example, "taste of paradise, female masseuse, 24 hours, outcalls available" with a photo of a seductive-looking woman in a flirtatious pose does not say "professional massage" to the reader. Another example of the type of advertising to avoid is "Angela's magic hands, full body sensual massage, beautiful female masseuses, 'it doesn't get any better than this,'" with a photo of a woman's hands with long nails. "Jeannie Pampers, 'get pampered at your own place'" is less obvious but still suggestive.

Photos should show professional massage with good draping. If using photos of actual clients, get written permission to use their photos or names. Professional associations and photo dealers may have stock photos that can be used in ads.

Giving the wrong impression in advertising can result in unwanted calls from people looking for prostitution. Have colleagues, family, or friends review your ads to evaluate their professional image. What seems cute or clever to you may give the wrong impression about your massage therapy practice.

Credentials

Credentials are professional designations or titles given to massage therapists by organizations such as schools, certification commissions, licensing agencies, and other legitimate institutions. Credentials should be represented honestly in advertising. The general public, clients, employers, and other health professionals rely on credentials to assess a person's training and qualifications.

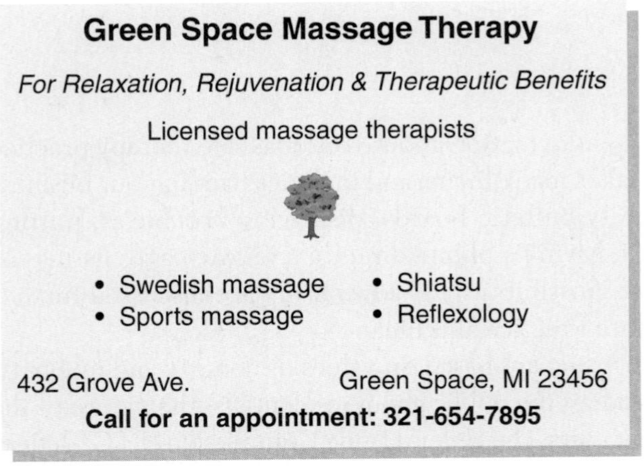

▶ **Figure 10–1** Massage therapy advertising should convey a professional image.

Green Space Massage Therapy

For Relaxation, Rejuvenation & Therapeutic Benefits

Licensed massage therapists

- Swedish massage
- Sports massage
- Shiatsu
- Reflexology

432 Grove Ave.   Green Space, MI 23456

Call for an appointment: 321-654-7895

Obviously, it is unethical to lie about your credentials. It is more likely that a massage therapist would mislead the public by being vague about qualifications or by wording his or her qualifications incorrectly in an advertisement. The ethical question to ask is "Will the public be misled about my qualifications if I use this wording?" Since massage therapists are recognized health professionals, they should display their credentials using the same conventions as other similar professions.

The credential received upon graduation from an entry-level massage program is usually a *certificate of completion* or a *diploma*. The correct way to word that credential in advertising would be "Graduate of ABC Massage School" or "Diploma from ABC Professional Massage Program."

Certification and *certified* are perhaps the most ambiguous terms used as credentials by massage therapists. Being "certified" is currently used to mean anything from completing a weekend workshop in some massage technique, to finishing a 500-hour program, to completing extensive training in a specialty, passing an examination, and keeping up with continuing education. This can be confusing to the general public.

A person from the general public who hears that someone is "certified" in some massage system expects it to be backed by considerable training and acquired expertise. In addition, other health professions generally reserve the term *certification* for lengthy programs aimed at competence in a specialty.

National certification and *board certification* are understood as being conferred after one completes a program of study and passes a written and/or performance examination. Adherence to a code of ethics and continuing education are often required. This level of certification is given by an independent, nonprofit organization or commission whose mission is to provide these credentials for the benefit of the public. Passing a profession's "boards" is often a prerequisite for getting an occupational license.

PRACTICAL APPLICATION

Knowing the correct ways to maintain a professional image and advertise your massage therapy practice is often a matter of knowing what *not* to do. In your community, observe what other massage therapists do to promote their massage practices. Keep your eyes and ears open for examples of good and bad advertising, professional and unprofessional images, appropriate and inappropriate use of credentials, and the use of guarantees, endorsements, and claims made in advertising.

Ask yourself whether the examples you find in your community reflect well or ill upon the massage practitioner. Take note of good examples that you might emulate, without violating another practitioner's copyright, trademark, or patent.

1. Find examples of deceptive advertising in a newspaper or magazine. What makes the advertisements misleading?

2. Find examples of professional and unprofessional advertising for massage in newspapers, magazines, and the phone book. What makes some examples unprofessional?

3. Find examples of credentials displayed correctly and questionably in advertising by massage therapists. What makes the use of credentials questionable?

4. Find examples of guarantees, endorsements, and claims made in advertising. Analyze their legitimacy. Should the massage therapist have such elements in his or her advertising? Would you?

So when is it ethical for a massage therapist to say that he or she is *certified*? Certification boards usually designate titles for those certified by their organization, for example, "Nationally Certified in Therapeutic Massage and Bodywork," or "Certified Rolfer" (Rolf Institute). Some use the word *registered* to mean much the same thing, as in "Registered Polarity Practitioner" (American Polarity Therapy Association). In any case, the title designates the practitioner as having acquired competence and continuing education in the subject, and using the title exactly as it is given is correct.

On the other hand, it is misleading to say that you are certified after having completed a weekend workshop in a certain technique, whether or not the presenter or organization giving the workshop says that you are certified. It is more accurate to say that you have completed so many hours of training in a particular subject. The certificate you receive at the end of the workshop is just that, a certificate of completion for the course of study.

The use of initials after a name is also a matter of judgment. Initials after a name are generally understood to signify an earned academic degree, board certification, or licensing. Academic degrees are AA, BS, MS, PhD, or some variation. NCTMB means Nationally Certified in Therapeutic Massage and Bodywork. In some states, LMT is used to designate Licensed Massage Therapist. In some Canadian provinces, RMT is used to mean Registered Massage Therapist. There are other variations for initials used by massage therapists, and it is wise to check on which designations are correct in your situation.

Initials are not meant to signify an occupation. The initials "MsT" (used to mean "massage therapist") and "CMT" (used to mean having a diploma from a massage program) are misleading. Information should be spelled out if using only initials would be misleading, for example, use the terms "massage therapist" and "graduate massage therapist." It may be more informative to spell out "licensed massage therapist" followed by the license number in states or local areas where licensing is required. Some states require a person's license number to appear on all advertising.

Guarantees and Endorsements

Honesty in advertising means describing the service or product truthfully and avoiding unfounded guarantees and claims. A **guarantee** is a promise that something will work as stated, usually with the implication that the money will be refunded if it does not.

The problem with making guarantees is that no one can predict the outcome of a particular massage session or series of sessions. There are too many variables involved. Statements like "guaranteed to reduce stress" or "guaranteed relief after one session" border on fraudulent. Using a ploy like "guaranteed to work or your money back" is not appropriate for a professional health service.

Some have suggested that massage therapists might use "satisfaction guaranteed or your money back" to show confidence in their service. The therapeutic result is not guaranteed, but the client's satisfaction, which is easier to substantiate, is ensured (Benjamin & Sohnen-Moe).

Endorsements or testimonials are anecdotes from someone besides the massage therapist, usually clients, about how well the massage worked for them. The Federal Trade Commission (FTC, 1980) defines an endorsement as "any advertising message … which consumers are likely to believe reflects the opinions, beliefs, findings, or experience of a party other than the sponsoring advertiser."

Some examples of massage therapy endorsements are: "My tension headaches went away after one massage." "I shaved 10 minutes off my marathon time with sports massage." "My insomnia dissolved, and I sleep like a baby after receiving massage from ABC Massage." Endorsements may be made by individuals, organizations, or experts.

While these statements by particular clients may be true, they may also be misleading. The FTC (1980) states that endorsements "may not contain any representations which would be deceptive, or could not be substantiated if made directly by the advertiser." Making claims for massage therapy is discussed in more detail in a following section.

Endorsements are best used sparingly, if at all. They are not a substitute for the results of research on the effects of massage. Acceptable strategies for advertising are discussed on page 278 in Chapter 12: Private Practice and Finances.

Prices and Bait Advertising

If a price is stated in an advertisement, the massage therapist must honor it in most cases. Exceptions would be if it is an obvious typographical mistake by the printer of a one-time ad (e.g., $6 instead of $65 for an hour-long massage) and would present an undue financial hardship. A mistake on a brochure should be fixed by hand and/or by having the brochure reprinted. It is wise to add in print that prices are subject to change to allow for raising prices in the future, especially in a brochure that someone may keep for a period of time.

If offering a special price or discount, the conditions should be clearly stated. For example, include the time period for the offer (e.g., November 20 through December 24, 2008), the specific service covered, and special conditions like "daytime appointments only."

Bait advertising is unethical and illegal. Bait advertising is "an alluring but insincere offer to sell a product or service which the advertiser in truth does not intend or want to sell" (FTC, 2000). The purpose of bait advertising is to generate leads to potential customers, or to sell something else at a higher price, which is called bait and switch. For example, it would be unethical to advertise $10 for a 30-minute massage, and then pressure the client to switch to a $60 hour massage instead. Other ethical considerations related to pricing are discussed later in the chapter.

⤳ CLAIMS FOR MASSAGE THERAPY

Claims that massage therapists make for their work must be honest and truthful. This includes claims made in advertising or directly spoken to a client, and those stated explicitly or implied. Exaggerated claims, like promising a client that massage can cure pain in five sessions, are almost always unfounded and dishonest.

Furthermore, the FTC requires that claims made in advertising are substantiated claims, that is "that advertisers and ad agencies have a reasonable basis for advertising claims before they are disseminated" (FTC, 1984). Businesses are required to possess information substantiating claims like "research shows..." or "doctors recommend...".

Scientific research is perhaps the most reliable evidence for claims about the various benefits of massage. Legitimate claims may also be backed by knowledge in textbooks and articles, logical deduction from facts, and personal experience. However, claims are legitimately made for massage therapy itself and not for how it will affect any particular client.

Massage therapists are admonished to "accurately inform clients, other health practitioners, and the public of the scope and limitations of their discipline," and to "acknowledge the limitations of and contraindications for massage and bodywork and refer clients to appropriate health professionals" (NCBTMB, 2001). For example, a client who comes for massage to lose weight or "melt fat" would be better referred to a nutritionist or personal trainer.

CASE FOR STUDY

Harry the Natural Salesman

Harry is a natural salesman and promoter, and he is putting those skills to use in building his massage practice. In his advertising, he claims that his massage can cure a variety of modern-day ills and always includes six testimonials from satisfied clients. Harry figures that getting potential clients to make appointments is most important and that all of his customers can only benefit from getting massage.

Question:
Is Harry's style of advertising ethical?

Things to Consider:

▶ Are there any legal implications with Harry's style of advertising related to claims for massage and the use of testimonials?
▶ Would this style of advertising be permitted under massage therapy licensing laws?
▶ Do any consumer protection laws apply?
▶ If Harry's ads are successful in attracting clients, aren't they acceptable from a business point of view?

▶ How does his style of advertising live up to values of honesty, integrity, and professionalism?
▶ Is this situation covered in a code of ethics or standards of practice for massage therapists?
▶ Who might be affected by this style of advertising, either positively or negatively?
▶ What is Harry's major motivation with this style of advertising?
▶ What are the most important considerations in this situation?
▶ What decision would maintain the highest standards?

Your Reasoning and Conclusions
_____
_____
_____
_____

It is the responsibility of massage therapists to become knowledgeable about the potential effects and benefits of massage, and to stay up-to-date on the latest research and knowledge in the field. This can be accomplished through reading and studying journals, pursuing continuing education, and looking up research on various topics of interest. Massage therapists who practice critical thinking examine evidence for the benefits of massage, and do not accept everything they read or hear without question.

Qualify claims about massage therapy by citing sources of information. **Qualifying statements** that can be made when speaking to clients include "in a pathology and massage text it says …," "a recent research study found that …," "from my experience I've noticed that …," "according to the manufacturer, this product …," and "other clients have reported that …". Having to qualify statements forces massage therapists to become more aware of how they know what they know. It is wise to check out claims made by vendors selling something or claims for new or unique techniques. Do not make claims you cannot reasonably substantiate or that you know or suspect are false.

COPYRIGHTS, TRADEMARKS, AND PATENTS

Copyrights, trademarks, and patents offer legal protection for intellectual property rights. It is a matter of ethics that these protections be respected by individuals and businesses.

Copyright laws protect written, musical, and artistic works from unauthorized use and are designated by the symbol ©. Copyrights are administered in the United States by the U.S. Copyright Office at the Library of Congress in Washington, D.C. (www.copyright.gov).

According to copyright laws, a person cannot copy brochures, flyers, pamphlets, business logos, artwork, books or significant parts of books, and other materials written or prepared by someone else without the author's or copyright holder's expressed permission. A work receives copyright protection immediately from the time it exists in fixed form. Protected use includes reproduction, derivative works, and distribution of copies. Authors and artists may sign over copyright for their work to someone else, such as a publisher.

When developing advertising materials and other documents, copyrighted works may be used for ideas and for reference, but should not be copied exactly and used as one's own. For example, it would be unethical to take someone else's unique brochure and just replace that person's name with yours without permission.

Some brochures are available for purchase and have a space for printing a business name and contact information. It is all right to buy these brochures for distribution, but unethical to copy them rather than ordering more from the publisher.

Fair use of a copyrighted work is allowed. "Fair use" allows limited use of copyrighted materials for education and research purposes. This does not apply to whole works or significant parts of works such as whole chapters in a book. Any use that takes away from the copyright holder's potential market for selling the work is not fair use. For example, if an author creates drawings of self-massage techniques to give to clients for home care and makes them available for purchase in notepad format, it would be unethical and illegal for you to photocopy them for your clients. If, however, they are published in a book, and the author clearly states that they may be copied for clients, then this use does not violate copyright law.

Trademarks offer exclusive use of a name or symbol to identify unique goods and services, and use the symbol ™ or ® for registered trademarks. Trademarks distinguish a particular brand or company from others. Trademarks are handled by the U.S. Patent and Trademark Office in Washington, D.C. (www.uspto.gov). States in the United States and Canadian provinces may also have laws that protect trademarks like names and logos for businesses that operate within their jurisdictions.

Trademarks include unique business names like "Wellspring Massage Therapy" or "Morristown Spa and Massage," along with the logo or identifying design used on documents and in advertising. Trademarks for services are also called *service marks* (sm). The business that uses the name or logo first and consistently on materials associated with the business has the right to the trademark. Most states have offices where the names of businesses can be researched to see if they are already in use. It is wise to register the name of your practice or business to protect it from use by someone else.

Artwork for logos and text for advertising may be in the public domain, meaning that they are commonly available or have been created for public distribution. Books of stock logos and clip art are available at printing companies, and professional associations may have text and designs for advertising available for general use. Using words and artwork in the public domain is an ethically safe and economical alternative to developing your own unique materials.

Massage and bodywork systems like Rolfing®, Jin Shin Do®, and Feldenkrais Method® are registered trademarks. Massage therapists may not use trademarked names in their advertising or descriptions of their work unless they hold credentials from the trademarked organizations that allow them to use the designation.

Patents are protections for inventions and include utility and design patents. The inventor of a massage tool, machine, or other product related to massage may apply for a patent from the U.S. Patent and Trademark Office. Patented inventions may not be copied by others for sale.

FEES AND PRICING

The exchange of money is an integral part of massage therapy practices and must be done with honesty and integrity. Key principles are fair compensation, clarity, and consistency.

Fair compensation is determined partially by the usual rate for massage in a particular location. What are others charging? Generally speaking, massage costs more in big cities than in rural areas or areas with lower costs of living. A house call usually costs more than in-office massage. A massage therapist with more training and/or experience may command a rate at the higher end of the scale than one just out of school. In many ways "fair" is determined by what the market will bear, that is, what people are willing to pay.

Once established, a pricing policy should be clearly stated in promotional materials, and posted prominently in the place of business. Simplicity is best, but different rates for different session lengths (usually 30, 60, or 90 minutes), or sessions for which special training is required (e.g., lymphatic drainage massage or sports massage) are appropriate.

Be sure that policies regarding when payment is expected and what form it can take (cash, check, credit/debit card) are clear. Tell clients before a session begins what rate will be charged. If a session goes longer than expected, it is the massage therapist's responsibility, and the client would not ordinarily be charged extra.

CASE FOR STUDY

Lilly's Pricing System

Lilly is just beginning to build her massage therapy practice. She worries about being competitive with other massage therapists in the area and has difficulty asking for money from clients. The going rate for massage seems so high to her. She never publishes her rates and changes her rates according to what she thinks the client can afford or will be willing to pay.

Question:

Is Lilly's pricing system ethical?

Things to Consider:

▶ Are there any legal implications for Lilly's pricing system? Do local licensing laws require posting rates?
▶ Does Lilly have the right to charge what she wants for her massage?
▶ How does her system of pricing live up to values of fairness and integrity?

▶ Is this situation covered in a code of ethics or standards of practice for massage therapists?
▶ Who might be affected by her system of pricing?
▶ What is Lilly's major motivation for this pricing system?
▶ What are alternative pricing strategies?
▶ What are the most important considerations in this situation?
▶ What decision would maintain the highest standards?

Your Reasoning and Conclusions

_____

_____

_____

_____

Consistent pricing is a matter of fairness. Charging one person less than another can be complicated, even when offering discounts for friends and family. Treating discounted sessions with less professionalism is unethical.

Special pricing like sliding scales and prepaid plans require careful thought. Sliding scales are problematic and are avoided by most practitioners. If a sliding scale is adopted, establish objective guidelines, for example, based on a person's or family's income. Prepaid plans can be good for marketing, but be sure to state the terms clearly. An example of a prepaid plan is a package of six prepaid sessions for the price of five sessions. Make time limits clear, like "must be used within one year" or by a certain expiration date.

Charging more for a massage when an insurance company is paying is considered unethical and may also be illegal. While it is true that practices using third-party payments have more paperwork to complete, those costs are typically absorbed in general operation costs.

TIPS AND GIFTS

Tips are gratuities (i.e., given in gratitude) over and above the cost of a massage session given directly to the massage therapist. Whether a tip is given and the amount is determined at the discretion of the client. Accepting tips in an ethical way calls for some careful thought.

Soliciting or accepting tips for massage therapy poses ethical questions not relevant to other service occupations. Complicating factors are that massage therapy is given in a variety of settings with different customs related to tipping (e.g., spas, salons, medical settings, and private offices), that massage therapists may have independent practices or may be employees, and that massage involves a therapeutic relationship with clients, which presents special responsibilities.

Accepting tips can be ethical if they do not negatively influence the therapeutic relationship, if they are truly optional, and if tippers and non-tippers receive the same level of care. Tips are most appropriate in settings where it is customary to give gratuities for services such as at salons, spas, hotels, and resorts.

In places where tipping is customary, owners of the business are usually not tipped. Employees or independent contractors who receive less than the cost of the massage are commonly tipped. In private massage practices, where the practitioner sets and keeps the full price of the massage, tips should not be expected.

Tips for massage are problematic in settings such as medical clinics, chiropractic offices, and private practices. Tipping health professionals is not customary. Tipping may be confusing and awkward for clients in settings considered to be health care related, rather than personal service or recreation related.

It is appropriate to let clients know if tipping is customary in a certain setting. A sign that states "Tips appreciated" lets clients know that it is a place where tips are accepted. However, clients must never feel that they need to give a tip to receive high-quality service. Tips should never be solicited personally by massage therapists.

Turn down tips that have expectations attached and tips that are too large. Tips that seem too large (e.g., $20 for a $60 massage) may involve transference on the part of the client or may be an attempt to gain favor. Such tips cross professional boundaries and should not be accepted. On the other hand, a client who offers a larger than usual tip in appreciation for pain relief or doing well in a big race after receiving sports massage may simply be expressing his or her gratitude, and accepting the tip causes no harm. These are judgment calls for the massage therapist to make. It is acceptable to adopt a "no tipping" policy in a private practice.

Gifts are a similar situation. Nonmonetary gifts that are tokens given in appreciation or at special times like the holidays may be appropriate to accept. Gifts given to gain favor compromise the therapeutic relationship and cross boundaries, and should be politely refused. Never accept a gift from a client whom you suspect has a romantic interest in you. Gifts with high monetary value are also inappropriate to accept. Trust your intuition to tell you that something does not seem right, or ask advice about it from a colleague or friend who understands the professional implications involved.

According to the IRS, tips are taxable income and must be reported when filing income tax returns. Monetary gifts would be considered tips. Keep a record of all tips received.

⟶ SELLING PRODUCTS

Some massage therapists sell products in conjunction with their massage practices. Massage-related products include massage oils and lotions, tools for self-massage like foot rollers, support pillows, hot and cold packs, and books and videos. Having products for sale can be a valuable service to clients and is not unethical as long as clients do not feel pressured to buy them from you. Your role as a massage therapist would be to inform clients about the benefits of products with the opportunity to buy them, if desired. There are clearer boundaries if products for sale are not displayed in the massage room, but are in a reception or sales area (Figure 10–2 ◀).

Selling products is often part of a spa or salon business, and employees may be expected to "push" the products for sale. This is problematic for massage therapists, who are cautioned not to use the power differential in the therapeutic relationship for their personal gain. As stated above, educating clients and making products available is acceptable; however, talking clients into products they may not want or need is not.

Be particularly aware of your conflict of interest if you are part of a multilevel marketing program. It is not ethical to use your massage clients to meet sales goals. Clients who feel pressured into buying products outside of their interest in receiving massage may also feel taken advantage of and seek massage elsewhere.

Be especially mindful if you are selling nutritional supplements, herbal preparations, or vitamins. Do not confuse being trained in selling a product by its manufacturer or distributor with having professional education in nutrition. To keep clear boundaries between your massage practice and nutritional sales, make sepa-

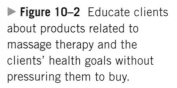

▶ **Figure 10–2** Educate clients about products related to massage therapy and the clients' health goals without pressuring them to buy.

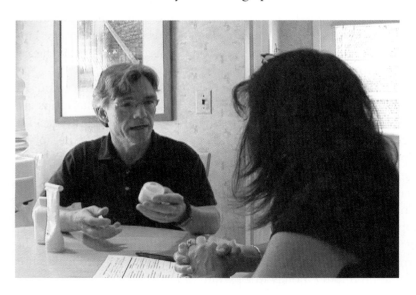

rate appointments to talk to clients about these other products, preferably in a space different from the massage office.

Know that your massage clients may see you as a health expert and may therefore give unwarranted trust in your judgment about nutrition. Make it clear that you are not an expert in nutrition unless you have additional academic training and credentials in that field. If clients feel that you are prescribing supplements for a specific medical condition, you may be perceived as practicing medicine without a license. You may also be liable if the client has a negative reaction to a product you sold to him or her.

INSURANCE BILLING

Some insurance companies cover massage therapy in their policies. Massage therapists who accept clients using insurance to pay their bills need to be educated about relevant company policies and procedures. It is dishonest and illegal to misrepresent the nature of treatment or the number of sessions given to a client. Keep adequate records to substantiate charges billed. It is unethical, and may be illegal in some places, to charge insurance companies more than clients who are paying out of pocket.

Since massage therapists are not considered primary health care providers (PHCPs), a diagnosis from a PHCP is usually necessary for insurance billing. These referrals are for a specific pathology, and massage billed to an insurance company must be related to treatment for the stated condition. "According to standard insurance definitions, treatment is warranted until the condition is corrected or maximum improvement is made" and also includes instruction for self-care and prevention of future occurrences of the same problem (Benjamin & Sohnen-Moe, 2003, p. 207). Massage sessions for maintenance and prevention are not usually included in insurance plans and would not be billed as treatment.

REFERRALS

It is expected that massage therapists make referrals to other health professionals when clients have needs outside of the therapists' scope of practice, or when massage may not be the best treatment for a specific condition. A client's needs may also be beyond a particular massage therapist's training or expertise, and referral to a massage therapist with advanced or specialized training might be best for the client.

Keeping a list of other health professionals (including doctors, chiropractors, naturopathic physicians, physical therapists, athletic trainers, and massage therapists) that you believe are competent and ethical is a good practice. When making referrals, give the client two or three names from which to choose. Become familiar with websites that list certified practitioners of specific massage and bodywork systems, or that list massage therapists and their specialties. Refer clients to those sites if appropriate.

It is unethical for health practitioners to reward each other for referrals in a quid pro quo manner with either money or gifts. For example, it would be unethical for a chiropractor to give a massage therapist $10 for every referral he or she makes to the chiropractor. This violates the principle of avoiding conflict of interest. Massage therapists are advised to "refuse any gifts or benefits which are intended to influence a referral, decision or treatment that are purely for personal gain and not for the good of the client" (NCBTMB, 2001).

The same principles apply when accepting referrals. Do not accept clients on referral that have conditions outside of your scope, and do not reward referrals made to you. Clients should be able to trust that referrals are made in their best interests and not for monetary gain. A thank you note for referrals is an appropriate acknowledgment. However, because of confidentiality issues, you might consider omitting the name of the client and just give a simple "thank you for a recent referral."

CLIENT BASE

Building a base of regular clients is the foundation of success for massage therapists, whether they are in private practice or employed somewhere like a spa. Clients will come back to massage therapists whom they respect and trust, and who give them good service.

There are a few ethical pitfalls in attracting and keeping clients. Previous sections have discussed making false claims and exceeding scope of practice. Another pitfall is trying to build yourself up by speaking poorly of another massage therapist. A wise person once said, "You don't make yourself taller by cutting down your neighbor." It is better to concentrate on the quality of what you offer than criticize a colleague to a client.

If you are employed somewhere like a spa or clinic, the clients you see there are shared by you and the larger business. It is considered unethical, and may be a violation of an employment agreement, to solicit clients seen at an employer's place for your private practice. For example, it would be unethical to say to a client, "Why don't you come for massage at my home office instead of here?" The temptation is there, since you might make more money by seeing a client in your own space.

The issue of "stealing" clients can be a murky one, since clients have free choice regarding from whom they receive massage. They also can get attached to their massage therapists, much the same as they do to the people who cut their hair. What if a regular client requests to see you at your place for the sake of convenience? If your employment agreement explicitly prohibits seeing the company's clients at another place, then this would be unethical.

What if you are leaving an employer and your clients want to keep seeing you for massage? It would be unethical to actually make an appointment for your private practice while on your employer's premises. However, providing information about your practice, if directly asked by a client, would in most circumstances be all right. Then the client can take the initiative to call you if he or she prefers to continue as your client. The key principles here are "no solicitation," the "client's initiative," and any prior employment agreement. In complex cases like these, it is best to apply the ethical decision-making model described on page 191 in Chapter 8: Foundations of Ethics to determine the most ethical path.

DEFAMATION

Defamation is a legal term for injury to a person or an organization's reputation. Defamation is known as *libel* if written and as *slander* if spoken. It is highly unethical to defame the character or reputation of a client or another massage therapist or health professional.

Defamation can also result in a civil lawsuit if the person defamed experiences a loss of some kind. A court may award a plaintiff monetary damages if the statements were untrue and/or made with malice or intent to harm. To avoid such issues, do not repeat malicious gossip.

CASE FOR STUDY

Rochelle and Client Choice

Rochelle started out giving massage at a local beauty salon as an independent contractor. There was a verbal agreement that she could use a spare room for appointments and split the receipts 60/40 with the salon owners. After a while, Rochelle decided that she would leave the salon and take a job at a local spa that offered better working conditions and employee benefits. She would receive a bit less income from each massage, but she figured that it was to her advantage overall. Another massage therapist is taking Rochelle's place at the salon. Massage rates are a little higher at the spa than at the salon.

Question:

Is it ethical for Rochelle to solicit her salon clients to come to the spa for massage instead of to the salon?

Things to Consider:

- ▶ Are there any legal implications in this situation?
- ▶ Was there an explicit or implicit agreement with the salon about whose customers the massage clients were?
- ▶ What values are involved in a decision to solicit those clients?
- ▶ Is this situation covered in a code of ethics or standards of practice for massage therapists?
- ▶ Who might be affected by Rochelle's solicitation, either positively or negatively?
- ▶ What is Rochelle's major motivation for soliciting these clients?
- ▶ What are alternative courses of action?
- ▶ What are the most important considerations in this situation?
- ▶ What decision would maintain the highest standards?

Your Reasoning and Conclusions

_____

_____

_____

_____

Defamation laws differ slightly in different jurisdictions but usually include accusations of criminal conduct and allegations that negatively affect a person's business or profession. Stating that a person has a disease or has engaged in certain sexual activity, thus damaging his or her reputation, may also be defamation.

Descriptive statements and opinions about situations are two different things. For example, it would be better to say to a coworker that a client came for massage smelling like beer and talking with a slur rather than to call him a "drunk" or "lush." If the descriptive statement was made in confidence as a matter of information to protect other massage therapists, or to describe to a supervisor why you refused to work with a client at a specific appointment, it might not qualify as defamation with damages. A court of law would make its own judgment.

Remember that a client may ask to see his or her records, so what is written in them needs to be thought out carefully to avoid accusations of libel. It is an especially sensitive situation to report perceived misbehavior by a client, or to record something not related to the massage itself that was told in confidence in a session. It is wise to stick with accurate objective descriptions and tell a coworker or colleague immediately after something unusual happens.

It is also defamation to criticize or malign another massage therapist or health professional. If you do not trust the competence of a colleague, and for some reason wish to reveal your view to someone else, state the facts and then your opinion separately. For example, "Two of my clients have complained about massage therapist 'G' using too much pressure and bruising them. I believe that she is being insensitive."

SAFETY AND WELFARE OF CLIENTS

Massage therapists are responsible for the safety and well-being of their clients during massage sessions and while clients are on the premises. It is unethical to put clients in danger through carelessness.

Provide regular maintenance for massage tables, chairs, and other equipment. Make sure surfaces are sanitary and massage procedures hygienic. Massage offices should be well lighted and free from obstacles that could cause accidents.

Massage therapists are guilty of negligence if an accident or injury is caused by their carelessness. If the cause is something a trained practitioner is expected to know, the massage therapist may be guilty of malpractice.

To protect themselves and their clients financially, massage therapists need to carry accident (slip and fall) insurance, as well as professional liability insurance. Carrying certain types of insurance may be a condition for maintaining a license to practice.

REPORTING UNETHICAL BEHAVIOR

What should massage therapists do when they suspect another massage therapist of unethical behavior? What kinds of actions are important to report? How much evidence is enough to accuse someone of wrongdoing? To whom do they report their suspicions? These are some important questions to ask before accusing someone of something that may affect that person's future as a massage therapist.

Before reporting suspected unethical behavior, be clear about the facts of the case and reasonably sure that something unethical happened. If the unethical behavior is relatively minor, and the person unaware that he or she is behaving unethically, talking to the offender about the situation may be the best response. For example, if someone starts talking inappropriately about a client, make a statement such as "This seems like gossip to me. We'd better not continue this conversation."

Reminding a coworker or colleague of an ethical principle may be enough to stop the unethical behavior. For example, if coworkers are leaving client files open on a desk, remind them that files are confidential and must be kept secure. Friendly reminders are usually accepted well.

If, however, the situation involves physical or emotional harm to a client, or to another health professional, then more official action may be required. Professional associations, certification commissions, and licensing agencies have procedures for reporting misconduct by professionals. Unethical conduct can result in disciplinary action against the offender, which ranges from letters of reprimand, to probation, to losing a membership or license. These actions would follow due process, investigation, and a hearing.

Passing along secondhand information is less desirable than convincing the person harmed, or a firsthand witness, to file a complaint. However, if the allegations are serious enough, and there is strong evidence for them, then they could be reported with or without firsthand information. The organization or agency receiving the report can determine if it wants to follow through with a hearing.

Where does someone report suspected unlawful behavior? If there is legal jurisdiction, then the licensing agency would be contacted. If it involves a business practice like deceptive advertising or a payment dispute, then a complaint can also be filed with the Better Business Bureau. The Federal Trade Commission has a complaint procedure in place for consumer protection (www.ftc.gov). Local and state governments may also have procedures for consumer complaints.

CRITICAL THINKING

If your state has occupational licensing, explain in writing the process for reporting misconduct by a massage therapist. Then answer the following questions:

1 In your state, what constitutes professional misconduct?

2 What disciplinary actions might happen to a massage therapist who is proven to have engaged in misconduct?

3 How do the standards of practice and code of ethics for massage practitioners protect both the practitioner and the consumer?

Chapter Highlights

▶ Business ethics are moral and legal considerations related to commercial transactions.

▶ Business practices and consumer protection laws give ethical principles legal force.

▶ A massage therapy practice blends professional aspects related to client relationships with business aspects of the operation; in this sense, a client is also a customer.

▶ Massage therapists must comply with local and state laws including occupational licensing laws, zoning ordinances, and business license and establishment license requirements.

▶ Design advertising to be professional and avoid deception.

  ● Display credentials honestly and correctly.
  ● Limit guarantees or promises about massage therapy, and use endorsements and testimonials sparingly.
  ● Advertised prices must be honored, discounts defined clearly, and bait advertising avoided.

▶ Claims for massage therapy must be honest and truthful, and backed up by research, if possible.

  ● Qualify claims by citing sources of information like textbooks or experience.

▶ Copyright, trademark, and patent laws protect intellectual property rights. Never claim another person's work as your own, and do follow principles of fair use.

  ● Massage therapists may not use trademarked names for massage and bodywork unless they hold proper training and authorization.

▶ Accepting tips or gifts is acceptable under certain circumstances.

  ● Tips are taxable income to be reported when filing income tax returns.
  ● Refuse tips and gifts if there are unethical expectations attached, and never accept gifts from clients who may have romantic intentions.

▶ Selling products as part of a massage practice may be ethical if done properly.

  ● Educating clients about useful products is acceptable, but pressuring them to buy is not.
  ● Do not use clients to meet sales quotas.
  ● Special care about scope of practice is warranted when selling nutritional products.

▶ When billing insurance companies for massage services, follow company policies and procedures and report treatment given honestly.

  ● It is unethical, and may be illegal in some places, to charge insurance companies more than clients who are paying out of pocket.

▶ Refer clients to other qualified health professionals for treatment beyond the scope of a massage therapist's own knowledge and skills.

  ● Receiving money or gifts from another health professional for referrals is considered a conflict of interest and is unethical.

▶ When building a client base, emphasize the quality of your service, rather than criticizing other massage therapists.
▶ Do not solicit clients of an employer's business for your own private practice.
▶ Defamation—that is, injury to another's reputation—is called libel if written and slander if spoken. Defamation can result in a civil lawsuit if the person defamed experiences a loss.

  ● It is safer to keep to descriptive statements of something that happened rather than give interpretations or opinions.
  ● Clients are entitled to see their records, so massage therapists should be especially careful about what is written in them.

▶ It is unethical to put clients in danger through carelessness or negligence.

  ● Keep premises and equipment clean and well maintained.

▶ Report suspected serious unethical behavior by other massage therapists to proper authorities, such as a state licensing agency or the local police.

Exam Review

Learning Outcomes

Use the learning outcomes at the beginning of the chapter and shown here as a guide to the major topics covered. Perform the task given in each outcome, and share your results with a study partner. Check off the tasks as you complete them.

  ❏ Follow consumer protection laws.
  ❏ Present your credentials honestly.
  ❏ Make truthful claims for massage therapy.
  ❏ Abide by copyright and trademark laws.

❏ Set fair policies related to money.
❏ Sell products with integrity.
❏ Make and take referrals properly.
❏ Increase client base ethically.
❏ Report unethical behavior appropriately.

Key Terms

To study key terms listed at the beginning of the chapter, choose one or more of the following exercises. Writing or talking about ideas helps you better remember them, and explaining them to someone else helps deepen your understanding.

1. Write a one-sentence definition of each key term. Put the term in a general category, and then distinguish it from other terms in that category. For example, "A *guarantee* is a promise that something will work as advertised." Or, "*Copyright* laws protect written, musical, and artistic works from unauthorized use." Try to capture the essence of each term in a concise statement.

2. Make study cards by writing the key term on one side of a 3 × 5 card and a concise definition on the other side. Shuffle the cards and read one side, trying to recite either the explanation or term on the other side.

3. Pick out two or three terms and explain how they are related. For example, explain how endorsements and deceptive advertising might be related.

4. With a study partner, take turns explaining key terms verbally.

5. Make up sentences using one or more key terms. Variation: Read your sentences to a study partner who will ask you to explain unclear statements.

Memory Workout

The following fill-in-the-blank statements test your memory of the main concepts in this chapter.

1. Business ethics are moral and legal considerations related to _____ transactions.

2. Massage therapists can mislead the public by being _____ about their qualifications or by wording their qualifications _____.

3. Information should be _____ out completely if using initials after a name would be misleading.

4. The FTC states that endorsements "may not contain any representation which would be _____, or could not be _____."

5. Advertising something for a certain price, and then pressuring the client/customer to buy something more expensive, is called _____ advertising.

6. Claims about massage should be qualified by citing _____ of information.

7. Massage therapists may not use _____ names for forms of bodywork, unless they have earned the appropriate credentials.

8. Charging more for a massage when an _____ company is paying the bill is considered unethical.

9. Tips that should be turned down are ones with _____ attached, or that are too _____.

10. Do not confuse being trained in selling a nutritional product by its manufacturer or distributor with having _____ _____ in nutrition.

11. It is unethical for health professionals to _____ each other for referrals.

12. It is unethical to _____ clients seen first at an employer's business.

Test Prep

The following multiple-choice questions will help to prepare you for future school and professional exams.

1. Consumer protection laws are designed to
   a. Ensure a minimum level of training for professionals
   b. Regulate where certain types of businesses can be located
   c. Protect the public from unsafe products and deceptive advertising
   d. Protect employees from unfair employment situations

2. When a seller makes a promise that something will work as stated, with the implication that the money will be refunded if it does not, it is called
   a. Endorsement
   b. Guarantee
   c. Testimonial
   d. Bait advertising

3. Which of the following is the most ethical method of advertising to clients that you have graduated from a massage therapy program?
   a. Spelling out "Graduate of ABC Massage Therapy School"
   b. Using the initials "GMT" after your name to designate "graduate massage therapist"
   c. Using the initials "CMT" after your name to designate "certified massage therapist"
   d. Any of the above

4. Which of the following offers legal protection for the exclusive use of a name or symbol to identify unique goods and services?
   a. Copyright
   b. Trademark
   c. Patent
   d. Licensing

5. When is it ethical to pressure massage clients to buy goods you have for sale?
   a. When you must meet a sales goal
   b. When you are sure that they will benefit from the product
   c. When you need to reduce inventory
   d. Never

6. Slander is
   a. Gossiping about someone
   b. Publicly criticizing someone's behavior
   c. Causing injury to someone's reputation by something written
   d. Causing injury to someone's reputation by something spoken

7. If an accident or injury results from carelessness, it is called

   a. Libel   c. Unfortunate

   b. Negligence   d. An act of God

8. When is it ethical to give reduced service to a client who never leaves a tip?

   a. At spas where tipping is customary   c. When saving energy for clients who do tip

   b. When a "tips accepted" sign is clearly visible   d. Never

Video Challenge

Watch the appropriate segment of the video on your CD-ROM and then answer the following questions.

Segment 10: Business Ethics

1. What are the ethical principles related to advertising discussed in the video?

2. What do the massage therapists in the video say regarding when accepting tips is ethical and when to turn them down?

3. What types of products might massage therapists sell to clients? What are some ethical principles related to selling products mentioned in the video?

Comprehension Exercises

The following exercises provide questions for you to answer and tasks you can do to enhance your understanding of the material presented in this chapter.

1. What types of laws must massage therapists be aware of for building ethical practices? What is the overreaching ethical principle related to laws?

2. What does the law say about making claims for a product or service? How do you qualify claims made for massage? Give an example.

3. When is it *not* ethical to accept tips from clients? What is the ethical principle related to soliciting tips?

4. What are the main ethical issues related to massage therapists selling products as part of their practices? Under what conditions is it ethical for a massage therapist to sell products to clients?

For Greater Understanding

The following exercises are designed to give you a deeper understanding of the subjects covered in this chapter. Action words are underlined to emphasize the active nature of this approach to learning.

1. Tell the class or a study partner about a time you were treated unfairly or dishonestly in a business transaction. Analyze what happened in ethical and legal terms. Were consumer protection laws or any other laws broken?

2. Speak to the class or a study partner about a time you were given a gift that didn't feel right to you (i.e., with expectations attached or too costly given

your relationship with the person). <u>Analyze</u> the person's motivation and your response. Was the outcome positive or negative? Would you act differently today?

3. <u>Tell</u> the class or a study partner about a time you felt pressured to buy something. <u>Analyze</u> the motivation of the seller and how you felt being pressured.

4. <u>Obtain</u> a copy of an employment agreement for a massage therapist at a spa or clinic. <u>Analyze</u> provisions for soliciting clients, and discuss it in terms of fairness or unfairness.

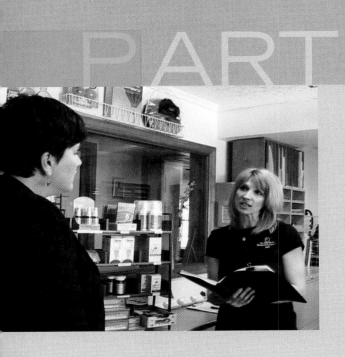

PART V

▶ **Chapter 11**
Career Plans
and Employment

▶ **Chapter 12**
Private Practice
and Finances

| CAREER DEVELOPMENT

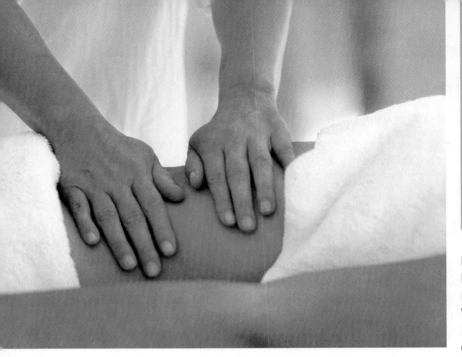

11

Career Plans and Employment

LEARNING OUTCOMES

After studying this chapter, you will have information to:

1. Develop career plans for the first year after graduation.
2. Create a vision and identity for a massage practice.
3. Identify the benefits and drawbacks of employment and self-employment.
4. Design a résumé, business card, brochure, and website.
5. Locate and secure employment as a massage therapist.

KEY TERMS

Employee	Mission statement	Résumé	Sole proprietor
Income goal	Practice identity	Self-employed	Vision
Independent contractor	Private practice		

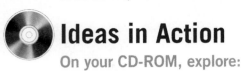

Ideas in Action

On your CD-ROM, explore:

▶ Developing a vision
▶ Employment interview

▶ Getting started in your career
▶ Interactive video exercises

⤷→ FOLLOW YOUR DREAM

Career plans begin with a dream—imagining the possibilities for your future as a massage therapist. Making that dream come true takes planning, effort, and perseverance. Career plans provide direction to achieving success step-by-step.

As described in Chapter 1, there are many career possibilities for massage therapists. Some work full time and some part time. Some look for certain settings such as spas, health clubs, integrative health care, or private practice. Some prefer to focus on specific populations like athletes, older adults, people with certain diseases, or those in rehabilitation from musculoskeletal injuries. Others focus on a specific type of massage and bodywork, such as Western massage, Asian bodywork therapy, reflexology, or chair massage. Many choose eclectic practices with a variety of clients and types of massage. There are many options.

A good place to begin career plans is to formulate your practice vision and identity. Focus for now on the first year after graduation. You can always revise the plan later on as you become more experienced and your vision evolves, but it is important to make a decision and choose a place to start.

⤷→ VISION

All aspects of your practice flow from your vision. Your **vision** is how you see your practice in its broad scope. It includes whether you work full time or part time, your practice format, the setting you are working in, your clients, what kind of massage you offer, and your income goals. The clearer the vision, the more likely you will be to achieve your career dreams one year after graduation and for each year of your practice into the future. A worksheet for outlining your practice vision is provided in Figure 11–1 ◀.

Part-Time or Full-Time Work

Massage therapists can have successful careers working full time or part time. Full-time work can be thought of as earning most or all of your income doing massage therapy. However, it is not as simple as a 40-hour workweek. For a private practice, figure full-time work in terms of client load at about 15–20 clients per week, spending 90 minutes on setup, massage, and cleanup for an hour appointment. That comes to 22 to 30 hours per week. Add in another 1–2 hours per day for related activities, like client notes, bookkeeping, and marketing your practice. Full-time employment may be 4–5 days per week, seeing several clients each day at a place like a spa, health club, or other facility.

It is important to keep in mind that because massage therapy is physically and emotionally demanding, taking more than 20 clients per week for 1-hour massage can put you at risk for injury, stress, and burnout. While some massage therapists may be able to handle more clients per week safely, massage therapists starting out are wise to build their stamina gradually and learn their limits. Take control of your own

Vision of Massage Therapy Practice for

_____
Name of massage therapist / Practice

Dates _____ to _____
         Month/Day/Year   Month/Day/Year

Size

      Full time—hours/clients per week _____

      Part time—hours/clients per week_____

Format

      Employee (preferred setting) _____
      Self-employed (private practice—sole proprietor/independent contractor)
      Combination

        _____ % employed (# days/clients per week _____)

        _____ % self-employed (#days/clients per week _____)

Mission Statement

_____

_____

_____

_____

Annual Income Goal

<$5,000   amount $ _____

$ 5,000–10,000   amount $ _____

$10,000–20,000   amount $ _____

$20,000–30,000   amount $ _____

$30,000–40,000   amount $ _____

$40,000–50,000   amount $ _____

>$50,000   amount $ _____

◀ **Figure 11–1** Vision worksheet.

well-being and set a schedule that is full yet reasonable. Figure on at least one day of rest per week and a minimum of 2–3 weeks of vacation per year. When you plan your budget for the year, figure in your scheduled holidays and vacation time.

Part-time work as a massage therapist can be a fulfilling way to supplement other income. Some massage therapists choose part-time work because they have another job that they do not want to give up, family responsibilities, or other time commitments. Part-time work ranges anywhere from 1–10 clients per week and accounts for part of your income or part of a total household income. You might work 2 nights at a spa, or take a few private clients per week. There are a variety of options for the part-time massage therapist.

Some massage therapists start out working part time while keeping a steady job doing something else, and then gradually develop a full-time practice. Some work part time in two different careers or jobs, or part time while pursuing advanced education. Formulating a career plan takes into consideration whether working full time or part time as a massage therapist is the goal, and how best to go about making that happen. Flexible scheduling is a major benefit of a career in massage therapy.

CASE FOR STUDY

Roberta and Her Dream Practice

Roberta has participated in sports all her life, from junior soccer to high school volleyball. She loves to work out and enjoys being around athletes. Her dream practice as a massage therapist is to work with athletes either in a health club, professional sports setting, or private practice.

Question:
What can Roberta do to increase her chances of achieving her dream practice after graduation?

Things to Consider:

▶ What expertise will potential employers and clients look for on her résumé?
▶ Could her grades in any particular subjects be important to a potential employer?
▶ How important might it be for her to keep up her own fitness level?

▶ What part-time jobs might she get for general experience in sports settings?
▶ What kind of volunteer work might she do to demonstrate experience with sports massage to a potential employer?
▶ What type of specialty training might she seek out?
▶ How can she create a professional identity to match her dream?
▶ What might her mission statement look like?

Ideas for Realizing Roberta's Dream Practice

_____

_____

_____

Employment or Private Practice

Practice formats include regular employment and self-employment in private practice. Many massage therapists have a combined practice, for example, part-time employment combined with a private practice for a full-time career. Each practice format has its upsides and downsides.

Regular employment can be found in spas, resorts, integrative health care clinics, and other settings that offer massage. The Internal Revenue Service (IRS) glossary says that an **employee** "works for an employer. Employers can control when, where, and how the employee performs the work" (www.irs.gov). Employers set prices, assign work schedules, book clients, provide equipment and supplies, advertise services, and generally take care of the business side of the practice. Employers may also dictate the type of massage offered to clients, set a dress code, or impose other restrictions. Massage therapist employees perform massage as scheduled and, in some cases, may be required to do other work such as paperwork, cleaning, or staffing a reception desk.

The upsides of regular employment are a stable hourly wage; low or no expenses for space, equipment, and supplies; potential for health insurance and vacation benefits; and having much of the business of massage taken care of by the employer. In addition, employers pay a portion of Social Security taxes (FICA). Downsides include no control over massage fees, less time flexibility, and less control over the schedule and work environment. Employees do not take home all of the fees that clients pay, but also do not have the extra expenses, responsibilities, and risks that self-employed massage therapists do.

You are considered **self-employed** if you carry on your practice as a sole proprietor or an independent contractor. Self-employment is sometimes referred to as being in **private practice**.

As a **sole proprietor,** you are the legally recognized business owner—the employer and employee rolled into one. This form of practice offers maximum flexibility for creating your own workspace, choosing clientele, controlling the type of massage offered, setting the schedule, and determining fees. You also have sole responsibility for building an adequate client base, complying with government regulations, completing paperwork and bookkeeping, and paying required taxes. Being a sole proprietor requires being a self-starter and self-motivator, and taking responsibility for getting things done.

An **independent contractor** performs services for another person or business, but is not an employee. Independent contractors are self-employed. They are contracted to accomplish a certain result, but are not under the direct control of an employer. An example of an independent contract situation for a massage therapist would be if a business hired a massage therapist to come to its office or workplace to give chair massage to employees on Employee Appreciation Day.

Some businesses use the independent contractor format rather than taking on the added expense of hiring massage therapists as employees. This applies to massage therapists who hire other massage therapists in order to expand their practices. The United States has labor laws that define when this is legal and when it is not, that is, when persons can be considered independent contractors and when they must be treated as employees.

Just declaring someone an independent contractor does not make him or her one in the eyes of the law. The courts have developed a strategy called the "dominant impression test" to distinguish between employees and independent contractors. No one factor determines status, but several factors taken together are considered for their overall effect. The following are some factors that help define employment:

- ▶ Instructions given about when, where, and how to perform the work
- ▶ Training provided
- ▶ Integration into the business operation
- ▶ Services rendered personally by the worker
- ▶ Set work hours and schedule
- ▶ Oral or written reports required
- ▶ Significant tools, material, and equipment furnished
- ▶ Right to discharge the worker at will
- ▶ Work performed on the business premises
- ▶ Ongoing relationship
- ▶ Working for or supplying services to only one business

The National Employers' Association offers a discussion of this issue in an article called "Employers beware, you can't have your cake and eat it too!" It looks at the implications of different provisions of the Labor Relations Act (www.neasa-sa.com).

Why is it important for massage therapists to understand the difference between employees and independent contractors? One reason is to know if you are being treated fairly and legally by a potential employer. Massage therapists can be taken advantage of by employers who are trying to avoid the responsibility and expense of having additional employees. Another reason is that if you want to expand your business by hiring other massage therapists, you will want to know the applicable labor laws. The U.S. government imposes monetary penalties on businesses that misrepresent employee status. Consult a lawyer for advice on whether a dominant impressions test for a certain situation points to employment or an independent contractor arrangement.

How do you determine which format is best for you starting out in your career? Only you can decide, but these are some factors to consider. Look for employment if you want to focus on clients rather than business tasks, or if you are looking for steady work with some benefits. Employment gives you immediate income with minimal or no startup costs. Also, if you have little work or business experience, you can learn the basics by working for someone else first.

Consider self-employment if you are self-motivated and like your independence. It helps to have prior business experience, good contacts or a natural ability to network, and the necessary skills to build a business from the ground up. Startup money is important to get a practice off and running. Private practices are not built in a day, but hard work and perseverance can lead to satisfying results.

Some massage therapists have short-term and long-term plans, which might entail starting out with part-time employment while building knowledge and skills with an eye toward building a private practice in the future. Table 11–1◀ compares different practice formats.

Mission Statement

A useful approach to clarifying your vision is to write a **mission statement**. A mission statement consists of 1 to 3 sentences defining the purpose of your practice and your main strategy for achieving competitive advantage. It answers the questions, "What is the focus of this practice?" and "Why would clients come to me (or why would an employer hire me) instead of someone else?"

TABLE 11–1

Comparison of Employment and Self-Employment Requirements, Upsides, and Downsides

Practice Format	Requirements	Upsides	Downsides
Employment	▶ Successful interview ▶ Meet employer expectations and obey policies ▶ Cooperate with coworkers ▶ Be reliable in attendance ▶ Satisfy customers and employer	▶ Stable hourly wage ▶ Low overhead ▶ Employer pays portion of FICA ▶ Employer advertises and schedules clients ▶ Employer handles government regulations such as business or massage establishment license ▶ Potential health insurance and vacation benefits ▶ Shared client base building with employer	▶ No control over fees, schedule, environment ▶ Less time flexibility ▶ Imposed dress code
Self-Employment Sole proprietor Independent contractor	▶ Business skills ▶ Self-motivation ▶ Discipline ▶ Perseverance ▶ Patience ▶ Ability to satisfy clients	▶ Control over fees, policies and procedures, and type of massage offered ▶ Create own environment ▶ Personal choice about clientele ▶ Set own schedule	▶ Income less predictable ▶ Expenses for space, equipment, and supplies ▶ Keep own records ▶ Build own client base ▶ Provide own health insurance ▶ Pay self-employment tax

A good mission statement narrows your focus and keeps you on a straight path toward your goal. A personal mission statement can lead you to employment in a particular setting or working with a certain type of client. A mission statement for a private practice serves as a reference point for the many decisions that must be made, and it defines who you are as a massage therapist. In a combined practice, your mission statement may have two different parts, or you may maintain a coherent mission throughout your practice. Some examples of mission statements follow.

Employed

My mission as a massage therapist is to apply my training to help clients achieve optimal wellness within the spa environment. Continuing education and active membership in professional associations keep my knowledge and skills about massage and bodywork in spas up-to-date and responsive to consumer trends.

My mission as a massage therapist is to apply my skills as part of an integrative team of health professionals in a medical practice environment. Advanced training in manual methods of pain management and musculoskeletal conditions provide me with the knowledge and skills necessary to treat patients in rehabilitation.

Self-Employed

My mission as a massage therapist is to apply my knowledge and skills to help clients achieve optimal wellness. Affordable massage therapy is offered in a clean, pleasant, and relaxing environment. This is a community-centered and family-based private practice welcoming people of all ages.

My mission is to help clients heal from illness and injury through massage therapy. Advanced approaches to healing through manual therapies are applied in a caring and competent manner. Collaboration with other health professionals ensures safe and effective treatment.

The mission of Office Oasis Massage is to relieve the stress of office workers by providing high-quality chair massage at a convenient time and place. In addition to relaxation, therapeutic applications focus on muscular aches and pains resulting from sitting at a desk for a major part of the workday. We create an oasis for rejuvenation in the midst of the workplace.

The mission of Gold Medal Sports Massage is to improve athletes' performance, and to prevent and treat sports-related injuries through massage therapy. Athletes receive personal attention from highly skilled sports massage professionals who understand their needs and competitive drive. We earn the athletes' confidence by producing observable results.

Since your mission statement directs your path, it is worth taking time to create one that truly reflects your current interests and talents. Write several drafts of your statement until it seems right for you at this time in your career.

Income Goal

An **income goal** specifies how much money you need or want from the practice in a certain time period, such as a year. This figure will guide you in many important choices, like whether to work full time or part time, whether to accept a certain job, or how many clients need to be scheduled per week. Income goals go hand in hand with mission statements in filling out the vision of a viable massage therapy practice.

Since massage therapists work both part time and full time, the range for potential income is wide. Income goals should be as realistic as possible. For example, a person in private practice has to build a client base, so the income for the first year or two will probably be less than it will be once the practice matures.

Projecting your personal expenses for the first year helps you determine how much money you need to bring in. That involves calculating, month by month, expenses like rent, food, transportation, health care, personal services, recreation, loan payments, and other essentials. Be as realistic and detailed as possible. Since the cost of living differs in different parts of country, and for cities and smaller towns, these projections will vary for different people.

For the first year, figure in startup costs for the practice. Startup costs will be discussed in detail on page 285 in Chapter 12: Private Practice and Finances. Take into consideration the income from another job or business and whether you share personal expenses with someone else. When all things are considered, determine how much you need to make from the massage therapy practice to pay the bills and have some discretionary money.

↪ IDENTITY

Practice identity flows from your vision and is the image you project to the world. It includes things like business name and logo, credentials, résumé, business cards and stationery, and a website. It includes your dress and office decoration. Even the color and quality of your sheets and the music you play reflect your practice identity.

Business Name and Logo

Your business name should take into consideration your vision and your potential market. It could be as simple as your name, for example, Robin P. Jones or Alex Lipinsky. A practice name could include your location, for example, Granite City Massage Therapy. Or it might contain some natural characteristic you want associated with your practice, for example, sky, water, clouds, rain, or earth. It might suggest the type of massage and bodywork you offer, such as quiet space, workplace oasis, or relief center. If you are choosing a business name that is not your own name, check with state or local authorities and the U.S. Patent and Trademark Office to make sure the name is not already taken (www.uspto.gov).

A *logo* is a symbol that identifies you and your practice at a glance. Your logo could be original artwork that you commissioned, paid for, and trademarked, or it could be chosen from clip art in the public domain. Printers usually have books of clip art from which people can choose a design or graphic for their business cards and stationery. Some people use stylized versions of their initials for their logos. Your name and logo are used on business cards, stationery, brochures, and your website.

Credentials

Information about credentials and the ethics related to their use are found on page 24 in Chapter 2: The Massage Therapy Profession, and page 231 in Chapter 10: Business Ethics. Remember that credentials are titles awarded for achievements and meeting professional standards. Use them correctly to advertise yourself to potential clients, other health professionals, and the general public. Credentials can be sought and earned to build an identity in concert with your mission.

Résumé

A **résumé** is a written summary of education, experience, achievements, professional memberships, and other information relevant to application for a job, volunteer position, or other occasion where someone wants a snapshot of your identity. A résumé contains selected pieces of information and not your entire personal history. It is formatted so that the reader can easily scan it at a glance for pertinent information.

It is important to have an up-to-date résumé on hand. In addition to accompanying job applications, résumés can be displayed on websites for massage therapy practices, among other uses. Figure 11–2 ◀ shows typical categories and content for massage therapists' résumés.

The basic elements of a résumé include general information like name, address, phone number, and e-mail and/or website address. Current practice is *not* to include your age, year of birth, marital status or family information, or Social Security number.

A detailed résumé contains dates, places, degrees, job titles, and credentials. It shows the depth of your knowledge and skills, past responsibilities and accomplishments, areas of expertise, and other elements for your identity as a massage therapist.

Education and training are listed in reverse chronological order. This section lists dates of attendance or graduation, school name and place, name of the course of study or program, and the degree or certificate earned. Program accreditation can be indicated. Sometimes formal education like college attendance is separated from massage therapy training.

Work experience is also listed in reverse chronological order. This section lists dates, employers' names, job titles and responsibilities, and special achievements. It is often useful to list military service and record. Massage therapy experience and other types of work may be separated into two different sections.

Credentials, including occupational licenses and specialty certifications, professional memberships, and special awards and achievements, are listed to build your identity further. Potential employers will be looking for required licenses and training in desired specialties. Professional memberships show a level of commitment to the profession, and awards indicate outside recognition of your achievements.

Volunteer experience is important for those with limited work experience and also shows an altruistic commitment to the community. Volunteer work relevant to massage therapy includes activities such as outreach programs, and officer or committee work in professional associations. Community volunteer experience might include work with the American Red Cross, a local food pantry, or an animal shelter.

Optional information includes hobbies, leisure activities, and other interests. These further define you as a person and may help your résumé stand out in a pile of otherwise similar résumés.

Résumé Design. Good résumés are simple in design and concise—one or two pages. They use a consistent format for margins and headings, and leave plenty of white space to avoid looking crowded. The font chosen for the text is easily readable. Word processing features like bold, italic, underlining, and capital letters are used conservatively to prevent too much visual distraction.

Remember that résumés are designed to be read at a glance. The main divisions within a well-organized résumé stand out and are easily located. Reverse chronological order is used for items like education and work experience, so that the most recent items are on top, and work history is traced backward by skimming down the list.

Unfamiliar abbreviations, symbols, or initials after a name are avoided, and entries are spelled out fully for the reader. For example, the initials *LMP*, used in some states, should be spelled out as *Licensed Massage Practitioner*. The same applies to organization

▶ **Figure 11–2** Sample of résumé content.

Name
Mailing Address
City, State, Zip Code
Telephone Number
E-mail Address/Website

RÉSUMÉ

[Optional: Mission Statement or Employment Goal]

EDUCATION (reverse chronological order)

Certificate/Date	School Name Massage Program Name City/State
Degree/Date	College Name City/State Major/Minor
Diploma/Date	High School Name City/State

EMPLOYMENT (reverse chronological order)

Dates	Employer or Self-Employed City/State Job title/Responsibilities
Dates	Employer or Self-Employed City/State Job title/Responsibilities

PROFESSIONAL AFFILIATIONS, LICENSE, CERTIFICATIONS, HONORS

Date	Massage License, State, Number
Date	Certification Name, Organization, City/State
Date	Professional Organization Membership, Level
Date	Award, Organization

VOLUNTEER EXPERIENCE

Date	Organization City/State Responsibilities
Date	Organization City/State Responsibilities

LEISURE ACTIVITIES

Activities

References available upon request.

names; for example, *AMTA* should be spelled out as *American Massage Therapy Association*, and *ABMP* as *Associated Bodywork and Massage Professionals*.

Grammatical style is consistent, especially elements like verb tense and punctuation. Grammar, spelling, and typographical errors are avoided by looking over the résumé carefully. Remember that your résumé is part of your identity and should reflect your best efforts.

Building an Impressive Résumé. The résumé can serve as a vehicle for planning professional growth. A look at your current résumé can bring to mind ideas for what education, work or volunteer experience, certification, or other additions would make it more attractive to a potential employer or client. Seek opportunities that demonstrate professional development and add them as they are completed. Use your mission statement as a guide. Keep the résumé in electronic form so that it can be updated easily and as often as needed.

Be sure that everything that appears on your résumé is true, and there is nothing misleading. Honesty and accuracy are expected in an ethical massage therapist.

Business Cards and Stationery

Business cards may be the single most important marketing device for building a client base. Business cards give clients and prospective clients essential information about you and how to contact you for appointments. They reflect who you are as a massage therapist.

A business card packs a lot of information into 2.5 × 3 inches of space. A typical card has your name and/or business name, address if you have an office, phone number to call for appointments, and other contact information such as e-mail address and website. It may list the type of massage and bodywork you offer and important certification and license information. The design may include a logo or graphic element. A sample business card design is shown in Figure 11–3◀.

As with résumés, readable and simple business cards are best. Make fonts large enough for everyone to read. Do not let elements and color detract from the essential information. However, a unique and attractive design may make a favorable impression.

Remember that most clients want to think that their massage therapist is professional, trustworthy, and competent. A well-designed business card communicates that impression.

A spa, health club, clinic, or other business that employs massage therapists may provide standard business cards with its name and logo. Since you still have to build a client base at a place of employment, business cards are important to have available there, too.

Although stationery may not be important for massage therapists who are employed full time, anyone in private practice should have stationery on hand for official correspondence. The design, color, and general impression should match business cards, brochures, and website elements to present a coherent identity.

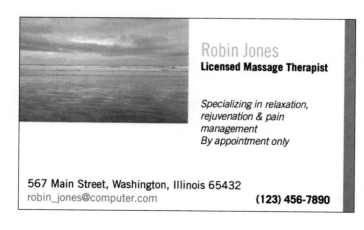

◀ Figure 11–3 Sample of a business card design.

Robin Jones
Licensed Massage Therapist

Specializing in relaxation, rejuvenation & pain management
By appointment only

567 Main Street, Washington, Illinois 65432
robin_jones@computer.com   **(123) 456-7890**

Brochures and Websites

Brochures and websites give potential clients more detailed information about massage therapists and their private practices. With word processing programs and digital photography, a massage therapist can create attractive brochures that reflect a practice identity. A simple tri-fold brochure can be printed on standard 8.5 × 11 heavyweight paper and copied in color.

A typical brochure for a massage therapy practice might have a cover page with the name and/or business name, address, phone number to call for appointments, and other contact information such as e-mail address and website. Photos of the massage therapist, the reception area and massage room, and other relevant images can be included. Other ideas include descriptions of the type of massage and bodywork offered, more detail on credentials, possible goals for massage sessions, policies, appointment times, and fees. Plan on updating a brochure about once per year.

Websites serve the same general purpose as brochures and may be more accessible to potential clients. Someone thinking about making an appointment with you may want to check your website for a better sense of you and your practice. Potential employers may also check out your website. Websites can hold more information than brochures, such as complete résumés, testimonials, fuller explanations of services, and more photos. They can have special features like links to other sites that have information about the type of massage therapy you offer.

Developing technology is making website creation more user-friendly and economical. Check out websites for other massage therapists as you plan your website design to see what the options are. Make sure that your website reflects your practice identity and that your image and information is consistent throughout your marketing materials. Some professional associations offer website hosting as a service to members. More information about marketing a private practice can be found on page 277 in Chapter 12: Private Practice and Finances.

GETTING EMPLOYMENT

Getting employment as a massage therapist is a step-by-step process that begins with finding the job opening and then interviewing successfully. It entails locating openings, filling out job applications, submitting résumés, writing cover letters, presenting references, getting interviews, and interviewing well.

CRITICAL THINKING

Analyze the identity or image of several different massage practices in your area. Look at résumés, business cards, brochures, and websites.

1 What do they say to potential clients about the massage therapist and his or her practice?

2 Is the image presented consistent with the reality of the practice?

3 Can you think of ways to create a more attractive identity for this practice?

4 What ideas would you consider using to create the identity of your own future practice?

Your school's placement department may have a listing of local employers and openings for massage therapists. Job postings for massage therapists can also be found in places like local newspapers, professional journals and magazines, and some websites listing employment opportunities. Networking with other massage therapists can lead to hearing about job opportunities.

As you survey the job market, think about the vision for your practice and whether it leads you toward certain types of jobs or settings. If possible, narrow your search to the types of jobs that best fit your career plan. You can also be proactive in identifying where you would like to work, and then inquiring about how to go about getting a job there.

Once a potential job situation is identified, your focus is on getting a job interview. Steps to the interview typically involve filling out a job application and/or submitting a résumé and references.

A job application is a preprinted form used by companies to get essential information for screening job applicants. It gives employers a standard format to more easily compare applicants and narrow down the pool before looking at résumés. Even though much of the information asked for may be on your résumé, do not write in "see résumé." The purpose of the form is for employers to easily see relevant information to determine if they want to look at your résumé. If the application is incomplete, they may not look any further. Fill in all information neatly and accurately. An employer may also want to see if you can read and follow directions, and how good your written communication skills, like grammar and spelling, are.

If the application asks why you want the job, take time to think about your answer. Let the employer know that you understand the job requirements, that you are familiar with the company and want to work there, and that you are a good match for the job. Be honest about your schooling and credentials. Misrepresentation is not only unethical but may have legal consequences. Many states require massage therapists to disclose prior criminal offenses to obtain licenses. Do not lie about past convictions on your job application. That is fraud and would later be grounds for immediate dismissal.

A potential employer may also ask for your résumé. If possible, submit it with a cover letter written in business letter format on good stationery. In the letter, introduce yourself, detail your qualifications, and state your interest in the job. Try to find out who is actually doing the hiring, and address the letter to that person. Show your knowledge about the company and the nature of the job. An employer will be impressed that you did your homework. Be sure to include your contact information and good times to call you.

References are good to have. These are people who know you personally, can recommend your work, and give a prospective employer information about you. References can be former employers, coworkers, people from volunteer and community work, teachers, or anyone who can give relevant information about your work, character, and factors relevant to the job. Never use family members as references. Later in your career, satisfied clients may also be willing to write letters of recommendation.

Keep two to three letters of reference on hand to include with a résumé or take to an interview. Prospective employers may want to call your references personally for verification and for further information. It is a good idea to call your references to ask their permission to use their names and to tell them what job you've applied for and when they might expect to be contacted by the employer.

Your answering machine or voice mail message should be one that you would want a prospective employer to hear. Remember that employers may call to arrange an interview or to ask questions.

Once prospective employers know that you are a job candidate, they notice how you dress and act. The impression you make stays with you. Even before a job interview, appear neat and well groomed to a potential employer, for example, when dropping off a résumé or inquiring about a place such as a spa or clinic (Figure 11–4 ◀).

A direct call to a manager or person hiring for a job may be useful. You can inquire if your information was received and if you need to send anything else. This gives the person a chance to hear your voice and talk to you personally.

Successful Job Interviews

Job interviews are a two-way street. The massage therapist is evaluating whether the job offers what he or she is looking for, and the employer is determining whether the massage therapist has the knowledge and skills for the position and will fit well into the work environment.

Before going for an interview, write down questions you would like answered about the job, benefits, pay, and other important factors. The following are things you might want to consider.

▶ What types of clients/patients come to the spa/clinic/office? What are they looking for from massage therapy? Does that fit your knowledge and skills, mission and identity?

▶ What exactly will your duties be? Will anything else in addition to doing massage therapy be required?

▶ How many massages will you be expected to do in one day? How much time will you have between massages?

▶ What paperwork is involved? Are SOAP notes required?

▶ Will you interact with other health professionals?

▶ What is your likely schedule? What days and times?

▶ What is the dress code? Are uniforms required and provided?

▶ What are the policies about sick days and vacations?

▶ Who will your supervisor be?

▶ What are the terms of your wages? Is this true employment or would you be an independent contractor? How often are you paid? Is there a policy about tips?

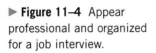
▶ **Figure 11–4** Appear professional and organized for a job interview.

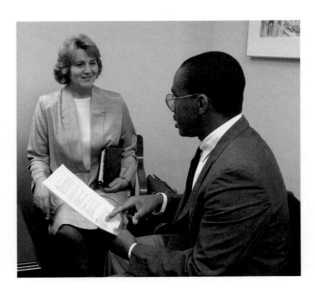

▶ Are there any benefits (e.g., health insurance, 401K or other retirement plan, vacation pay)?
▶ Do they have an employee policy manual?
▶ Are there any additional perks (e.g., use of spa or health club, free parking)?

To further prepare for the interview, plan what you will wear. Choose clothes that fit well into the environment in which you would be working. Find out in advance if you will be expected to give the interviewer a massage. If so, arrive dressed appropriately or be ready to change into proper clothes for giving massage.

Review the materials you sent to the employer. Bring copies to the interview so that you can refer to them if you forget something. Bring letters of recommendation if you did not send them before. Also bring your massage therapy license if one is required in the employer's area. Arrange any papers you bring to the interview neatly in a folder so that you appear organized. To boost confidence and practice your verbal responses, role-play the interview with another massage therapist or friend.

On the day of the interview, arrive a little early to settle in and relax. Greet the interviewer by name if you know it. Be prepared to answer the following common interview questions:

▶ "Tell me a little about yourself and your background in massage."
▶ "How did you hear about this job?"
▶ "What types of massage therapy are you trained in?"
▶ "What makes you qualified for this job?"
▶ "Why do you want this job?"
▶ "How do you think you'll fit in here?"
▶ "When are you available to work?"
▶ "What are your salary requirements?"

A massage therapist often is asked to give a massage to the interviewer or someone else connected to the employer. This is reasonable since the employer is hiring the massage therapist for his or her skills. Before the massage session, ask if the employer or hiring person would like you to do a health history interview, or if the person receiving the massage has a file you can review. Even if the employer or interviewer says to go ahead with the massage without a health history, do a brief verbal screening for contraindications and ask the person to clarify what he or she wants from the massage. It is important to know the employer or interviewer's expectations so you can plan the session accordingly. He or she may be looking for specific things in your massage.

Be very careful in responding to questions and requests. A potential employer may be testing to see how well you keep professional boundaries, or how you handle inappropriate behavior. Be confident and act professionally at all times.

Illegal Interview Questions. It is wise to be informed about interview questions that courts have determined to be discriminatory in nature and illegal to ask. Federal and state laws attempt to ensure that job candidates are hired based solely on their qualifications for the job. Discrimination in hiring is prohibited based on certain factors such as marital status, family responsibilities, plans for pregnancy, child care arrangements, age, gender, sexual orientation, nationality, ethnic background, and disability. Comments about one's weight, height, and grooming are also not appropriate. See the National Labor Relations Board (www.nlrb.gov) and the U.S. Equal Employment Opportunity Commission (www.eeoc.gov) websites and similar agencies in your state for further information on illegal hiring practices.

Appropriate questions are directly related to job qualifications and are usually general in nature. The following are acceptable questions:

▶ "Do you have any responsibilities that will limit what days or times you can work?"
▶ "Are you prepared to perform four or five massages in a day?"
▶ "If you are hired, could you provide verification of your right to work in the United States?"
▶ "Do you have training in working with the elderly?"

If you think the interviewer has asked an illegal question, you have various options for responding. It may have been an innocent mistake by an untrained interviewer or a truly discriminatory inquiry.

Depending on the situation, you can steer your answer more toward what you think the interviewer is trying to get at or what you want the person to know about you. For example, a good response to "How old are you?" might be "After I finished high school I completed my massage training and am well prepared for the responsibilities of this job." Or you could respond, "Is there an age requirement for the job?" This question steers the interviewer back to job qualifications.

If you feel there is potential for illegal discrimination for some reason, it is wise to practice your responses to illegal questions. Planning ahead and good communication skills will help you complete job interviews with confidence.

After the Interview. If the job is offered to you after the interview, your possible responses are yes, no, or I have to think about it. Before you accept a job offer, be sure that the job meets your requirements in terms of your vision and income goals. If you have done your homework and are sure the job is everything you have been looking for, do not be afraid to say yes right away. If you have any doubts, take time to talk it over with friends or family and think about your decision.

If the job is not offered to you right away, feel free to call back in a day or two to see how things stand. They may have hired someone else or may have more interviews to do. Calling to inquire shows continued interest and keeps your name visible.

PRACTICAL APPLICATION

Role-play job interviews with a study partner or friend. Use specific job postings to add some reality to the exercise. Write out expected questions and even some illegal questions for your interviewer to ask. Practice your responses aloud. Rehearse your responses until you have confidence in your ability to answer them well.

Keep in mind that the purpose of a job interview is not only to answer questions posed by the interviewer, but also to ask questions that will allow you to determine if the job you are applying for is right for you. What questions will you ask your interviewer to find out more about the job expectations, the working environment, clients, benefits, etc.?

Now switch roles with your study partner.

1. Critique each other's answers to the interview questions. Constructively brainstorm together about how your answers could be improved.

2. Take careful note of which types of questions were the most difficult to answer and plan to practice these until you are satisfied that you can answer them well.

If you do not get the job, call and ask if the employer or hiring person would share with you why you were not hired, or what would have made you a more desirable candidate. The company may have found someone more qualified, or who was available for more days or hours. Take it as a learning experience to increase your chances of success in the future.

Chapter Highlights

▶ A massage therapist's career plans begin with formulating the vision and identity of a future practice.

- The practice may be full time or part time and may consist of regular employment, self-employment, or a combination of the two.
- The mission statement defines the purpose of the practice and the main strategy for achieving a competitive advantage.
- Income goals specify how much money is needed or wanted from the practice in a certain period of time, such as a year.

▶ Practice identity flows from the vision and is the image projected to the world.

- Business cards present a lot of information in a small space and are important for building a client base.
- Brochures and websites are useful for displaying more detailed information.

▶ Getting employment as a massage therapist entails locating openings, filling out job applications, submitting résumés, writing cover letters, presenting references, getting interviews, and interviewing well.

- A résumé summarizes relevant education, experience, and professional achievements and is essential when looking for employment.
- A cover letter for a résumé should explain why you are qualified for the job and reflect your suitability for the place of employment.
- References provide outside verification of your past performance and give you credibility.

▶ Job interviews are for massage therapists to evaluate whether the jobs offer what they are looking for and for employers to determine if the massage therapists have the qualifications for the positions.

▶ Preparation for an interview involves writing your questions about the job and practicing answers to probable questions from the interviewer.

- Giving a massage is often part of a job interview for massage therapists.
- Project confidence and be professional at all times. Be aware of illegal questions from interviewers and respond tactfully.

▶ Accept a job offer right away if you are sure you want it, but do not be afraid to say no or ask for time to think about it if you are not sure.

- Call the employer if you do not hear back from the company within a few days.
- If you do not get the job, try to find out why, and consider it a learning experience for future success.

Exam Review

Learning Outcomes

Use the learning outcomes at the beginning of the chapter and shown here as a guide to the major topics covered. Perform the task given in each outcome, and share your results with a study partner. Check off the tasks as you complete them.

- ❏ Develop career plans for the first year after graduation.
- ❏ Create a vision and identity for a massage practice.
- ❏ Identify the benefits and drawbacks of employment and self-employment.
- ❏ Design a résumé, business card, brochure, and website.
- ❏ Locate and secure employment as a massage therapist.

Key Terms

To study the key terms listed at the beginning of the chapter, choose one or more of the following exercises. Writing or talking about ideas helps you better remember them, and explaining them to someone else helps deepen your understanding.

1. Write a one-sentence definition of each key term. Put the term in a general category, and then distinguish it from other terms in that category. For example, "*Independent contractor* is a form of self-employment in which a person performs services for another person or business, but is not an employee." Or, "A *résumé* is a document that summarizes education, work experience, and professional achievements and is used in seeking employment." Try to capture the essence of each term in a concise statement.

2. Make study cards by writing the key term on one side of a 3 × 5 card and a concise definition on the other side. Shuffle the cards and read one side, trying to recite either the explanation or term on the other side.

3. Pick out two or three terms and explain how they are related.

4. With a study partner, take turns explaining key terms verbally.

5. Make up sentences using one or more key terms. Variation: Read your sentences to a study partner who will ask you to explain unclear statements.

Memory Workout

The following fill-in-the-blank statements test your memory of the main concepts in this chapter.

1. Employees do not take home all of the _____ paid by clients, but also do not have the _____ that self-employed massage therapists have.

2. You are considered self-employed if you carry on your practice as a sole _____ or an independent _____.

3. A mission statement consists of one to three sentences defining the _____ of your practice and your main strategy for achieving _____ advantage.

4. A well-designed business card communicates the impression of the massage therapist as _____, _____, and _____.

5. Massage therapists in private practice should have official _____ on hand for written correspondence.

6. Websites serve the same general purpose as _____, and may be more _____ to potential clients.

7. A job application is a preprinted form used by companies to get essential information for _____ job applicants.

8. Misrepresentation on a job application is not only unethical, but may have _____ consequences.

9. References are people who know you personally and who can _____ your work.

10. When giving a massage as part of a job interview, it is important to know the interviewer's _____ so you can plan the session accordingly.

11. Federal and state laws attempt to ensure that job candidates are hired based solely on their _____ for the job.

12. Not getting a certain job can be taken as a _____ experience to increase your chances of success in the future.

Test Prep

The following multiple-choice questions will help to prepare you for future school and professional exams.

1. Which of the following offers immediate income with minimum startup costs?
   a. Sole proprietor
   b. Employee
   c. Independent contractor
   d. Private practice

2. Which of the following is *not* part of a mission statement for a massage therapy practice?
   a. Focus of the practice
   b. Purpose of the practice
   c. Income goal
   d. Competitive advantage

3. A logo is
   a. Part of your practice identity
   b. A symbol that identifies your practice at a glance
   c. Original or clip art
   d. All of the above

4. On a résumé, education and work experience are typically listed in
   a. Chronological order
   b. Reverse chronological order
   c. Alphabetical order
   d. Order of importance

5. The single most important marketing device for building a client base will most likely be your
   a. Diploma
   b. Résumé
   c. Business card
   d. Brochure

6. Which of the following would *not* be appropriate to list as your references as part of a job application?
   a. Family members
   b. Teachers
   c. Former employers
   d. Satisfied clients

7. Which of the following is *not* appropriate for a prospective employer to do during a job interview?
   a. Ask about your qualifications for the job
   b. Ask for a sample massage session
   c. Ask about your marital status and children
   d. Ask about your ability to work a certain schedule

8. If you have limited job experience, which of the following would likely impress a prospective employer the most as evidence of your character and sense of responsibility?
   a. Music or other collection
   b. Professional image you project
   c. Good grades in school
   d. Volunteer work in the community

Video Challenge

Watch the appropriate segment of the video on your CD-ROM and then answer the following questions.

Segment 11: Career Plans and Employment

1. What were the initial visions of the massage therapists interviewed in the video of their future practices? How did they change with time?

2. What does the massage therapist in the video say about having small goals? How did that lead her in the direction she wanted to go?

3. According to the video, how should you prepare for a job interview?

Comprehension Exercises

The following exercises provide questions for you to answer and tasks you can do to enhance your understanding of the material presented in this chapter.

1. What is the purpose of developing a vision of your future massage therapy practice? What are the essential elements of that vision?

2. Compare employees and independent contractors. What does the government look for in determining which category best fits a particular job? What is the dominant impression test?

3. What are some questions you might have for a potential employer during a job interview? Why would you be asking questions at this time?

For Greater Understanding

The following exercises are designed to give you a deeper understanding of the subjects covered in this chapter. Action words are underlined to emphasize the active nature of this approach to learning.

1. <u>Write</u> a mission statement for your future massage therapy practice. Take into account your current interests, talents, and employment goals. <u>Write</u> your mission statement in positive language so that it may inspire you and keep you on track to meet your overall career goals.

2. <u>Develop</u> a personal budget for a year listing projected expenses and total income, including income from various jobs and contributions from spouse or family. Given your circumstances, <u>determine</u> how much money you need to make from your massage therapy practice to cover bills and have some discretionary income. This is your income goal for your massage therapy practice.

3. <u>Develop</u> a list of job opportunities for massage therapists in your area. How many job postings could you find? How many fit your vision for your practice?

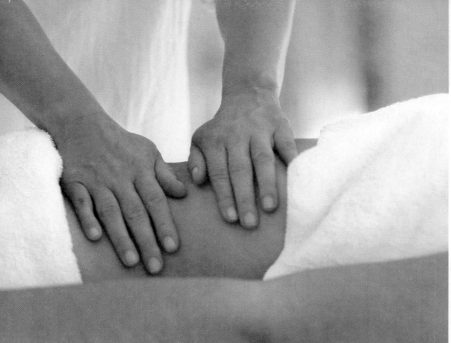

12

Private Practice and Finances

LEARNING OUTCOMES

After studying this chapter, you will have information to:

1. Develop a business plan for a private practice in massage therapy.
2. Create a marketing strategy to build a client base.
3. Organize a massage practice office.
4. Enter into contracts with knowledge and forethought.
5. Establish policies for practice management.
6. Create a filing system for keeping client records.
7. Project startup costs for a massage therapy practice.
8. Project first-year income and expenses.
9. Design a bookkeeping system for tax purposes.
10. Manage practice finances on a daily basis.

KEY TERMS

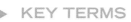

Business plan	Estimated tax	Promotions	Startup costs
Cash reserve	Fixed costs	Salary draw	Variable costs
Contract	Marketing	Self-employment tax	

Ideas in Action

On your CD-ROM, explore:

- ▶ Business plan
- ▶ Advertising
- ▶ First-year budget
- ▶ Bookkeeping
- ▶ Interactive video exercises

PRIVATE PRACTICE

A self-employed massage therapist is said to have a private practice. A private practice can be small and part time, with a few clients per week, or it can be large and full time and serve many clients each week. A private practice in massage therapy has much in common with other small businesses that sell products and services to the public. For example, a massage therapy practice is regulated as a business and has responsibilities for keeping financial records for tax purposes. It also markets services to the public to build a client base. This chapter provides an overview of the business side of having a private practice in massage therapy.

BUSINESS PLAN OVERVIEW

A **business plan** spells out the details of putting the practice vision into operation. A business plan has four major parts: description of the business, marketing, management, and finances. The major elements of a business plan for a massage therapy practice are summarized in Figure 12–1◀. Further information about developing a business plan is available from the U.S. Small Business Administration (www.sba.gov). The remainder of this chapter discusses these elements in more detail.

DESCRIPTION OF THE BUSINESS

The vision and identity developed in your career plan (see page 252 in Chapter 11: Career Plans and Employment) lays the foundation for the description of your private practice, that is, your business. The mission statement is a good opening for the description. Express the size of the business in terms of whether it is full time or part time, how many clients are planned on average per week, and the total number of clients per year. State your income and profit goals. Looking at the income and profit goals in relation to the number of clients is essential. Remember that income from clients minus business expenses and taxes is the real profit from the practice. It is the profit that you put into your pocket. Do the math to see if your expectations are realistic. Finances are discussed in more detail later in the chapter.

Legal Structure

The concept of sole proprietor was introduced in Chapter 11: Career Plans and Employment, on page 255, to distinguish employment from self-employment. Sole proprietor is the most common legal structure chosen for massage therapy practices, especially when starting out. Other choices are partnership and corporation. Major differences in the three structures have to do with who owns the business, who takes profits and losses, who is responsible for legal matters, and what taxes apply. Figure 12–2◀ summarizes the characteristics of the three possible legal structures.

Private Practice Business Plan

Section 1: Description of the Business
▶ Vision
- Mission
- Size (full time or part time; number of clients per week or month)
- Income and profit goals
- Legal structure (sole proprietor, partnership, corporation)

▶ Location
- Home, space rental, or traveling practice
- Applicable ordinances and zoning laws

Section 2: Marketing
▶ Market research
▶ Client sources
▶ Advertising and promotions
- Business card
- Brochure
- Website
- Other

Section 3: Management
▶ License, insurance, contracts
▶ Policies
▶ Office space
▶ Appointments
▶ Client records

Section 4: Finances
▶ Startup budget
▶ First year budget
▶ Bookkeeping
▶ Taxes
▶ Banking

◀ **Figure 12–1** Business plan for a private practice in massage therapy.

It is outside of the scope of this book to delve deeply into the pros and cons of partnerships and corporations for massage therapy practices. If you want to know more, someone experienced in business, such as a lawyer or accountant, can help sort out the issues. Information is also available from the U.S. Small Business Administration (www.sba.gov).

For the purposes of this text, a sole proprietor legal structure will be assumed. A sole proprietor makes all decisions, takes all profits and losses, is personally liable for lawsuits, and pays income taxes on business profits as personal income.

Location

Location can make or break a business. Marketing research can tell you where your potential clients are, and how much competition will be in a certain area. Municipal ordinances regulating massage therapy and local zoning laws may limit where a massage therapy business may be located.

Options for massage therapy practice locations include a home office, space in a commercial building or within another business space, and a storefront. Each of these places has advantages and disadvantages.

Many massage therapists have satisfying practices in their homes. The main advantages here are low overhead and a short commute. Home-based practices

▶ **Figure 12–2** Comparison of legal structures for private practices.

Options for Legal Structures*

Sole Proprietor

- ▶ Owned by one person who makes all decisions and who takes all profits and losses.
- ▶ Owner is personally liable for any lawsuits that arise from the business.
- ▶ Registered in the state as a sole proprietor.
- ▶ Owner pays income taxes on the business profits as personal income.

Partnership

- ▶ Two or more owners who make decisions and share profits.
- ▶ All partners are liable for lawsuits that arise from the business.
- ▶ Legal contract called a "partnership agreement" defines the responsibilities of each partner.
- ▶ Partners pay income taxes on their share of the profits as personal income.

Corporation

- ▶ A corporation is a legal entity or "person" under the law and is composed of stockholders operating under one company name. Stockholders own the corporation and elect a board of directors to manage the company.
- ▶ The corporation is liable for lawsuits that arise from the business. Stockholders have limited liability and cannot have their personal assets taken to pay a judgment from a lawsuit.
- ▶ Corporations are registered by states in the United States and must abide by that state's laws related to corporations. Laws differ in different states.
- ▶ Main disadvantage in some types of corporations is that corporate profits are taxed twice—once as a corporation and again as dividends to individual stockholders on their personal income tax.
- ▶ Types of corporations
  - *C Corporation* sells ownership as shares of stock; limited liability for stockholders; income taxed twice.
  - *Subchapter S Corporation* limits the number of stockholders to 75; has limited liability; income taxed only once as personal income of the owners.
  - *Professional Corporation* for professionals in practice together; special rules apply.
  - *Nonprofit Corporation* or 501c (3) set up with mission to improve society; tax exempt; no profits shared by stockholders.
  - *Limited Liability Company* (LLC) combines best features of partnerships and corporations; limited personal liability; income taxed once.

*See U.S. Small Business Administration [www.sba.gov] and U.S. Internal Revenue Service [www.irs.gov] for more information about legal structures for businesses.

require a separate space dedicated to massage and, ideally, separate entrances and bathrooms. Mixing of personal and business space should be avoided. Having strangers in their homes may not appeal to some massage therapists. In addition, zoning laws may prohibit home businesses, or a variance may be required. Despite all the potential difficulties, home-based practices can be quite successful with careful planning.

Renting space is another option. A room in an office building or within another business may be all you need. Rooms within spas, salons, health clubs, and medical offices can offer a nice reception area and give valuable exposure to potential clients. Sometimes massage therapists rent rooms to other massage therapists. If an acceptable schedule can be worked out, sharing space with another massage therapist can be a good startup alternative. Note that this is not a legal partnership, but simply a space-sharing arrangement.

Storefront rental is a larger financial commitment. The advantage is that foot traffic in the area may result in more clients as people walk by and see your business signs. You can design the space as you like it and even rent space to other massage therapists or other compatible businesses. It is also a more complex situation, complete with a landlord, more possible legal restrictions, more initial financial outlay for altering the space to fit your needs, more upkeep expenses, and usually a greater monthly financial liability. A storefront may be a good option for a suburban or small-town practice.

An alternative to having a fixed location is to have an on-the-road practice in which you go to your clients' locations. You can see private clients in their own homes, or in places like hotels and resorts, nursing homes, or the workplace. An individual client may contract with you for massage, or you may have an arrangement as an independent contractor to provide massage to patrons or employees of another business in its space. A traveling practice eliminates overhead for space, but requires a means of transportation and possibly special equipment for easy transport.

↪ MARKETING

A market is defined as "a group of people with the potential interest of buying a given product or service." **Marketing** is the process of identifying these potential customers and meeting their needs and wants. In marketing yourself, you identify potential clients who want what you have to offer.

In a sense, everyone is a potential client, so you must decide to whom to market your services. Options are to try to appeal to a broad, diverse market or to narrow your focus to a group with specific needs. When starting out, it might be wiser to market to a broader audience and narrow your focus later, if you want to, once your client base has grown.

Marketing also takes into consideration your competitive advantage, which is the reason people would come to you for massage instead of someone else. Factors that may give you an advantage are quality, expertise, price, location, variety of services, special skills, convenience, or environment. From the business point of view, it is useful to think of clients as customers or consumers.

Market Research

Market research is the process of collecting relevant information for identifying and reaching potential customers. The following are basic market research questions for massage therapists.

- ▶ Who are my potential clients? Who is interested in receiving the massage therapy that I offer?
- ▶ What do they hope to gain by receiving massage?
- ▶ Who in the area can afford massage?
- ▶ How do potential clients find out about massage therapists in the area?
- ▶ Who else is providing massage in the area? Who do they seem to be targeting or attracting?
- ▶ Is there an untapped or underserved market in the area?
- ▶ What are my strengths and/or preferences in massage therapy, and how do they match up with potential markets?
- ▶ How can I develop my own niche or loyal client base?
- ▶ Who is the target audience for my massage practice?

Answers to these questions are found in a variety of sources. To begin with, the Wellness Massage Pyramid discussed on page 5 in Chapter 1: A Career in Massage Therapy offers insight into the broad range of possibilities as to why people might need or want massage therapy. Consumer research conducted by associations and organizations provides insight about massage consumers. An example is the annual *Massage Therapy Consumer Survey Fact Sheet* from the American Massage Therapy Association (www.amtamassage.org).

Magazine and journal articles can show what the general public is looking for from massage therapy and the latest trends. Organizations or support groups for people with certain illnesses or disabilities may promote massage to their members. The local library or phone book has information about who in a geographic area is already providing massage and whom they are targeting, as well as potential competing practices at spas, salons, health clubs, YMCAs, integrative health care facilities, chiropractic offices, and other places.

Once potential clients are identified, you can make decisions about how best to reach them, and position your practice as the best choice for their needs.

Building a Client Base

A primary source of clients in a personal service like massage is word of mouth, that is, recommendations from other clients, friends, and family. Referrals from health professionals like personal trainers, chiropractors, physical therapists, and doctors can also be important.

Professional associations and independent groups offer special massage therapist locator services to the general public. Potential clients often check the Internet to locate massage therapists in their areas, and so subscribing to one of these services may be beneficial.

Networking in the community helps potential clients get to know you. Many massage therapists join their local chamber of commerce, or service clubs like Rotary International and Lions Clubs International. Besides being supporting members, massage therapists give presentations about massage to these community organizations. Special interest groups such as sports clubs, senior centers, and support groups are also open to having speakers come to talk to them. Good presentation skills are useful in marketing private practices.

Getting your name and face out to the public is the key. People need to know that you are in the area and how to contact you for an appointment.

Advertising and Promotions

Advertising is a paid public announcement providing information about a product or service to potential customers. Ads may be in print or electronic media and range in size from what can fit on the side of a pen to an outdoor billboard.

The purpose of advertising is to attract potential clients to a specific business or person, and convince them that their needs or wants can be fulfilled by the service advertised. Ads remind potential clients of needs or wants and may even create a desire for the service that did not exist before. Ads convince potential clients that a certain business or person is the right one to fulfill their desires.

The most cost-effective advertising investments for a startup massage practice are business cards, brochures, websites, and phone directory yellow pages ads. In smaller towns, ads in the local newspaper may be worthwhile. Visible signs with basic information also let potential customers know that you are in the area. Perhaps the most expensive and least effective advertising for most small practices are big-city newspapers and television and radio ads, unless there are local channels or stations that serve the immediate area in which your practice is located.

Advertising opportunities can be found in a variety of public places. For example, a public sports facility may have advertising space around a lobby bulletin board, or a local movie theater may show ads for community businesses on the screen before the feature starts. Some fundraising groups sell space in ad books or souvenir programs and encourage their supporters to do business with sponsors who bought ads. These types of advertising build awareness of your existence and can make your name familiar in the community over a period of time. Buy such ads in places where you think your potential clients will see them. When someone thinks of massage therapy, your name will come up in association.

Promotions are ways to encourage people to pick up the phone and make those appointments. Promotions include giving discounts to new clients for their first massage, or a discounted package for a series of sessions, for example, five sessions for the cost of four. Some massage therapists offer seasonal discounts around the holidays, or for special groups like teachers, police, and firefighters. Gift certificates can also bring in new clients.

Advertising and promotion ideas abound in a free market environment. A lot can be learned from becoming more aware of how other businesses market their services. Some may work for a massage therapy practice and some may not.

In any case, care must be taken in marketing and advertising to avoid unethical practices. Many of the ethical pitfalls in this area of business were discussed in Chapter 10: Business Ethics. To summarize here: Tell the truth and avoid deception, be professional, do not make guarantees, use testimonials sparsely, list prices honestly, and honor copyright and trademark rights. Figure 12–3◀ lists some ideas for building a client base.

MANAGEMENT

Management involves activities necessary to keep the business running smoothly. Obtaining licenses and insurance, defining policies, and negotiating contracts are examples. Massage office design and upkeep, making appointments, and maintenance of client files are also important management functions. All the behind-the-scenes

◀ **Figure 12–3** Ideas for building a client base.

Building a Client Base

Sources of Clients
- ▶ Word of mouth from other clients, friends, and family
- ▶ Referrals from other health professionals
- ▶ Referrals from massage therapist locator services
- ▶ Networking in the community (chamber of commerce, service groups, special interest groups)

Advertising
- ▶ Business cards
- ▶ Signs on a place of business
- ▶ Yellow pages phone book
- ▶ Website
- ▶ Brochure
- ▶ T-shirts, caps, pens, bags, or other objects with name and contact information for a business
- ▶ Refrigerator magnets with business name and information
- ▶ Signage on cars and vans
- ▶ Printed signs for placement on bulletin boards or in windows
- ▶ Advertisements in newspapers, magazines, or newsletters
- ▶ Direct-mail coupons
- ▶ Announcements on local radio or television stations

Promotions
- ▶ Discount for new clients
- ▶ Packages of sessions at special price
- ▶ Seasonal promotions
- ▶ Discount for special groups
- ▶ Gift certificates

operations that make it possible for the massage therapist to provide a therapeutic experience for clients falls into the category of management. This section discusses some of the basic management details of a massage therapy practice.

Licenses and Insurance

Certain licenses may be required to start a private massage practice. First, an occupational license to practice massage therapy must be obtained from the state or local government where applicable. This applies to employment as well as to having a private practice.

Second, a business license may be required by a city or county. Some places have special massage establishment licenses and space requirements. Zoning may limit where a massage business can be located. Before you sign a rental contract, make sure that massage is legally allowed in that location and get the required permits. See Chapter 10: Business Ethics, on page 228 for more information about zoning ordinances and licensing.

Insurance protects you financially. *Professional liability insurance* covers you for liability for incidents arising from the massage therapy itself. Criminal acts or actions outside of the scope of massage therapy as legally defined are usually excluded. Injuries occurring when practicing without a required license may also not be covered. Read your professional liability insurance policy to clearly understand what it includes.

Premise liability insurance, also called "slip and fall" insurance is for accidents to clients and visitors on the business premises not related to massage. *Renters' insurance* covers the cost of equipment, supplies, and other objects lost or damaged due to fire, theft, or flood.

Contracts

Setting up a private practice usually entails some legal agreements or contracts. Examples are rental agreements, phone and Internet service, credit cards, linen service, cleaning service, and bills of sale. Independent contractor agreements are used when a massage therapist provides massage services to another business. It is important to understand the basic elements of contracts to ensure that agreements entered into support your business plans and expectations.

A **contract** is an official written agreement between two or more people. The terms of a contract may be upheld in court if one party is considered to have breached or violated the agreement. Lawsuits arise when agreements are either not clear or have not been kept.

A contract must have a clear statement of the terms of the agreement, that is, person A agrees to this, and person B agrees to that. The length of the agreement should be specified from beginning date to ending date. What happens if one party breaches the agreement may be clarified, such as arbitration or mediation. Grounds for termination and method of termination should be spelled out. Acknowledgment of understanding of the agreement, the date of the agreement, and parties to the agreement and their signatures appear on the contract. Guidelines for legal agreements include:

▶ Always put contracts in writing and have them signed and dated by all legally responsible parties.
▶ Never sign a significant contract, for example, partnership, rental, or lease without a lawyer looking it over first.
▶ Always read contracts before you sign them, so that you know what you are agreeing to. You will be held responsible whether you have read it or not.
▶ If you write the contract, use the simplest language possible so all parties understand what they are agreeing to; avoid legalese when possible.

▶ Have legal counsel review the contract if it involves a significant amount of money.

▶ Don't be afraid to suggest changes to a contract presented to you. If all parties agree to a change, simply strike out the words you do not want, write in alternate terms if appropriate, and have each party initial the change.

▶ For a contract involving a lot of money, add a witness, who is a neutral party, to the signing of the agreement.

Massage therapists who work as independent contractors usually have a stock contract that they fill in for different situations. This contract is an agreement by a massage therapist to provide massage services for a separate legal entity. It states the fee per massage session or time worked, date(s) of service, place, and how and when payment is made. It may stipulate conditions such as how clients are solicited and scheduled, reporting mechanisms, and type of massage provided. There may be a cancellation provision. Both parties sign the contract and keep copies for future reference.

Verbal agreements may be legally binding but are hard to enforce. People may have different understandings of the agreement, or may remember details differently. Always get agreements related to your business in writing and signed. Laws related to contracts vary by state.

Practice Policies

Practice policies clarify expectations and specific points of the agreement between the massage therapist and the client. Policies set the ground rules for what happens given a particular situation. They should be given to clients and signed as part of the general client intake.

There are many types of policies. Pricing policies list fees for different services, and posting them may be required by law. Payment policies specify when payment is due; for example, before or after a session. Method of acceptable payment is clarified; for example, cash, check, debit card, or credit card. Other financial policies include insufficient funds/returned check policy and an insurance reimbursement policy. Some massage therapists have a satisfaction or money-back guarantee.

Late arrival policies clarify what happens when clients come late for appointments. One approach is that clients pay for the time periods they have scheduled. If clients are late, their massages end at the originally designated times, and the clients owe the originally agreed-upon fees. Another approach may be that a client who is over 30 minutes late for an appointment does not receive a massage and is charged as if he or she were a no-show.

A cancellation policy may be that 24-hour notice is required or $25 will be charged for the missed appointment. It may also be that no penalty is incurred if the time slot is subsequently filled. A missed appointment policy may be that clients pay in full for missed appointments, or alternatively, that clients pay 50 percent of the original fee for missed appointments.

Conduct policies clarify to clients that the massage provided is a nonsexual massage, and that any attempt to sexualize a session will be grounds for termination of the massage without a refund of fees. Hygiene policies might specify that clients are expected to come for massage clean and free of strong scents from products like perfumes and cologne, or that clients are expected to shower immediately prior to a massage.

A health history disclosure and update policy might be that clients agree to disclose medical conditions and medications as requested to screen for contraindications. They might also be expected to keep the massage therapist updated on any changes in conditions and medications.

A termination policy might state that the massage therapist reserves the right to terminate a session if he or she believes that the safety or health of the client or massage therapist would be threatened if the session were continued. A confidentiality and privacy policy reiterates that the massage therapist will not talk to anyone, including health care providers and insurance companies, without the client's permission. It also states that client health and session records will be kept secure and only seen by those needing to see them.

A scope of practice statement defines what type of massage therapy is offered and for what purposes. It is good to make clear that the massage therapist applies massage within his or her scope of practice and will refer clients as needed to an appropriate massage therapist or health care professional. Explanation of scope of practice is often followed by a consent form.

Waiver of liability can be attached to a policies document. In waivers, clients agree to hold the massage therapist harmless for unpredictable negative reactions or results. This may benefit the massage therapist in the event of a lawsuit, but waivers do not usually hold in cases of proven negligence.

Clearly stating policies in writing promotes greater understanding of expectations and defines important aspects of the therapeutic relationship. Signed copies should be kept in clients' files, and additional copies be given to them to take home. A summary of types of policies important to a massage therapy practice appears in Figure 12–4◀.

Massage Practice Office Space

Massage practice offices have some common requirements whether in the home or in a commercial building. There should be space set aside for a reception area, massage therapy room, business office, and bathroom.

The reception area is where clients are greeted and can wait if they are early for an appointment. A reception area typically has one or two chairs, a small table, a lamp, and decorations. Framed certificates may hang on the wall. The area should be inviting, comfortable, and partitioned off from the massage therapy room.

The massage therapy room must be large enough for all of the equipment and supplies needed for massage sessions. At a minimum, it should hold a massage table and sitting stool on wheels, with adequate space for movement around the table. Storage cabinets hold linens, lotions, and other supplies, and a covered container keeps dirty linens separate. An accessible tabletop is necessary for lubricants, small

▶ **Figure 12–4** Types of policies important for a massage therapy practice.

Financial Policies
  Pricing/fees
  Payment due
  Methods of payment
  Insurance reimbursement
  Insufficient funds or returned checks
  Satisfaction or money back guarantee

Client Behavior Policies
  Late arrival
  No-show or missed appointment
  Cancellation
  Conduct or unacceptable behavior
  Hygiene
  Health history disclosure and update

General Practice Policies
  Schedule of days and times for appointments
  Services and types of massage therapy offered
  Scope of practice
  Referral
  Termination
  Confidentiality
  Consent for massage applications
  Waiver of liability

hand tools, hot packs, and other objects used during massage. A stepping stool may be useful for short or less mobile clients to get onto the table.

The room should also have a chair and clothes rack for clients' belongings. A small wall mirror is useful for clients to check their hair or makeup after massage. Anatomy charts, certificates, or artwork may be hung on the walls. The floor covering should be easily washable.

Office space is set aside for working on and keeping financial records, client files, and other aspects of the business side of the practice. Office furniture includes a desk and chair and a locking file cabinet. Basic office equipment includes a phone and answering machine, with optional computer, printer, and copier. Storage space is needed for office and cleaning supplies. Figure 12–5 ◀ shows a basic layout for a massage therapy office.

A bathroom should be accessible for client use. Some massage ordinances also require showers. Check local massage ordinances for requirements related to massage establishments.

Appointments

Making and keeping appointments is an important time-management function. A massage therapist should have a separate appointment book for his or her private practice. This can also serve as a supporting document for tax purposes.

An appointment book can be the pencil-and-paper variety, or be in electronic form. A drawback of electronic record keeping is the potential for a glitch that wipes out

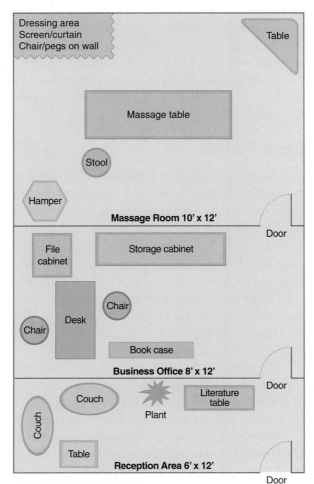

◀ **Figure 12–5** Basic office area.

PRACTICAL APPLICATION

Visit several massage therapy practices and carefully observe the offices. Sketch their office spaces using approximate dimensions. Answering the following questions will help you focus on the elements that constitute a well-designed massage therapy office space.

1 What colors, smells, lighting, or other factors do you remember from your visits to massage therapy offices? Which ones made a favorable or unfavorable impression on you?

2 What was it about the offices' atmosphere, comfort, and safety practices that impressed you?

3 Which elements did the offices have in common?

4 What were the elements that left you with a positive impression?

Now design your own massage office space. Include reception area, massage room, business office, and location of bathrooms. Incorporate elements that will positively influence clients coming to you for massage.

---

appointment information. On the other hand, a traditional appointment book can be lost. Keeping a backup of all electronic information is vital for responsible record keeping.

Generally, the days of the week and times appointments are scheduled should be consistent and a matter of policy. Resist the temptation when starting out to take appointments whenever clients want them. If clients are informed of your days and times of operation, they generally find a time that works for them. Switching appointment times to fit clients' schedules should be kept to a minimum.

Leave at least 30 minutes between appointments if you have one massage room in a location. If traveling to an appointment, plan enough time for travel plus setup and takedown.

Client Records

Create a folder with essential information for each regular client. File folders with fasteners at the top keep papers in order. On one side of the folder, attach a cover sheet with contact information such as name, address, phone number, and e-mail address. A signed policy agreement and waiver, and HIPAA (Health Insurance Portability and Accountability Act) confidentiality statement, if applicable, are underneath. On the other side, fasten the initial health history form and SOAP notes for subsequent sessions. Financial records are usually kept in separate files from session records (Figure 12–6 ◀).

Client records must be kept secure and locked to ensure client confidentiality, and in some cases may require compliance with HIPAA regulations (www.hhs.gov/ocr/hipaa). See page 218 in Chapter 9: Therapeutic Relationship and Ethics, for more on HIPAA requirements.

Electronic systems are available for client records. Computer programs for keeping client files have been developed and can be found on the Internet and advertised in professional journals. Back up electronic files daily for preservation in case of file corruption and use passwords for client record security.

Keep accurate, honest, adequate client records. Keep client records secure and confidential. Abide by laws related to record keeping, for example, those set forth by HIPAA. Schedule record keeping into your practice time. Doing paperwork is an important part of a massage therapy practice.

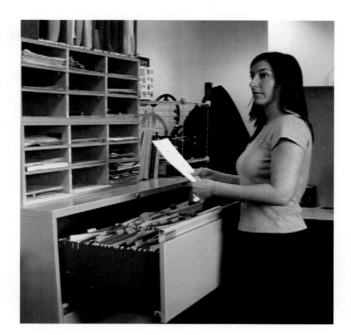

◀**Figure 12–6** Client files are kept in alphabetical order in locked file cabinets.

FINANCES

The financial viability of a massage therapy practice is fundamental to its success. That means setting income goals and profit projections, budgeting for income and expenses, tracking money coming in and going out, and paying taxes. Once you understand the basics of business finances and put them into practice, it can be rewarding to watch your massage therapy business grow and prosper.

Income and profit goals are part of the vision for your private practice. *Gross* income means how much money is collected from clients, while *net* income is what is left over after expenses and taxes. After subtracting expenses from income, a negative number means the business had a *loss* for the year, and a positive number shows your *profit*. The concept is simple, but keeping expenses low enough in relation to income in order to generate a profit is the challenge of having a private practice. More about planning for profit is discussed later in the chapter in the section on figuring the first-year budget.

Startup Costs

Startup costs are the initial expenses involved in setting up a massage therapy practice. Many of these costs are incurred before the first client walks in the door. Startup costs include buying basic equipment like a massage table and related equipment, linens, and lotions; getting a license to practice; securing professional liability insurance; printing business cards; purchasing basic office supplies; establishing phone service and an answering machine; and paying a security deposit and first month's rent. Other costs fall into the "nice to have" category rather than the essential things. Nonessential expenses can be put off until money is available.

Startup costs are related to the type of private practice being developed. Some types of practices have lower startup costs than others. Typical startup cost categories for a massage practice are listed in Figure 12–7◀.

Startup cash may come from a variety of sources. Some massage therapists use their personal savings, or borrow from family members. Some work at other jobs with steady income and start out as part-time massage therapists, gradually building their practices. A smaller number of massage therapists take out loans from banks or credit

▶ **Figure 12–7** Typical startup cost categories for a massage therapy practice.

Typical Startup Cost Categories

Licensing costs
Occupational license (application, exam, fingerprinting, other)
Massage establishment license
Business permit or license

Professional association membership

Insurance
Professional liability
Premise liability ("slip and fall")
Health insurance
Auto insurance
Other insurance

Business checking account

Communication services
Phone installation or connection
Computer connection to Internet

Massage equipment
Massage table and accessories
Massage chair and accessories
Heater for hot packs
Freezer for cold packs
Other equipment

Office furniture and equipment
Light fixtures
Computer and printer
Sound system for music
Answering machine

Supplies
Linens (sheets and towels)
Oils
Hot and cold packs
Appointment book/system
Forms and folders for client records
Miscellaneous office supplies
Decorations for office

Marketing and advertising
Business cards
Brochures
Website
Stationery

Legal and professional fees
(e.g., lawyer, bookkeeper, accountant)

Office setup
Security deposit
First month's rent
Communications installation
Utilities deposit

Other

unions. Some startup costs can be covered by credit cards, but these often incur high interest payments that eat into profits. Starting out with the least amount of debt at the lowest interest rate is a good financial goal.

First-Year Budget

The first-year budget forecasts income and expenses for the initial 12 months of operation. Month-by-month budgeting is usually the most useful. Develop a

CRITICAL THINKING

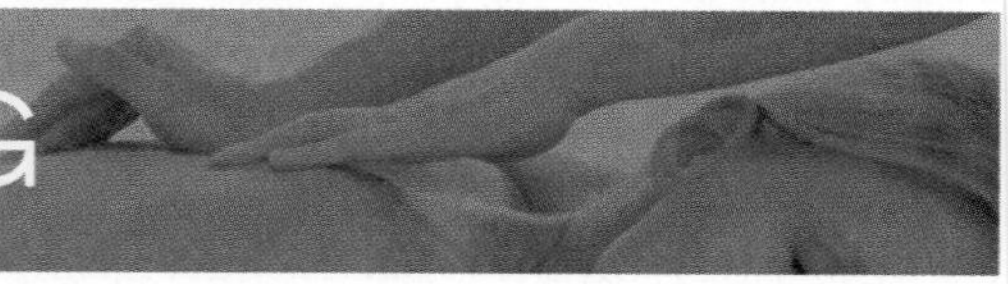

Write a business plan for your future massage therapy practice. Refer back to your notes about your practice identity and mission statement in writing your business plan. Present your plan to the class and solicit feedback and suggestions. Review and revise your plan as you think of better approaches.

Now list the startup costs for a private practice you currently have in mind. Ask yourself these questions:

1 How do you plan to get the money needed for the startup?

2 Are there any ways to reduce startup costs to increase your profits in the beginning?

month-by-month chart or spreadsheet that shows monthly expenses and projected income from the practice.

Projecting income for the first year can be tricky. Income will be a factor of the number of clients seen per week multiplied by the fees collected per session. Research the going rate for massage in your area. When starting out, you might want to consider staying on the lower side of the cost range to attract clients, especially if there is a lot of massage available in your area. On the other hand, if you are one of a few massage therapists, or if you have a unique service, you may want to charge the average rate or more.

Expect a gradual growth in clients and massage sessions over the 12-month period. Figure no more than 6 clients per week in the first 6 months, gradually working up to 10 to 15 per week by the end of the year. Be conservative. Allow for cancellations. It is better to have more income than predicted. Remember to plan for vacation time, holidays, and sick days during the first year. Projecting 4 weeks of down time is recommended.

Projecting monthly expenses allows you to determine how much income you need to break even, or make a profit, in any given month. **Fixed costs**, sometimes called *overhead*, are expenses you have whether you see clients or not, for example, rent and utilities. Fluctuating operating expenses, or **variable costs**, like laundry and massage supplies, depend on the number of clients seen.

Some experts recommend putting enough money in the bank to cover at least 3 months' fixed costs before you start your practice. This is called a **cash reserve** and should be figured in startup costs (Mariotti, 2007). Ideally, a cash reserve should be built up and maintained throughout a practice to cover unforeseen events like illnesses or family emergencies. Deficits in one month can be made up in subsequent months, or profits in one month can help offset expected expenses in coming months. By the end of the year, hopefully, income will outpace expenses to yield a profit.

A **salary draw** is the money taken out of the practice monthly for your personal use. Some experts recommend not expecting a salary draw for the first 6 months of a new practice. This allows for income to be put back into the business to cover operating expenses and build the cash reserve. To make this possible, some massage therapists build up savings, borrow money, depend on spouses or family for support, or keep part-time jobs to cover personal expenses until their practices start turning a good profit.

Keeping expenses low is paramount. Income minus expenses predicts your cash flow, or how much cash you have on hand at any one time. If your expenses outpace your income, and you have no savings to back you up, your practice will eventually fail. Careful monitoring of income and expenses can help you make adjustments as your practice evolves. Consider the first-year budget as a working plan for developing the business side of your practice. A sample spreadsheet for developing a first-year budget appears in Figure 12–8◀.

Income Taxes

Massage therapists pay income tax on the profits from their private practices, in addition to taxes related to employment. This means that they must keep accurate records of income from their private clients, as well as receipts from business expenses.

The following information is an overview of the subject of income taxes; however, a professional tax preparer is recommended for specific questions about any individual situation. The Internal Revenue Service (IRS) has informational booklets on matters related to taxes that are updated every year (www.irs.gov). Some IRS publications and forms that massage therapists may find useful are listed in Figure 12–9◀.

PROJECTED INCOME

Source	Jan	Feb	Mar	April	May	June	July	Aug	Sept	Oct	Nov	Dec
Massage fees												
Tips												
Miscellaneous												
Monthly Totals												

PROJECTED EXPENSES

Expense	Jan	Feb	Mar	April	May	June	July	Aug	Sept	Oct	Nov	Dec
Loan payment												
Rent												
Phone												
Utilities												
Bank fees												
Linen service												
Cleaning												
Bookkeeper												
Insurance												
Memberships												
Continuing Education												
Business travel												
Estimated taxes												
Salary draw												
Miscellaneous												
Monthly Totals												

▲ **Figure 12–8** Sample budget spreadsheet form for first year of business.

The *tax year* for sole proprietor businesses like massage therapy practices is the calendar year beginning January 1 and ending December 31. *Taxable income* is the total income from a massage therapy practice minus qualified business expenses. All fees collected, as well as tips, are considered taxable income. For employed massage therapists tips are also taxable income.

▶ **Figure 12–9** Useful IRS publications and forms.

IRS Publications*

- ▶ Your Federal Income Tax–For Individuals (Publication 17)
- ▶ Starting a Business and Keeping Records (Publication 583)
- ▶ Tax Guide for Small Businesses (Publication 334)
- ▶ Instructions for Schedule C or C-EZ
- ▶ Business Expenses (Publication 535)
- ▶ Tax Withholding and Estimated Tax (Publication 505)
- ▶ Reporting Tip Income (Publication 531)
- ▶ Employee's Daily Record of Tips & Report to Employers (Publication 1244)
- ▶ Travel, Entertainment, Gift & Car Expenses (Publication 463)
- ▶ Business Use of Your Home (Publication 587)

Forms for Filing Income Taxes

- ▶ Form 1040 Individual Income Tax Return
- ▶ Schedule C Profit or Loss from Business (sole proprietorship)
- ▶ Schedule SE (Form 1040) Self-Employment Tax
- ▶ Form 1065 (partnership)
- ▶ Form 2553 Election by a Small Business Corporation
- ▶ Form 1120S U.S. Income Tax Return for an S Corporation

*IRS forms and publications can be obtained online from www.irs.gov, or by calling the IRS toll free number, or from the U.S. Post Office during tax season. Tax laws are changed yearly so obtain the latest publication available.

CASE FOR STUDY

Jim and His Startup Plans

Jim wants to build a private massage practice after graduation, but realizes that will take money he does not have right now. He is willing to get part-time employment as a massage therapist as he builds his own business. His mission is "to apply my knowledge and skills to help clients achieve optimal wellness. Affordable massage therapy is offered in a clean, pleasant, and relaxing environment. This is a community-centered and family-based private practice welcoming people of all ages."

Question:
What strategies can Jim use to minimize startup costs and build his own private practice over time?

Things to Consider:

▶ How can Jim decide how many days to devote to employment and how many to building his private practice during the first year?

▶ Employment in what type of setting(s) would contribute most to his long-range plans for his private practice?
▶ What are the options for his initial private practice location to minimize overhead?
▶ How can he build a solid client base for his private practice successfully and ethically?
▶ In what ways can he best and most cheaply get his name out into the community?
▶ What could his contingency plans be if (a) his private practice grows more rapidly than expected or (b) his private practice grows more slowly than expected?

Ideas for Accomplishing Jim's First-Year Goals

_____

_____

_____

Massage therapists who do not sell products usually use the *cash method* of accounting. Under the cash method, income is reported in the tax year it is received, and expenses are deducted in the tax year they are paid for. A different system called the *accrual method* is sometimes used by businesses. In the accrual method, income is reported in the tax year it is earned, even though payment may be received in a later year, and expenses are deducted in the tax year they are incurred, whether or not they are paid in that year. (See IRS Publication 583, *Starting a Business and Keeping Records.*)

Qualified business expenses reduce the amount of taxable income. Most expenses related to maintaining a practice/business are deductible, for example, equipment and supplies, office rent, continuing education, and license fees. Mileage to and from clients' homes or other travel may be deductible; however, travel to and from a place of employment is not deductible. Keeping good records and receipts related to business expenses is essential for an accurate calculation of deductions. Check with a tax preparer for further information on allowed deductions. (See IRS Publication 535, *Business Expenses.*)

Form 1040 is used to file U.S. income taxes for individuals and covers both employment and self-employment. Form 1040 is a summary form to which other forms and schedules are attached, for example, W-2 forms to report wages and tips from employment. Schedule C reports small business income and expenses. Form 1099 is similar to a W-2 form from an employer but is used to report income as an independent contractor.

Various other forms are attached to the 1040 form as needed to complete the filing. A tax preparer can help you figure out which forms are required for a specific case. (See IRS Publication 17, *Your Federal Income Tax for Individuals.*)

Self-employment tax (SE tax) is a Social Security and Medicare tax for individuals who work for themselves. It applies to Social Security coverage for retirement, disability, survivor, and Medicare benefits. SE tax applies if your net earnings from self-employment are $400 or more. SE tax is in addition to your regular income tax, and was about 15% in 2007. Some SE tax may be claimed as a business expense, but rules change yearly. (See Schedule SE [Form 1040], *Self-Employment Tax.*)

Estimated tax must be sent to the IRS four times a year in April, June, September, and January. Estimated tax payments, similar to withholding for employment income, estimate the tax that will be owed at the end of the year. Since you are your own employer, you have the responsibility for paying estimated tax. Estimated tax payments should appear on the budget as an expense. (See IRS Publication 505, *Tax With-holding and Estimated Tax.*)

Using a tax preparation professional is recommended unless you have all income from regular employment, or an otherwise simple tax situation. Costs for tax preparation are qualified business expenses.

Tax preparation is made easier with a good bookkeeping system. The tax preparer takes the numbers provided by you and fills in tax forms. An accountant who is a tax preparer can also give you advice on deductions and other ways to reduce income tax owed at the end of the year. Setting up a bookkeeping system is addressed later in this chapter.

Incomes taxes are an integral part of the financial planning of a private practice in massage therapy—not an afterthought. Good planning can reduce any confusion and stress surrounding bookkeeping and taxes. It is all part of the business side of having a massage therapy practice.

Bookkeeping

Bookkeeping involves keeping accurate records of income and expenditures for tax purposes and tracking payments made by clients, as well as calculating how the business side of the practice is doing financially. The bookkeeping system chosen for a specific practice depends on how large the practice is and how skilled the massage therapist is with numbers.

Bookkeeping Systems. One choice for bookkeeping is a simple handwritten ledger. The advantage of pencil-on-paper systems is that they are inexpensive and easy to learn. The process of making entries by hand can lead to a better understanding of how ledgers work. It is estimated that "half of all new businesses use hand-posted ledgers the first year, and some never see a need for anything else" (Kamoroff, 2003, p. 42). For most sole proprietor massage therapists, a handwritten bookkeeping system is adequate.

Published bookkeeping ledgers typically have a page for listing details of daily expenditures, and daily receipts or income. There is sometimes a section for expenditures broken down by category of deduction such as rent, postage, and telephone. Keeping running totals for expenditures and income provides a check of profits at a glance and is handy at tax time (Figure 12–10◀).

Often these record books include additional useful information like a tax calendar, allowable deductions, instructions for making entries, calculation of net worth, and tax information sheets. The *Dome Simplified Weekly/Monthly Bookkeeping Record* is an example of a handwritten system available from office supply stores.

Computer programs for bookkeeping are also available, for example, QuickBooks® (www.quickbooks.intuit.com). Some programs are designed specifically for massage therapists' needs. Computer programs do essentially the same things as hand-posted ledgers. Their advantages are that they are faster, provide clean-looking reports, and do the math for you. Some software programs integrate banking and bookkeeping and can generate totals and reports easily. Mastering the software may take some time, but for larger practices, bookkeeping by computer may make sense.

Accountants and bookkeepers can also be hired to help track finances. *Accountants are trained in the principles of setting up and auditing financial accounts and are

Week of _____ 2__ __ __
        Month/Day to Month/Day

Total Receipts for the Week*			
Day	**Notes — Fees & Tips**	**$ Amount**	
Sun			
Mon			
Tues			
Wed			
Thurs			
Fri			
Sat			
Total This Week			
Previous Total			
Total for Year to Date			

*A receipt book or notations in an appointment book serve as supporting documents for the daily receipt totals in the ledger.

Expenditures for the Week*				
Date	**Paid To**	**Check#/Credit**	**$ Amount**	

*Receipts for goods and services purchased, reflected in cancelled checks and credit card bills, are support documents for expenditures listed.

Expenditures by Deduction Category*					
#	**Category**	**Total This Week**	**Previous Total**	**Total for Year to Date**	
1	Rent				
2	Phone				
3	Utilities				
4	Linen service/laundry				
5	Equipment				
6	Massage supplies				
7	Office supplies				
8	Advertising				
9	Travel				
10	Professional dues				
11	Continuing education				
12	Miscellaneous				

*Expense categories are set up by an accountant or bookkeeper and reflect the usual expenses of the business.

◀ **Figure 12–10** Sample of a weekly bookkeeping ledger.

responsible for reporting financial results in accordance with government and regulatory authority rules. Accountants can set up bookkeeping systems and prepare taxes. *Bookkeepers* record day-to-day transactions in systems chosen by the business owner. They take care of the paperwork involved in recording expenditures and receipts, and may also balance the checkbook. Bookkeepers still have to be provided with necessary checks, bills, receipts, and other records from the business.

Tracking Client Payments. Massage fees collected plus tips received equal income from a private practice. A simple way to track client payments is to keep a handwritten receipt book. A typical receipt lists the amount of money received, method of payment (cash, check, or charge), date, service rendered, client's name, and the person who took the payment and filled out the receipt. The client gets one copy, while a carbon copy stays in the receipt book. The receipt book can serve as a supporting document for book-keeping and tax reporting purposes.

As a backup record, a daily accounting of income can be made right in an appointment book. For each appointment kept, write the amount the client paid plus tips. Also note when appointments are cancelled or missed. This provides a valuable cross-check and record of the daily activity of the practice.

One-write systems are useful for offices with more than one massage therapist, or for tracking payment histories of individual clients. These systems include a running daily income ledger for the office, individual client ledger cards that can be filed alphabetically, and individual receipts for each transaction. These are sometimes called pegboard systems.

There are also computer systems for tracking client payments. Whatever system is used, receipts should be entered into the bookkeeping system daily.

Banking

It is important to keep a separate business checking account for a private practice. It keeps personal and business finances clearly separate and makes bookkeeping simpler. There is also less chance of confusion if audited for income taxes.

Compare fees and features for business accounts before choosing a bank. Choose a bank convenient for making frequent deposits. Establishing a banking relationship may come in useful if seeking a business loan or for credit card processing in the future.

A few important rules apply to banking. First, pay all business bills by check, from a petty cash account, or a credit card designated for the business. Second, deposit all income, checks and cash, into the business account. Third, when taking money out of the business account for personal use, write a check to yourself payable to "cash" or write "personal draw" on the memo line. This way personal draws or withdrawals can be tracked more easily (Kamoroff, 2003).

Set aside time every month to balance the business bank account and review financial records. It is recommended that bank statements and cancelled checks be kept for at least 7 years.

→ CONCLUSION

The journey to becoming a successful massage therapist in some ways never ends. Beyond graduation loom the challenges of getting employment or setting up a private practice. But the reward of having meaningful and satisfying work that sustains you through the years is worth the effort.

Traditionally, careers in certain professions are launched with ceremony and pledges of dedication and ethical conduct. These festivities mark the end of initial training and the official beginning of the real work. It is instructive to analyze elements of oaths in some of the more established professions. They include loyalty and appreciation of teachers, statements of humility and compassion, and dedication to service and honor. They look to the future and to growth in the profession.

The following "invitation" is based on similar oaths from other health professions. It summarizes important ideas to keep in mind as you start out in your new chosen profession.

Invitation to Massage Therapists

Welcome into the ranks of therapeutic massage and bodywork professionals.

May you remember your days at school with fondness and appreciation.

May you honor your teachers and all who helped you through your training.

May you serve your fellow creatures with compassion and humility.

May you always hold the best interests of your clients above your own personal gain.

May you behave honestly and honorably in your practice.

May you continue to seek knowledge and skill in your profession—there is always more to learn.

May you join your colleagues in protecting the practice of massage therapy.

May you value always the healing benefits of touch.

And over all, may you find fulfillment and meaning in the work of your hands.

PJB

Chapter Highlights

▶ A self-employed massage therapist is said to have a private practice with a business side, much like other businesses.

▶ A business plan spells out the details of a practice and includes sections on business description, marketing, management, and finances.

▶ A business description explains the practice vision and identity, as well as legal structure and plans for location.

- Most massage therapists start out as sole proprietors, with office locations in the home, in a commercial space, or traveling to the clients' homes or workplaces to give massage.

▶ Marketing is the process of identifying potential clients and their needs or wants using market research.

▶ In building a client base, it is important to find ways to make yourself visible to the public and provide contact information.

- Business cards are a key tool for obtaining new clients.
- Paid advertising may help, as well as promotions, to encourage people to make appointments.

▶ Management includes activities necessary to run the business.

- Acquiring necessary licenses, insurance, and contracts lays the foundation.
- Written policies clarify expectations related to fees, hours of operation, payment, conduct, scope of practice, client health information and confidentiality, and other aspects of the client relationship.

▶ Massage practice spaces typically have a reception area, massage therapy room, office, and bathrooms.

- Spaces should be attractive, comfortable, safe, and comply with local ordinances.

▶ Appointments may be listed by hand in an appointment book or in electronic form.

▶ Client records with basic information, health histories, and session notes are kept well organized and secure.

▶ A good financial goal is to start out in practice with the least amount of debt as possible at the lowest interest rate.

▶ Planning a first-year budget helps forecast income and expenses and is essential for making good financial decisions.

- Tracking monthly income and expenses closely is essential for financial viability.
- Keeping fixed and variable costs to a minimum maximizes profits in the end.
- A salary draw is the money taken out of the business for your personal use.

▶ Income taxes must be paid annually on profits from the business.

- Taxable income for a sole proprietor is the total income (fees and tips) from the practice minus qualified business expenses.
- Estimated taxes are paid to the IRS four times per year by massage therapists with private practices.
- The IRS publishes many useful instruction booklets.
- Hiring a professional tax preparer is recommended for massage therapists with private practices.

▶ Bookkeeping systems record financial transactions related to the practice.

▶ Keep financial records up-to-date and accurate.

- Set aside time every month to balance the business bank account and review financial records.

Exam Review

Learning Outcomes

Use the learning outcomes at the beginning of the chapter and shown here as a guide to the major topics covered. Perform the task given in each outcome, and share your results with a study partner. Check off the tasks as you complete them.

❑ Develop a business plan for a private practice in massage therapy.
❑ Create a marketing strategy to build a client base.
❑ Organize a massage practice office.
❑ Enter into contracts with knowledge and forethought.
❑ Establish policies for practice management.
❑ Create a filing system for keeping client records.
❑ Project startup costs for a massage therapy practice.
❑ Project first-year income and expenses.
❑ Design a bookkeeping system for tax purposes.
❑ Manage practice finances on a daily basis.

Key Terms

To study key terms listed at the beginning of the chapter, choose one or more of the following exercises. Writing or talking about ideas helps you better remember them, and explaining them to someone else helps deepen your understanding.

1. Write a one-sentence definition of each key term. Put the term in a general category, and then distinguish it from other terms in that category. For example, "*Marketing* is the process of identifying potential customers or clients, and meeting their needs and wants." Or, "*Fixed costs* are expenses incurred whether clients are seen or not, also called *overhead*." Try to capture the essence of each term in a concise statement.

2. Make study cards by writing the key term on one side of a 3 × 5 card and a concise definition on the other side. Shuffle the cards and read one side, trying to recite either the explanation or word on the other side.

3. Pick out two or three terms and explain how they are related.

4. With a study partner, take turns explaining key terms verbally.

5. Make up sentences using one or more key terms. Variation: Read your sentences to a study partner who will ask you to explain unclear statements.

Memory Workout

The following fill-in-the-blank statements test your memory of the main concepts in this chapter.

1. Income from clients minus business expenses equals the real _____ from the practice.

2. The main advantages of a home practice are low _____ and a short _____.

3. Marketing is the process of identifying potential _____, and meeting their needs and _____.

4. Advertising is a _____ public announcement providing information about goods and services to potential _____.

5. Discounts and gift certificates are examples of _____ to attract clients.

6. _____ may result when agreements and contracts are either not clear or have not been kept.

7. Clearly stating _____ in writing promotes greater understanding of expectations and defines important aspects of the therapeutic relationship.

8. Reception areas should be _____ _____ from the massage therapy room.

9. Starting out with the least amount of _____ at the lowest _____ rate is a good financial goal.

10. Money put away to cover fixed costs when starting out, or later in case of emergency, is called a cash _____.

11. Money taken out of the practice for personal use is called a _____ _____.

12. Taxable income includes all fees collected plus _____ received.

Test Prep

The following multiple-choice questions will help to prepare you for future school and professional exams.

1. The most common legal structure for massage practices starting out is
   a. Sole proprietor
   b. Partnership
   c. Limited partnership
   d. Corporation

2. A primary source of clients in a personal service like massage is
   a. Newspaper advertising
   b. Radio advertising
   c. Word of mouth from satisfied clients
   d. Direct mail advertising

3. Insurance that covers you for liability for incidents arising from massage therapy itself is called
   a. Premise liability insurance
   b. Catastrophic insurance
   c. "Slip and fall" insurance
   d. Professional liability insurance

4. How often should electronic files and records be backed up?
   a. At least once a week
   b. At least monthly
   c. Daily
   d. Biweekly

5. Money left over after expenses are paid is called
   a. Gross income
   b. Net income
   c. Profit
   d. Both b and c

6. Expenses incurred whether you see clients or not are called
   a. Fixed costs
   b. Variable costs
   c. Startup costs
   d. Reserve

7. When you are self-employed, estimated tax payments must be sent to the IRS
   a. Two times a year
   b. Four times a year
   c. When taxes are filed
   d. When requested in writing

8. In addition to regular income tax, massage therapists in private practice pay an additional tax to cover Social Security and Medicare. This tax is referred to as
   a. Reserve tax
   b. Variable tax
   c. Net income tax
   d. Self-employment tax

Video Challenge

Watch the appropriate segment of the video on your CD-ROM and then answer the following questions.

Segment 12: Private Practice and Finances

1. What do the massage therapists interviewed in the video say about who helped them get started in their practices? What kind of help did they get?

2. What ideas for marketing and advertising a massage therapy practice are presented in the video?

3. What does the video say about the importance of figuring start-up costs and developing a first-year budget?

Comprehension Exercises

The following exercises provide questions for you to answer and tasks you can do to enhance your understanding of the material presented in this chapter.

1. List the four sections of a business plan, and explain what information goes into each section. Why is a business plan important for starting and maintaining a successful massage therapy practice?

2. Define *market research*. List at least five useful market research questions.

3. Explain why a good bookkeeping system is essential for a massage therapy practice. What are the elements of a good bookkeeping system?

For Greater Understanding

The following exercises are designed to give you a deeper understanding of the subjects covered in this chapter. Action words are underlined to emphasize the active nature of this approach to learning.

1. Interview a massage therapist with a successful practice. Question him or her about the most useful things learned about the business side of massage therapy. Ask the individual to share his or her biggest mistakes and best advice.

2. Conduct market research for the area in which you plan to open a private practice. Who is already practicing in the area? What kind of massage therapy are they offering? How do they advertise their services? What type of competitive advantage might you develop?

3. List the startup costs for a private practice you currently have in mind. How do you plan to get the money needed for the startup? Are there any ways to reduce startup costs to increase your profits in the beginning?

4. Develop a first-year budget for a private practice you currently have in mind. Use a month-by-month format. List all fixed and variable expenses you can think of. Determine your cash flow for each month.

APPENDICES

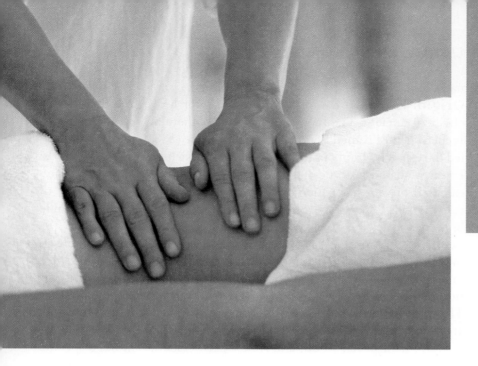

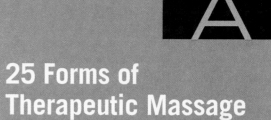

25 Forms of Therapeutic Massage and Bodywork

The therapeutic massage and bodywork forms described below are some of the major systems practiced today. Descriptions include a summary of their origins and history, techniques and applications, the theory on which they are based, and some resources for further information. Noncommercial websites are listed when available, and books for forms that do not have relevant websites (e.g., Ayurvedic massage) are also cited. Readers are encouraged to check the Internet for websites appearing after publication of this text.

Many of the forms of massage and bodywork listed are root systems from which other forms or spin-offs have been derived. Because the field of massage therapy is an emerging profession with a large entrepreneurial component, there are several trademarked forms, e.g., Rolfing®. Spin-offs of originals may also be trademarked, or there may be generic spin-offs without trademarks.

For further explanations of these and other forms of massage and bodywork, see *Discovering the Body's Wisdom* by Mirka Knaster (New York: Bantam Books, 1996).

1. Alexander Technique

Origin: Alexander Technique was developed by an Australian named Frederick Matthias Alexander (1869–1955), who practiced in London in the early 1900s. Alexander, a Shakespearean actor, cured himself of loss of voice through correction of faulty posture in the head and neck. He later worked with other actors and public speakers using the same method to improve their vocal abilities.

Technique: Alexander Technique is a form of contemporary bodywork in which a teacher guides the student through various movements like sitting, walking, and bending. The emphasis is on achieving balance in the head–neck relationship, called Primary Control. Poor habitual patterns are replaced by light, easy, simple, and integrated movement.

Theory: Proper body alignment and movement patterns are achieved by heightened kinesthetic awareness, and conscious movement.

Websites: Alexander Technique (www.alexandertechnique.com)
Alexander Technique International (www.ati-net.com)
American Society for the Alexander Technique (www.alexandertech.org)

2. Aromatherapy Massage

Origin: The use of natural plant essences for health and therapeutic effects is ancient. The modern term "aromatherapie" was coined by a French chemist named Rene Maurice Gattefosse (1881–1950) as he studied the use of fragrant oils for their healing properties in the 1920–1930s. Later, Madame Marguerite Maury (1895–1968) started prescribing essential oils for her patients, and is credited with the modern use of essential oils for massage. She wrote an important aromatherapy guide in French in 1961 that was translated into English in 1964.

Technique: Aromatherapy massage involves the use of essential oils in massage oil blends for their therapeutic effects. Techniques of Western massage, Ayurvedic massage, and other systems of soft tissue manipulation may be used in the application of aromatherapy massage oils.

Theory: Essential oils are highly concentrated aromatic extracts that are cold-pressed or steam distilled from plants such as grasses, leaves, flowers, fruit peels, wood, and roots. Each essential oil has a specific therapeutic effect such as relaxing, boosting immune system, relieving congestion, or soothing muscular aches and pains. Common massage blends contain essential oils such as peppermint, lavender, citrus, tea tree, and rosemary.

Website: National Association for Holistic Aromatherapy (www.naha.org)

3. Ayurvedic Massage

Origin: Ayurvedic massage is one of the healing practices of ancient India. Vedic scriptures of India dating back to 3000 BCE describe healing practices including massage with oil.

Technique: Ayurvedic massage techniques include rubbing, kneading, squeezing, tapping, and pulling or shaking the body. Emphasis is given to massage of the head and feet. Sessions are invigorating and the recipient changes position several times. Pressure is applied to *marmas,* or pressure points on the body.

Theory: Ayurvedic massage is based in traditional Ayurvedic medicine of India. Massage is thought to remove obstructions to the flow of *vayu* (wind) through *siras* or wind-carrying vessels to reduce pain, relieve tension, and encourage more natural breathing patterns. Massage oils are chosen according to body type, the atmosphere and the season.

Reference: *Ayurvedic Massage: Traditional Indian Techniques for Balancing Body and Mind* by Harish Johari (Rochester, VT: Healing Arts Press, 1996).

4. Clinical Massage Therapy

See Medical Massage

5. Craniosacral Therapy (CST)

Origin: Craniosacral therapy stems from the work of an osteopath named Dr. William Garner Sutherland (1873–1954) in the early 1900s. Dr. Sutherland developed the basic theory of CST, including cranial suture movement, rhythmic motion of cerebrospinal fluid (i.e., Breath of Life), and the relationship between craniosacral rhythm and health. John E. Upledger, D.O., has continued development of this work, and added the concept of SomatoEmotional Release (SER) of negative emotions stored in traumatized tissues. The Upledger Foundation was established in 1987 to study CST.

Technique: Craniosacral therapy is a form of contemporary bodywork that uses gentle compression to realign the skull bones and stretch related membranes to balance the craniosacral rhythm (CSR), and improve function of the nervous system.